In vitro methods in toxicology

Edited by

C.K. ATTERWILL
Head of Investigative Toxicology
Smith Kline & French Research Ltd
and
C.E. STEELE
Head of Reproductive Toxicology
Smith Kline & French Research Ltd

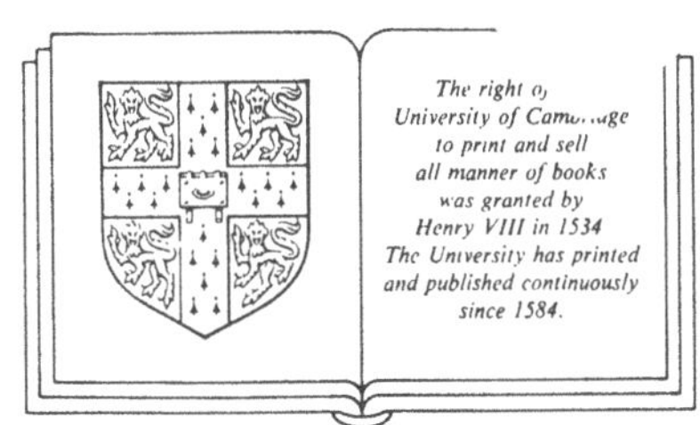

CAMBRIDGE UNIVERSITY PRESS
Cambridge
New York New Rochelle
Melbourne Sydney

CAMBRIDGE UNIVERSITY PRESS
Cambridge, New York, Melbourne, Madrid, Cape Town, Singapore, São Paulo, Delhi

Cambridge University Press
The Edinburgh Building, Cambridge CB2 8RU, UK

Published in the United States of America by Cambridge University Press, New York

www.cambridge.org
Information on this title: www.cambridge.org/9780521104753

First published 1987
This digitally printed version 2009

A catalogue record for this publication is available from the British Library

ISBN 978-0-521-32684-1 hardback
ISBN 978-0-521-10475-3 paperback

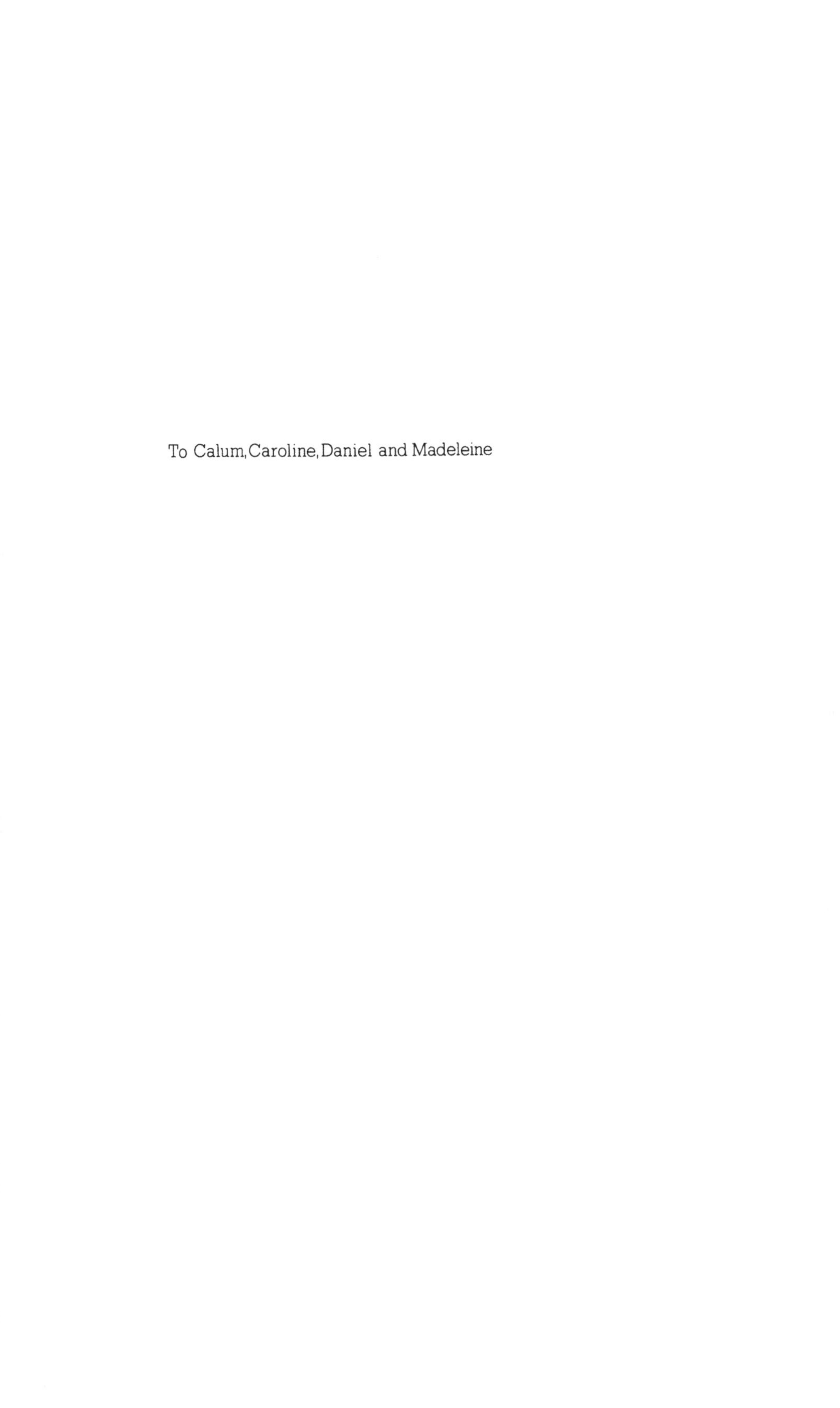

To Calum, Caroline, Daniel and Madeleine

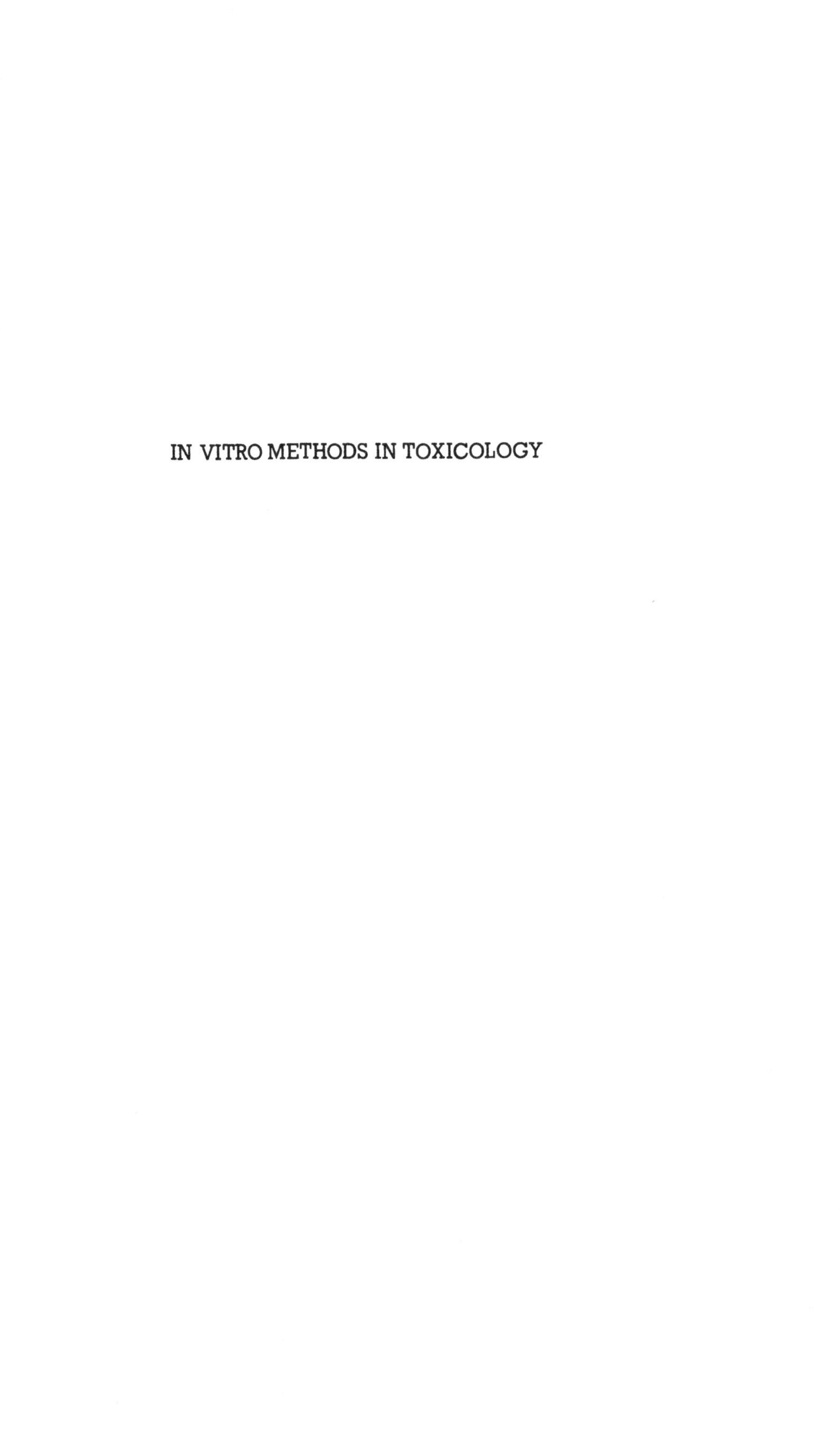

IN VITRO METHODS IN TOXICOLOGY

CONTENTS

CONTRIBUTORS

C.K. Atterwill, Smith Kline & French Research Limited, The Frythe, Welwyn, Herts AL6 9AR, UK

G.R. Betton, Smith Kline & French Research Limited, The Frythe, Welwyn, Herts AL6 9AR, UK

G. Bkaily, Faculty of Medicine, University of Sherbrooke, Sherbrooke, Quebec, Canada J1H 5N4

C.G. Brown, Smith Kline & French Research Limited, The Frythe, Welwyn, Herts AL6 9AR, UK

N.A. Brown, MRC Experimental Embryology and Teratology Unit, Woodmansterne Road, Carshalton, Surrey SM5 4EF, UK

R.C. Brown, MRC Toxicology Unit, Carshalton, Surrey SM5 4EF, UK

R. Chenery, Smith Kline & French Research Limited, The Frythe, Welwyn, Herts AL6 9AR, UK

A. Cockburn, Research Division, Beecham Pharmaceuticals, Honeypot Lane, Stock, Essex CM4 9PE, UK

D.L. Cockroft, ICRF Developmental Biology Unit, Zoology Department, South Parks Road, Oxford OX1 3PS, UK

P.A. Duffy, Imperial Chemical Industries plc, Pharmaceuticals Division, Mereside, Alderley Park, Macclesfield, Cheshire SK10 4TG, UK

O.P. Flint, Imperial Chemical Industries plc, Pharmaceuticals Division, Mereside, Alderley Park, Macclesfield, Cheshire SK10 4TG, UK

S.J. Freeman, Smith Kline & French Research Limited, The Frythe, Welwyn, Herts AL6 9AR, UK

D.A. Garside, Smith Kline & French Research Limited, The Frythe, Welwyn, Herts AL6 9AR, UK

E. Harpur, MRC Mechanisms of Drug Toxicity Research Group, Pharmaceutical Sciences Institute, Aston University, Birmingham B4 7ET, UK

W.R. Hewitt, Smith Kline & French Laboratories, 1500 Spring Garden Street, Philadelphia, PA 19101, USA

J.B. Hook, Smith Kline & French Laboratories, 1500 Spring Garden Street, Philadelphia, PA 19101, USA

P. Johnson, Smith Kline & French Research Limited, The Frythe, Welwyn, Herts AL6 9AR, UK

P.S. Lawrence, Unilever Research, Colworth House, Sharnbrook, Bedford MK44 1LQ, Beds., UK

G.B. Leslie, Smith Kline & French Research Limited, The Frythe, Welwyn, Herts AL6 9AR, UK

J.S.H. Luke, Smith Kline & French Research Limited, The Frythe, Welwyn, Herts AL6 9AR, UK

P.E. McKibbin, Central Toxicology Laboratory, Imperial Chemical Industries plc, Alderley Park, Macclesfield, Cheshire SK10 4TJ, UK

K. Miller, The British Industrial Biological Research Association (BIBRA), Woodmansterne Road, Carshalton, Surrey SM5 4DS, UK

S. Nicklin, The British Industrial Biological Research Association (BIBRA), Woodmansterne Road, Carshalton, Surrey SM5 4DS, UK

A. Poole, Smith Kline & French Research Limited, The Frythe, Welwyn, Herts AL6 9AR, UK

M. Richold, Unilever Research, Colworth House, Sharnbrook, Bedford MK44 1LQ, Beds., UK

M.A. Smith, Smith Kline & French Laboratories, 1500 Spring Garden Street, Philadelphia, PA 19101, USA

N. Sperelakis, University of Cincinnati, Medical Center, Mail Location 576, 231 Bethesda Avenue, Cincinnati, Ohio 45267-0576, USA

C.E. Steele, Smith Kline & French Research Limited, The Frythe, Welwyn, Herts AL6 9AR, UK

S.G. Volsen, The British Industrial Biological Research Association (BIBRA), Woodmansterne Road, Carshalton, Surrey SM5 4DS, UK

Preface

It became apparent on entering a commercial toxicology environment and attempting to establish in vitro laboratories that there exists no single, comprehensive text on currently available in vitro toxicological models. This gap in the literature was not due to a paucity of information since this field has been rapidly expanding, particularly in the last decade.

Current interest in this area is prompted by both new Home Office Animal Legislation and an awareness of a need for ethical and scientific alternatives to whole animal experimentation. We hope that this book will appeal to a wide audience including students of toxicology, practising toxicologists and pathologists, regulatory agencies, and those working in academia.

The book is divided into three sections. The first section deals with target organ toxicology and covers such diverse organs as the ear, heart, kidney and brain. This is followed by a second section of general and topical techniques including irritancy and genotoxicity testing. Finally, the various aspects of reproductive toxicology, including teratology and male and female fertility, are described in five separate chapters. All contributions are put into perspective by introductory and concluding chapters.

We would like to thank the Pharmaceutical Companies, and Government and University Departments who gave their staff the time and facilities to produce their contributions to this book. Special thanks are due to our own employers, Smith Kline & French Research Limited, and to the staff of Cambridge University Press.

CKA & CES
February 1987

INTRODUCTION

G.B. Leslie and P. Johnson

Smith Kline and French Research Limited, The Frythe,

Welwyn, Herts. AL6 9AR

The toxicology of drugs, potential drugs and other chemicals which might adversely affect humans or animals has been one of the most rapidly expanding areas of biological science during the last 25 years. This same period has seen the accelerating development of the techniques for cell and tissue culture *in vitro*. It is not surprising therefore that toxicologists have enthusiastically embraced these new techniques to develop their understanding of cellular mechanisms of toxicity and to provide screens for assessment of new compounds.

As might be expected the increased interest by toxicologists in *in vitro* techniques has also been reflected by the scientific literature. A review entitled "Tissue Culture and Toxicology" by R.C. Rofe (1971) proposed the comparison of the responses of a selection of human and animal tissues to compounds for which *in vivo* toxicological data already existed. A decade later saw the publication of two useful reviews by D. Neubert (1982) on the Use of Culture Techniques in Studies on Prenatal Toxicity and by J. Hooisma (1982) on Tissue Culture and Neurotoxicology. Reviews of *in-vitro* techniques as alternatives to animal tests include those of Balls and Clothier (1983) on Differentiated Cell and Organ Culture in Toxicity Testing and by A.M. Goldberg (1985) on An Approach to the Development of *In Vitro* Toxicological Methods. A new journal entitled "*In Vitro* Toxicology" begins publication in 1987.

It is evident from the increasing number of scientific meetings that this area of work has become of great interest and importance to scientists of many disciplines.

In recent years this has been exemplified in Europe by three International Workshops held on Tissue Culture Applications in Toxicology. The first of these held in Soesterberg, Holland in 1980 (Heilbronn 1980) identified the need for better education in *in vitro* toxicology and for comparison of results with those from *in vivo* studies. At the second in Hasselunden, Sweden, International Workshop on the Application of Tissue Culture in Toxicology (Toxicology *25* (1982) 1 *et seq*). There were several presentations on metabolic activation systems which are essential in attempting to emulate *in vivo* conditions in *in vitro* systems. The third workshop held in Urbino, International Workshop on the Application of Tissue Culture in Toxicology (Preface in Xenobiotica (1985) *15*, 8/9. 633-634). Italy focussed on cytotoxicity and teratogenicity and looked at the development of screening tests, the analysis of mechanisms of action and at studies on biotransformation.

In the USA Workshops have been held since 1975 (Berky & Sherrod 1976) and the Johns Hopkins Centre for Alternatives to Animals Testing (C.A.A.T.) have organised four rather specific symposia on *in vitro* toxicology. The 1982 symposium surveyed new methodological approaches to Product Safety Evaluation (Goldberg, 1983) and in 1983 looked at alternative approaches to reduce animal use in acute toxicity testing (Goldberg, 1984). Their 1984 symposium (Goldberg, 1985) considered *in vitro* alternatives to the Draize test in the measurement of irritancy and in 1986 the theme was 'approaches to validation'.

The New York Academy of Sciences organised a symposium on Cellular Systems for Toxicity Testing in 1982, the proceedings of which were published (Williams, Dunkel & Ray 1983).

In the UK two meetings were held in 1985. In March the Lord Dowding Fund organised a meeting held in London on Human Tissues and Tissue Culture in Biomedical Research (Human Toxicology (1985) 4 555-556) and in September several scientific organisations and companies sponsored a large and very successful meeting at Reading on Practical *In Vitro* Toxicology the proceedings of which are about to be published.

Thus it is apparent, with increasing scientific need for alternatives to animal experimentation, and increasing perception of the potential value scientifically, ethically and commercially of *in vitro* techniques in toxicology, that scientific effort in this area will increase dramatically over the next few years. It is important, however, that the potential for the reduction in, or avoidance of, whole animal experiments should not force irrational acceptance of unvalidated tests. It is also important that the value of some *in vitro* approaches should be recognised as complimentary to whole animal experiments at the current state of our knowledge.

The single most important advantage of *in vitro* tests, with a potential which has not yet been realised, is that they allow comparisons of the effects of cellular and organ exposure to drugs and chemicals to be entrapolated across species to include man himself through the use of human cell cultures from necropsy or biopsy material. In other words, such techniques have the potential to allow the toxicological evaluation of compounds in animals and man on an equal basis, which cannot be achieved in classical *in vivo* toxicological testing. However the difficulties experienced by many laboratories in obtaining human tissue cannot be ignored and are a serious impedance to progress in this area. The comparison across species may be extended further to the establishment of cultured cell lines which can allow scientists in different laboratories to compare results and permit the necessary standardisation which is fundamental to good scientific practice.

In the opinion of the authors it is essential to establish standards of methodology which will allow parallel assessment by independent laboratories of *in vitro* parameters of closest relevance to the *in vivo* situation. Certainly much is at stake, both in terms of safety and in terms of expensive commercial risk, in interpretations of *in vitro* data which may "kill" a perfectly valid development compound or alternatively allow an unacceptably toxic compound to proceed, with ultimate adverse effects in man.

This leads inevitably to questions on the predictive value of positive or negative results *in vitro*, but the weighting given to such tests can only be established with the experience of time and hard data, by relating *in vitro* observations to proven *in vivo* effects with well-studied compounds. It is clearly important that the aim of all laboratories should be to establish *in vitro* end-points which will bear the closest possible relationship to responses obtained *in vivo*. If this is not achieved *in vitro* parameters will not gain the required scientific and regulatory acceptance in relation to their relevance to ultimate safety *in vivo* in man.

Although there has been a predominance of work in the field

of genotoxicity (mutagenicity) testing, _in vitro_ approaches are moving into the field of immunotoxicology and will inevitably expand to the study of all potential target organs. However, the continuing debate concerning the validity of many genotoxicity tests, particularly in terms of their ability to predict potential carcinogens, emphasizes the rigorous evaluation which must be applied to new _in vitro_ approaches if they are to gain acceptance by the scientific community.

Following the thalidomide tragedy and the establishment of Regulatory Authorities to consider new drugs and other chemicals, the pharmaceutical and other industries set up more formal toxicological evaluation procedures. "In house" toxicology departments were soon supplemented by Contract Research organisations and a series of standard "Regulatory" tests became an international requirement for all new compounds which might be taken by man (and other animals) either deliberately or accidentally. The objective of these rather stereotyped studies was to identify the nature of the toxicity of a compound and to assess the potential risks by extrapolation from toxic responses at various dose levels to the therapeutic dose in man, the highest 'no-effect' dose in animals being used as the basis of the so-called 'therapeutic ratio'.

Although the therapeutic ratio is a valid concept, one of the fundamental guiding principles of the toxicologist is that he is _not_ trying to demonstrate that a potential drug or other chemical is non-toxic. The fact that _all_ chemicals are toxic has been well recognised for centuries. It was Phillipus Theophrastus Aureolus Bombastus Von Hohenheim (1492-1541), otherwise known as Paracelsus, who said "All substances are poisons; there is none which is not a poison. The right dose differentiates a poison and a remedy".

If we accept that all chemicals are "poisons" it follows that toxicologists are not looking at a compound to see whether it is toxic but to find out the degree of toxicity and the nature of the toxicity. What is important in the development of drugs is the ratio between the therapeutic and the toxic doses or blood levels and between the desired and unwanted effects. The "regulatory" tests achieve this to some degree.

Another important guiding principle for the toxicologist is that toxicology is essentially a predictive science. We study the nature of the toxic effect in order to assess the risk to man. Unfortunately, there have been sufficient instances of toxic effects arising only after wide exposure to man of compounds which have fully satisfied international regulatory requirements with regard to animal testing to question the predictability of "standard" tests for many substances.

The toxicologist is going to administer increasingly high doses of compound to experimental animals in order to identify target organs or other limiting toxicity. After this in collaboration with colleagues in other disciplines he has to make risk assessments and contribute to the development and selection of other candidate compounds. Once target organ or limiting toxicity is identified mechanistic studies are required and it is here that *in vitro* techniques are now becoming widely and increasingly used.

Subject to the validation which has been discussed above, these tests must surely take their place alongside, for example, biochemical or pharmacological tests *in vitro* at the subcellular, cellular or organ level which currently play their part with *in vivo* tests in forming an overall, and more complete, scientific picture of a new test compound.

Very often whole animal studies may not be appropriate for mechanistic studies because in many cases the adverse effect becomes apparent only after very long periods of chronic dosing.

It has often been possible to demonstrate that risk to humans is not likely once the mechanism of action of the adverse effect in the experimental animals has been understood. Sometimes the species specificity of toxic effects have been confirmed by utilising cell cultures from several species including humans. When the mechanism of an adverse effect seen in whole animals studies has been studied and is considered possibly to be predictive of risk in humans the compound may have its development curtailed. However, other candidate compounds may need evaluation in short term models designed to detect potential adverse effects when only small amounts of compound are available. _In vitro_ techniques are frequently the most appropriate means of doing this. In both economic terms and use of animals, such early comparative tests with different compounds in _in vitro_ systems must be attractive. The extension of this to multi-compound screening is a matter of individual research and development strategy. Such short term models may also be used in drug design, since when playing "molecular roulette", potency data in biological or pharmacological assays provide only part of the information required by the medicinal chemist. A modern cost effective approach to drug design must take into account toxicological potential as well as inherent biological activity.

We anticipate that the progress of the science of toxicology in the pharmaceutical, agrochemical and other similar industries will lead increasingly to mechanistic approaches to toxicology and increasing use of _in vitro_ techniques and models.

Contributors to this book have covered almost every area of toxicology and have utilised a full range of *in vitro* techniques ranging from mammalian cell lines, including human, at one end of the spectrum to abbatoir material (eyes) and classical pharmacological isolated organ techniques (hearts) at the other. Whether chicken eggs used for studies on chorio-allantoic membranes or whole rat embryos are *in vitro* or *in vivo* are moot points but they certainly represent humane alternatives to the use of whole animals and provide elegant investigational tools and models for toxicological study.

It is clear that this volume will provide a valuable reference for scientists involved in the toxicological investigation and evaluation of potential new drugs, agrochemicals, food additives etc. It should interest graduate and postgraduate students and research workers in toxicology as this subject becomes an integral part of the training of toxicologists, particularly since individual chapters cover not only the philosophy and strategy of the use of *in vitro* models but also give attention to detailed methodology.

References

M. Balls & R. Clothier. Differentiated Cell and Organ Culture in toxicity testing. Acta. Pharmacologica et Toxicologica (1983) 52 Suppl 2 115-137.

J. Berky & P.C. Sherrod (Editors). "In Vitro Toxicity Testing" in Proceedings of the 1st and 2nd Working Conference on Toxicity Testing In Vitro 1975/1976 (Philadelphia Franklin Institute Press)

A M Goldberg (Editor). Proceedings of the symposium on "Product Safety Evaluation: Development of New Methodological Approaches", Alternative Methods in Toxicology 1. (1983) Liebert, New York and Basel.

A M Goldberg (Editor). Proceedings of the symposium on "Acute Toxicity Testing - Are There Alternative Approaches? "Alternative Methods in Toxicology 2. (1984), Liebert, New York and Basel.

A M Goldberg (Editor). Proceedings of the symposium on "In Vitro Toxicology" Alternative Methods in Toxicology 3. (1985), Liebert, New York and Basel.

A.M. Goldberg. An Approach to the Development of in vitro Toxicological Methods. Fd. Chem. Toxic. (1985) 23 No 2 205-208.

E. Heilbronn Summing up of the International Workshop on the Application of Tissue Culture in Toxicology. Toxicology (1980) 17 269-272.

J. Hooisma. Tissue Culture & Neurotoxicology. Neurobehavioural Toxicology and Teratology (1982) 4 617-622.

D. Neubert. The Use of Culture Techniques in Studies on Prenatal Toxicity. Pharmac. Ther. (1982) 18 397-434.

P.C. Rofe. Tissue Culture and Toxicology. Fd & Cosmet. Toxicol. (1971) 9 685-696.

G.M. Williams, V.C. Dunkel & V.A. Ray. Editors. Cellular systems for Toxicity Testing. Annals of N.Y. Academy of Sciences. 407 (1983).

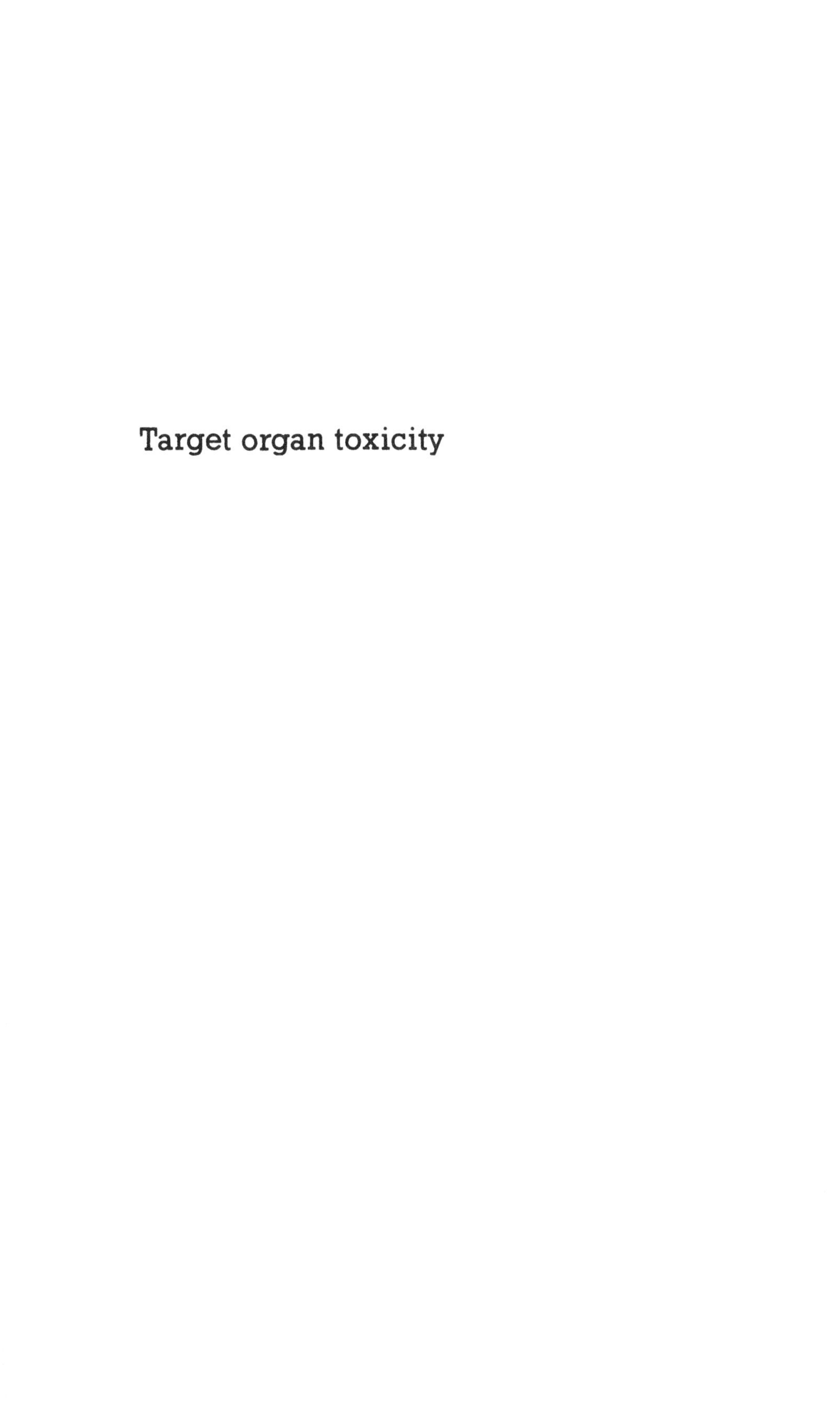

Target organ toxicity

IN VITRO METHODS IN RENAL TOXICOLOGY

M. A. Smith
Department of Investigative Toxicology, Smith Kline & French Laboratories, Philadelphia, PA 19101

W. R. Hewitt
Department of Investigative Toxicology, Smith Kline & French Laboratories, Philadelphia, PA 19101

J. B. Hook
Department of Investigative Toxicology, Smith Kline & French Laboratories, Philadelphia, PA 19101

INTRODUCTION

The kidneys are particularly susceptible to xenobiotic-induced toxic injury. This is due primarily to the unique structure and function of these highly dynamic organs. The nephron, the functional unit of the kidney, consists of the glomerulus and at least 12 morphologically and functionally distinct tubular segments. Individual nephron segments contain one or more cell types which are structurally and functionally related; and these cell types may differ in their susceptibility to toxicant-induced injury. Factors which may predispose the kidneys to toxicant-induced injury include: 1) the high rate of renal blood flow (approximately 25% of total cardiac output); 2) mechanisms for concentrating toxicants within the tubular fluid; 3) transport systems capable of concentrating toxicants within cells; and 4) a substantial capacity for xenobiotic biotransformation. The renal cortex receives 85 to 90% of the total renal blood flow. As a result, the renal cortex, which is 90% proximal tubular tissue, may be preferentially exposed to blood-borne toxicants. Proximal tubular cells contain several active transport systems for the secretion and/or reabsorption of xenobiotics. Toxicants may achieve high concentrations within proximal tubular cells if they are substrates for one or more of these transport systems. In addition, protein endocytotic mechanisms located in the luminal membrane of proximal tubular cells also may contribute to reabsorption and intracellular concentration of toxicants. The renal cortex contains cytochrome P-450-dependent mixed-function oxidases which are capable of activating xenobiotics to toxic, reactive intermediates. Singly, or in concert, these factors render the proximal tubule the most frequent target of chemical-induced toxicity in the kidney (Hook & Hewitt,1986).

In contrast to the cortex, blood flow to the renal medulla is relatively low and it might be expected that a smaller percentage of toxicants would reach the medulla. However, compounds present in the tubular fluid can pass through the loop of Henle and collecting duct and may be concentrated and trapped within the medulla via the renal counter-current exchange mechanisms. There is no detectable mixed-function oxidase activity within the inner renal medulla; however, the prostaglandin endoperoxide synthetase system is active in medullary (but not cortical) tissue and may mediate the bioactivation of compounds to toxic intermediates within the renal medulla. Thus, like the proximal tubule, medullary nephron segments may also be targets for the toxic effects of chemicals.

The development of methods to evaluate renal damage are complicated by the structural and functional heterogeneity of the kidneys. This review will focus on _in vitro_ methods which may be used to detect and quantitate renal dysfunction. These methods provide varying degrees of specificity for evaluating the localization of and mechanisms of toxicant-induced injury.

PRACTICAL ASPECTS

Isolated perfused kidney

The isolated perfused kidney is the only _in vitro_ method which allows renal function to be studied in the presence of an intact vasculature and normal anatomical relationships between nephrons. Unlike other _in vitro_ systems, the effects of a toxicant on intrarenal haemodynamics can be observed using an isolated perfused kidney. A rapidly recirculating perfusion system has been described in detail by Newton and Hook (1981). In this system a rat kidney is perfused via the renal artery at a constant pressure with an oxygenated modified Krebs-Ringer bicarbonate buffer. Glomerular filtration rate, fractional sodium excretion, water reabsorption, perfusate flow rate and perfusion pressure frequently are used as indices of organ function and as criteria for viability of the kidney. Alteration in these indices have been used to evaluate the direct, nephrotoxic potential of various chemicals including the antineoplastic agent cisplatin (Sumpio et al., 1985) and the aminoglycoside antibiotics (Collier, et al.,

1979). The isolated perfused kidney is also an excellent tool for examination of the filtration, secretion, reabsorption and metabolism of xenobiotics in an intact functioning organ free of systemic vascular influences and free from metabolic participation by other organs (eg., the liver). For example, renal metabolism of the analgesic acetaminophen (APAP) and the subsequent formation of reactive metabolites, independent of hepatic biotransformation, have been evaluated in the isolated perfused kidney (Emslie et al., 1981; Newton et al., 1983).

There are limitations when using the isolated perfused kidney for evaluation of toxicant action in the kidney [see table]. The difficulties in maintaining a viable preparation for more than 4 hours limit the duration of experimental observations. In addition, although glomerular and proximal tubular functions are satisfactory in the isolated perfused kidney, there is a reabsorptive defect in the distal tubule which is not yet fully characterized (Maack, 1980). This defect prevents the isolated perfused kidney from concentrating urine properly. Mitochondrial swelling and cellular disruption occurs in the cells of the thick ascending limb of Henle following perfusion for 90 minutes (Alcorn et al. 1980). This selective abnormality in thick ascending limb cells following perfusion may be related to the concentrating defect. The intrarenal disposition and potential toxicity of certain compounds may be altered by this distal defect. Thus, the isolated perfused kidney may be limited in its utility for evaluating nephrotoxic agents which affect the distal tubule or medulla. The time and expense involved in setting up the isolated perfused kidney often limits its routine use for toxicological evaluations. However, it can be used to answer questions pertaining to renal xenobiotic metabolism and the subsequent effects of potentially toxic metabolites on renal function.

Renal slices

Renal slices have been used frequently to evaluate the nephrotoxic effects of a variety of xenobiotics; the experimental methodology has been described by Hirsch (1976) and Berndt (1976). Ease of preparation and manipulation are the major advantages to using renal slices for evaluating nephrotoxicity. The effects of toxicants in specific regions of the kidney can be determined in slices prepared from cortical or medullary tissue (Smith et al., 1983; Rapp et al., 1980). Slices prepared from animals challenged with a toxicant can be used to provide more sensitive indices of xenobiotic-induced renal dysfunction than standard estimates such as blood urea nitrogen or serum creatinine concentrations. In addition, slices can be prepared from naive animals and exposed to the toxicant _in vitro_. Thus, the _in vivo_ and _in vitro_ effects of a toxicant can be compared in similar tissue preparations and it can then be determined if the effects of the toxicant are due to a direct action on kidney tissue or due to extrarenal effects. Renal slices have been prepared from a number of mammalian species, including mouse, rat, rabbit, hamster, guinea pig, dog, monkey and human. The wide range of species from which renal slices can be prepared, coupled with the ease of preparation, markedly facilitates interspecies comparisons of toxicant-induced renal dysfunction [see table]. Similarly, renal slices can be readily obtained from fetal, neonatal, adult and senescent animals, thus allowing comparison of age-related differences in the susceptibility of the kidney to chemical-induced damage.

Studies from several laboratories have demonstrated that the _in vitro_ renal cortical slice accumulation of organic ions such as p-aminohippuric acid (PAH) and tetraethylammonium (TEA) was among the most sensitive and versatile indicators of renal proximal tubular injury (Phillips et al., 1977; Kluwe, 1981; Kyle et al., 1983; Miyajima et al., 1983). The relative sensitivities of various renal function tests were compared after oral administration of biphenyl, carbon tetrachloride (CCl_4) and mercuric chloride ($HgCl_2$) to rats (Kluwe, 1981). The tests included determinations of urine specific gravity, pH and volume, as well as urinary excretion of glucose, protein, electrolytes and several enzymes. In addition, serum urea nitrogen, creatinine and electrolyte concentrations, creatinine clearance, kidney weight and the ability of renal cortical slices to accumulate PAH and TEA were assessed. The most useful tests for assessing nephrotoxicity were changes in kidney weight, urinary concentrating ability and _in vitro_ accumulation of organic ions. Consistent with Kluwe's report

(1981), depression of PAH and TEA accumulation in renal cortical slices following _in vivo_ administration of cephaloridine, $HgCl_2$ and potassium dichromate ($K_2Cr_2O_7$) were found to correlate well with observed changes in renal histopathology (Miyajima et al., 1983). In addition to slice PAH and TEA accumulation, slice oxygen consumption and gluconeogenic capacity have been used to determine the extent of proximal tubular injury following _in vivo_ or _in vitro_ exposure to $K_2Cr_2O_7$ (Kacew and Hirsch, 1981). Alterations in PAH and TEA accumulation and inhibition of gluconeogenesis by renal cortical slices were observed following _in vivo_ exposure to $K_2Cr_2O_7$. Incubating renal cortical slices with $K_2Cr_2O_7$ _in vitro_ resulted in decreased oxygen consumption and alterations in slice organic ion accumulation. In this study, the pattern of effects of $K_2Cr_2O_7$ after _in vitro_ exposure was similar to that observed after _in vivo_ administration of this toxicant.

Certain disadvantages have been associated with the renal slice technique. For example, kidney slices contain a heterogeneous population of tubules and there is a lack of adequate methodology for discriminating between toxicity to the proximal tubule versus other nephron segments contained in the slice. The renal cortical slice system is limited by the inability to distinguish toxicant effects that are specific for the thick ascending limb or the distal tubule. Some drugs, such as gentamicin, are transported across the luminal membrane _in vivo_ prior to causing nephrotoxicity. There is evidence that drugs in the incubation medium have limited access to the luminal side of slice cortical tubules since the lumens of the tubules are collapsed; hence, the basolateral membrane may be preferentially exposed to toxicants in slice preparations (Arthus et al., 1982). However, drugs such as the aminoglycoside antibiotic gentamicin can produce toxicity when incubated _in vitro_ with renal slices (Cohen et al., 1975). Since the mechanism of the uptake and toxicity of gentamicin _in vitro_ is as yet unknown, the relevance to _in vivo_ studies is still unclear. At present, slice preparations have a limited viability of 4 - 6 hours. This may pose some problems when determining the relevance of data gathered from short-term incubations, when toxicity _in vivo_ may take days to become manifest. To overcome this, some investigators choose to incubate slices with higher concentrations of toxicant in order to observe a response in a shorter period of time. This is a valid manoeuvre only if the tissue concentrations reached _in vitro_ are determined and compared to those obtained _in vivo_. Nonetheless, given the limitations of the system, renal slices still provide a simple and rapid means of evaluating nephrotoxicity _in vitro_ in a tissue preparation that maintains cell-to-cell and nephron-to-nephron interactions similar to those observed _in vivo_.

Renal tubule suspensions

Suspensions of renal tubules provide another method to study renal metabolism and toxicity _in vitro_. Tubule suspensions are most commonly obtained from rabbit or rat kidney, although tubule suspensions have been prepared sucessfully from kidneys of other species. Enzymatic digestion of tissue slices or fragments (Balaban et al., 1980) or mechanical disruption of kidney tissue (Meezan et al., 1973) are often used for preparation of fragment suspensions. Preparations of tubule fragments consisting of defined nephron segments have been obtained by density gradient centrifugation (Scholer & Edelman, 1979; Vinay et al., 1981; Cojocel et al., 1983; Chamberlin et al., 1984). There are disadvantages in using renal tubule suspensions for evaluation of nephrotoxicity. Renal tubules have a limited duration of viability. Experiments longer than 1.5 hours in duration may not be feasible with isolated renal tubules (Rasmussen, 1975). This limits experiments to the evaluation of the acute effects of nephrotoxic agents on tubule suspensions. If tubule suspensions are obtained from animals that have been exposed to a toxicant _in vivo_, the adverse effects of the toxicant on tubule function may be evaluated _in vitro_. However, preparation of tubule suspensions require the use of digestive enzymes, and/or substantial mechanical stress. Loss of damaged tubules from kidneys challenged _in vivo_ with a toxicant is highly likely when using these suspensions. Spurious results may be obtained due to selection of a population of relatively undamaged tubules during preparation. Although an intact epithelial structure can be maintained in suspension, the enzymatic treatment used to obtain the tubules can result in loss of the tubular basement membrane

(Chamberlin et al., 1984). Altered tubular handling of xenobiotics *in vitro* and hence, the nature of toxicities, may result.

Assessment of nephrotoxicity with renal tubule suspensions provides an advantage, however, over the isolated perfused kidney and renal cortical slices. Preparations of tubule fragments from specific nephron segments may be obtained, allowing the effects of toxicant-induced injury on specific nephron segments to be observed [see table]. For example, unlike renal slices, suspensions of thick ascending limbs or distal tubules make it possible to evaluate the effects of toxicants on these regions of the nephron. In addition, suspensions of renal tubules may be more economical than renal slices, since a larger number of experiments can be performed on tubule samples obtained from a single animal; reagent costs, however, are greater for suspensions than slices.

Renal cell suspensions

Methods similar to those used for the isolation of renal tubule fragments have been used to obtain suspensions of renal cells. Various methods have been employed to effect the separation of specific renal cell types from kidney tissue; however, the heterogeneity of the kidney makes this a difficult process [see table]. Isokinetic gradient centrifuga- tion, free flow electrophoresis, enzymatic digestion, density gradient centrifugation, flow cytometry and monoclonal antibodies have been used to isolate specific renal cell types (Kreisberg et al. 1977; Heidrich & Dew, 1977; Dworzack & Grantham, 1975; Eveloff et al. 1980; Endou et al., 1982; Smith & Garcia-Perez, 1985). Each of these methods are effective for obtaining desired cell types, however; there is considerable difference in the effectiveness of the cell separation and in the difficulty and expense involved with each method. For example, cell separation by flow cytometry is precise, but requires expensive equipment that is not readily available in most laboratories. Monoclonal antibodies can be used for selective cell separation, but require time consuming production of the antibodies prior to their use in cell separation. In contrast, density gradient centrifugation can be easily adapted by most laboratories for routine cell separation, but lacks the precision of flow cytometry and monoclonal antibody separation.

The difficulties encountered in preparing suspensions of specific cell types may have prevented investigators from using suspensions of renal cells in lieu of other _in vitro_ preparations. As with other _in vitro_ preparations, suspensions of renal cells can only be used for short-term studies. The cell suspensions are usually not viable for periods greater than 6 to 8 hours. In addition, data obtained from an isolated cell system may be difficult to interpret and relate to the intact kidney. Cells in suspension no longer have the same polarity as cells in a preparation of intact tubules. Since the distinct basolateral/apical "sidedness" of the cell is lost in a suspended cell system, compounds may not enter the cell in suspension via the same mechanisms as they do _in vivo_. In addition, the importance of cell-to-cell interactions in normal renal function cannot be accounted for in a cell suspension. However, if these limitations are considered when interpreting results, suspensions of renal cells may prove to be a useful tool to examine cell-specific biochemical differences and susceptibility to toxicants.

Renal cells in culture

The metabolic and functional aspects of renal epithelial cells have been examined _in vitro_ through the use of established cell lines and primary cell cultures. Perhaps the most well studied cell lines are the LLC-PK1 and MDCK which are derived from pig kidney and dog kidney, respectively. The LLC-PK1 cells express characteristics of proximal tubular epithelium and the MDCK cells express characteristics of distal tubular or cortical collecting duct epithelium (Gstraunthaler et al., 1985). Each cell line is morphologically similar to the supposed tissue of origin; the LLC-PK1 cells have pronounced microvilli on the apical membrane as is found on proximal tubular cells, whereas the MDCK cells have short blunt microvilli like those found on distal tubular cells. In addition, the LLC-PK1 cells express a profile of enzymatic activity much like that expressed by proximal tubular cells. The profile of enzymatic activity expressed by MDCK cells suggest that they are not of proximal tubular origin. Both cell lines have been well characterized biochemically and possess many of the transport functions of renal cells _in vivo_ (Handler et al., 1980). Other renal cell lines include the BHK baby hamster kidney fibroblast-like cells, MDBK bovine kidney epithelial cells and the BSC-1 African green monkey kidney epithelial cell line (Sakhrani & Fine, 1983). Primary cultures of renal cells have been prepared from glomeruli, proximal tubules, thick ascending limbs and collecting tubules obtained from rat and rabbit kidneys (Burg et al., 1982; Chung et al., 1982; Curthoys & Belleman,1979; Kreisberg et al., 1978; Sato & Dunn, 1984) and from human renal tissue (Wilson et al.,1985; Trifillis et al., 1985) [see table]. Depending on the cell type and the propensity toward fibroblast overgrowth, the primary cell cultures may remain viable for one to several weeks. Manipulation of nutrient medium components can affect the growth and viability of renal cells in culture (Gilbert & Migeon, 1977; Taub & Sato, 1980).

Renal cell culture offers advantages over other methods for assessing the effects of toxic agents on renal cells. Defined populations of cells from specific nephron segments can be isolated and grown in culture. Biochemical measurements and morphological alteration in response to toxicants can be observed easily within the same sample. Unlike isolated cells, cultured renal cells maintain their cell-to-cell interactions and the polarity that is observed *in vivo* (Ojakian and Herzlinger, 1984). In addition, cells in culture have had the opportunity to recover from the enzymatic digestion process and attach to a solid support, thus regaining the basement membrane damaged during isolation. Toxicants can be applied to basolateral or luminal surfaces and transcellular transport of fluid and ions can be readily assessed. The culture system is economical with regard to animal use. One rat can yield 40 to 60 culture dishes for experiments and only small quantities of toxicant need be added for study. Unlike the other *in vitro* systems, culture systems are viable for several days to several weeks, thus, it is possible to conduct toxicity studies of longer duration.

Cultured renal cells are not without their limitations, however. In contrast to slice or tubule systems, cell culture is expensive regarding time, reagents and the need for an appropriate facility and personnel trained in tissue culture. The decline in renal drug metabolizing enzyme activities over time could pose potential problems when evaluating compounds that rely on particular enzymes for detoxication or to express their toxicity. The rate of decline of drug metabolizing enzymes in cultured renal cells is similar to that observed with cultured hepatocytes and presents an obstacle to those wishing to conduct drug metabolism studies in culture (Sirica & Pitot, 1980; Smith et al., 1986). Cells cultured on flat culture dishes have only the apical side exposed to the toxicant in the medium thus, compounds that enter the tubular cells from the basolateral side may not express the same toxicity _in vitro_ as they do _in vivo_. This problem may be overcome by growing cells on suspended collagen disks. The use of renal cell lines for toxicity evaluation can present problems in extrapolating data obtained from cells that have been in culture for long periods of time to the intact animal. These cells may have de-differentiated in culture and may differ significantly from the tissue of origin. If used properly, however, cell culture systems do provide a unique way to observe direct renal cellular responses to toxicants.

EXPERIMENTAL EXAMPLES

Isolated Perfused Kidney

APAP is an antipyretic analgesic which can produce centrolobular hepatic necrosis and acute renal failure in humans following ingestion of a large overdose (Boyer & Rouff, 1971). APAP administration to rats resulted in acute tubular necrosis restricted to the straight segment of the proximal tubule (McMurtry et al., 1978). These authors postulated that, like the liver, the kidney was able to metabolize APAP via a cytochrome P-450-dependent mechanism to a reactive electrophilic species capable of binding to tissue macromolecules, once detoxication by glutathione (GSH) had been overwhelmed. Newton et al., (1982) determined that the kidney produced an electrophilic metabolite of APAP which could combine with and deplete renal GSH in a fashion similar to that observed in the liver. The formation of the electrophilic metabolite appeared to be dependent on renal cytochrome P-450 metabolism, since treatment with an inducer of cytochrome P-450 (polybrominated biphenyls, PBBs) enhanced renal GSH depletion by APAP, whereas treatment with a cytochrome P-450 inhibitor (piperonyl butoxide) reduced the GSH depletion produced by APAP. In subsequent studies, the isolated perfused kidney was used in conjunction with _in vivo_ toxicity studies to evaluate potential strain differences in the nephrotoxicity and metabolism of APAP by Fischer 344 (F344) and Sprague-Dawley (SD) rats (Newton et al., 1983). Strain differences in APAP-induced functional changes were observed _in vivo_, with the SD rat being less susceptible to APAP-induced nephrotoxicity than the F344 rat. These strain differences in susceptibility to APAP-induced nephrotoxicity were thought to be due to differences in renal cytochrome P-450 activation of APAP or the deacetylation of APAP to the nephrotoxic metabolite, p-aminophenol (PAP). Isolated kidneys from SD and F344 rats perfused with APAP, excreted PAP at similar rates and no differences were observed in the covalent binding of cytochrome P-450-mediated APAP metabolites in SD or F344 rats. Thus, the strain differences observed in APAP-induced nephrotoxicity could not be attributed to differences in the renal metabolism of APAP. Using the isolated perfused kidney in conjunction with _in vivo_ experiments allowed the relationship between strain differences in APAP-induced nephrotoxicity and renal APAP metabolism to be defined.

Renal slices

Chloroform ($CHCl_3$), a haloalkane well known for its ability to cause hepatotoxicity and nephrotoxicity, can be metabolized by the liver to a highly reactive toxic intermediate, phosgene, via a cytochrome P-450-dependent reaction (Pohl, 1979). However it was unclear if phosgene, or a metabolite of phosgene, formed in the liver was responsible for the production of renal injury. Renal cortical slices prepared from mice treated with $CHCl_3$ were used to evaluate renal $CHCl_3$ metabolism (Smith et al., 1983). As early as two hours after a subcutaneous injection of $CHCl_3$, nephrotoxicity could be produced and detected in male mice, but not in female mice. Renal cortical slices prepared from male mice treated with $CHCl_3$ demonstrated a decreased ability to accumulate organic ions, whereas slices prepared from female mice treated with $CHCl_3$ were unaffected. Renal cortical glutathione concentrations declined in male mice, but not in female mice, in a time course that paralleled the effects observed with organic ion accumulation. Significantly, $CHCl_3$ was equally hepatotoxic in both male and female mice. This suggested that perhaps a reactive metabolite was formed in situ in the kidneys of male mice, but not in female mice.

To address this question further, in vitro studies were conducted to characterize the renal metabolism of $CHCl_3$ (Smith & Hook, 1983). The same pattern for the time course and sex-related differences in $CHCl_3$-induced nephrotoxicity in vivo was observed in vitro. Preincubation of renal cortical slices from male mice with $CHCl_3$ resulted in a decreased ability of the slices to accumulate organic ions. In contrast, preincubation of slices from female mice with $CHCl_3$ had no effect on slice organic ion accumulation. Demonstration of a toxic response by renal slices incubated with $CHCl_3$ in vitro, indicated that the kidneys were able to metabolize $CHCl_3$ in situ to a toxic intermediate. Cleavage of the C-H bond has been shown to occur in the hepatic metabolism of $CHCl_3$ (Pohl, 1979) and may be a requisite metabolic step in the kidney as well. Further evidence for the renal metabolism of $CHCl_3$ was provided by the observation that preincubation of male kidney slices with deuterated $CHCl_3$ ($CDCl_3$), a less nephrotoxic compound, resulted in attenuation of the decline in organic ion accumulation. Incubation of renal slices with $CHCl_3$ under conditions which diminished the activity of renal cytochrome P-450 prevented the $CHCl_3$-induced decrease in organic ion accumulation. This observation provided further evidence that $CHCl_3$ may be metabolized in situ by the kidney to a nephrotoxic metabolite. These studies demonstrate how an in vitro system can be used to elucidate the mechanism of action of a nephrotoxic agent.

Renal slices from specific regions of the kidney can be used to differentiate the effects of toxicants on cortical or medullary tissue. Renal medullary slices have been used to confirm that benzidine, a urinary bladder carcinogen, could be metabolically activated in intact renal medullary tissue (Rapp et al., 1980). The toxic effects of benzidine are thought to be due to the metabolic activation of the compound to a reactive intermediate which then reacts with urinary bladder tissue. Zenser et al. (1979) demonstrated that renal medullary, but not renal cortical or hepatic microsomes could metabolize benzidine via a prostaglandin- mediated process to a reactive intermediate capable of binding to proteins. The prostaglandin endoperoxide synthetase-mediated cooxidative metabolism of benzidine was prevented by inhibitors of prostaglandin endoperoxide synthetase and stimulated by fatty acid substrates. The cooxidative metabolism of benzidine was demonstrated to occur in an intact tissue preparation such as renal inner medullary slices (Rapp et al., 1980). The cooxidative metabolism and subsequent tissue binding of benzidine in the medullary slices suggested that benzidine may be metabolically activated in the renal medulla.

Renal tubule suspensions

Suspensions of defined nephron segments may be useful in delineating nephron segment-specific processes that may mediate toxicity. For example, nonprotein sulfhydryl (NPSH) content, an indicator of renal GSH content, was not significantly different in proximal and distal tubule suspensions (Cojocel et el., 1983). In addition, proximal tubule suspensions contained high cytochrome P-450 activity, whereas distal tubule suspensions contained no measurable activity of cytochrome P-450. This would suggest a differential ability of proximal and distal tubules to metabolize xenobiotics and suggest that the proximal tubule would be more susceptible to toxicants that are activated to toxic, reactive intermediates by this enzyme system. Cojocel et al. (1983) also demonstrated that distal tubule suspensions deacetylated APAP to PAP and O-deethylated 7-ethoxycoumarin to 7-hydroxycoumarin to a lesser degree than did proximal tubule suspensions. In addition, proximal tubule suspensions appeared to have a greater capacity for glucuronidation than did distal tubule suspensions. These differences in xenobiotic metabolizing capability may play a role in cell specific mechanisms of nephrotoxicity (Cojocel et al., 1980).

Renal handling of energy substrates (lactate, glutamine and oleate), gluconeogenesis, organic ion transport and oxygen utilization all have been evaluated in renal tubule suspensions (Guder & Wirthensohn, 1979; Gullans et al., 1984; Huang & Lin, 1965; Balaban et al., 1980). Alterations in several of these functions have been used to assess toxicant-induced renal dysfunction *in vitro*. For example, tubule suspensions obtained from rabbits pretreated with dichlorovinylcysteine (DCVC) demonstrated a decreased ability to accumulate organic ions (Hassall et al., 1983). Similar effects on organic ion transport occurred when rabbit tubules were exposed to DCVC *in vitro*. The similarity of the effects produced by DCVC *in vivo* and *in vitro*, suggested that tubule suspensions would be useful in studying the mechanisms of DCVC nephrotoxicity. In subsequent studies, rabbit renal tubule suspensions were used to examine the biotransformation and resultant toxicity of the glutathione conjugate of DCVC (DCVG) (Hassall et al., 1984). Glutathione conjugates formed in the liver are transported to the kidney where they are presumably further metabolized to a nephrotoxic intermediate. Tubules isolated from rabbits pretreated with DCVG exhibited an impaired ability to transport organic ions; this also was observed in tubules from naive animals exposed *in vitro* to DCVG. *In vitro* metabolism experiments later demonstrated that DCVG was metabolized to the nephrotoxic agent DCVC by the tubules.

Renal cells in culture

Renal cell lines have not been used extensively in toxicological evaluation; however, the potential utility of these cell lines has been established. The LLC-PK1 cell line has been used to assess aminoglycoside-induced toxicity *in vitro* (Hori et al. 1984; Schwertz et al. 1986). Cells from the LLC-PK1 cell line have a fixed polarity and are able to form tight junctions. This enables the the cells to behave as an epithelial sheet and transport salt and water from the culture medium. The transepithelial transport of salts and water is regulated by cAMP and results in fluid accumulation between the culture dish and the cell monolayer, giving the appearance of domes across the surface of the cultured cells (Handler et al., 1980). Inhibition of dome formation by aminoglycosides in LLC-PK1 cells was used to rank-order the nephrotoxic potential of various aminoglycoside antibiotics. The rank-order of toxicity of aminoglycoside antibiotics *in vitro*, as indicated by a concentration-dependent inhibition of dome formation, was compatible with the rank-order of nephrotoxicity observed *in vivo*. Aminoglycosides decreased the intracellular content of cAMP and hence, dome formation, in a concentration-dependent manner. Aminoglycoside treatment also increased the release of brush border and lysosomal enzymes into the culture medium. In addition, treatment with aminoglycosides resulted in myeloid body formation, a morphological alteration similar to that observed _in vivo_. LLC-PK1 cell cultures were used to characterize further the phospholipid alterations induced by aminoglycoside antibiotics (Schwertz et al.,1986). Exposure of the LLC-PK1 cells to aminoglycosides resulted in myeloid body formation and elevation of total cellular phospholipid content. Phosphatidylcholine, phosphatidylinositol and polyphosphoinositide concentrations increased in a time-dependent manner after aminoglycoside treatment, with phosphatidylinositol concentration showing the greatest percentage increase. The responses of these cells to aminoglycosides were similar to those reported for _in vivo_ exposure to aminoglycosides (Feldman et al., 1982; Knauss et al., 1983). Schwertz et al.(1986) demonstrated that the increase in phosphatidylinositol content was due to aminoglycoside-induced inhibition of phosphatidylinositol degradation. These studies demonstrate that a response observed _in vivo_ can be produced in cultured renal cells and that these cells can be used successfully to study the mechanism of toxicity of compounds such as the aminoglycosides.

Primary cultures of renal epithelial cells have not been used routinely to study nephrotoxicity _in vitro_. The _in vitro_ toxicity of $HgCl_2$, $CdCl_2$ and cephaloridine in primary cultures of renal cortical epithelial cells has been examined to characterize the effects of various nephrotoxic agents in culture (Acosta et al., 1985). $HgCl_2$- and $CdCl_2$- induced alterations in cytoplasmic (lactate dehydrogenase) and brush border enzyme (alkaline phosphatase) activities were in accord with observed morphological damage. These enzymes were not sensitive indicators of cephaloridine-induced toxicity in culture. Instead, decreased plasma membrane (Na^+/K^+ ATPase) and mitochondrial enzyme (succinate dehydrogenase) activity proved to be the more sensitive indicators of cephaloridine-induced toxicity in the cultured cells. Primary renal epithelial cell cultures have also been used to evaluate metal toxicity _in vitro_ (Cherian, 1985). Divalent metals, such as Pb^{2+}, Hg^{2+}, Cd^{2+} and Zn^{2+}, exhibited different profiles for uptake into renal cells; Pb^{2+} and Hg^{2+} were taken up most avidly by the cells and also produced the greatest toxicity. The cellular uptake of Cd from Cd-metallothionein (Cd-MT) and from $CdCl_2$ was compared; uptake of Cd was greater from $CdCl_2$ than from Cd-MT, but the toxicity of Cd-MT was much greater than that observed with $CdCl_2$. Cherian (1985) suggested that the toxicity of Cd-MT occurred during its transport across the plasma membrane, while the toxicity of $CdCl_2$ occurred after it had entered the cell.

DISCUSSION AND CONCLUSIONS

The limitations of nephrotoxicity evaluation *in vitro* make it necessary to ask well defined questions regarding the interactions of the toxicant with the renal tissue, for there is some question as to the validity of using *in vitro* systems for evaluating nephrotoxicity (Bach et al., 1985). Correlation of *in vitro* responses to toxicants with those observed *in vivo* must be made in order to validate the *in vitro* systems. Toxicant distribution may not be the same *in vitro* as it is *in vivo*; thus, the responses of the tissue to the toxicant may be altered. The renal vasculature is very important in renal responses to toxic injury, yet the isolated perfused kidney is the only *in vitro* system that has the potential to mimic the *in vivo* situation with respect to the anatomical relationship of the nephrons and intrarenal vasculature. However, the isolated perfused kidney does not maintain the same degree of normal renal function as is observed *in vivo*.

In vitro methods of evaluating nephrotoxicity provide several advantages over existing *in vivo* methodology. *In vitro* systems allow the effects of potential nephrotoxic agents to be assessed directly on renal tissue without the interference of hormonal, metabolic or compensatory responses of the intact animal. Experimental conditions can be rigidly controlled with *in vitro* systems; the concentrations of toxicants and durations of exposure to toxicants can be easily manipulated *in vitro*. Small quantities of chemicals may be used for test purposes; this may be of particular value when test compounds are limited by availability or expense. Except for the isolated perfused kidney, most *in vitro* systems are economical and allow many samples to be obtained from one animal so that the number of animals required for experiments is reduced. Tissue from a single animal can yield enough sample to test multiple compounds at various concentrations and time points. By choosing specific cell types, tubule segments or regional slices for study, the effects of toxicants can be examined in defined areas of the kidney. The ease with which the environment and duration of exposure to a toxicant can be controlled in *in vitro* systems facilitates their utility in performing mechanistic studies of renal toxicants. If the limitations of *in vitro* systems are not overlooked, they can be valuable tools to answer specific questions about direct renal responses to nephrotoxic insult.

REFERENCES

Acosta, D., Sorensen, E.M.B., Anuforo, D.C., Mitchell, D.B., Ramos, K., Santone, K.S. & Smith, M.A. (1985). An *in vitro* approach to the study of target organ toxicity of drugs and chemicals. In Vitro Cell. Devel. Biol. 21, 495-504.

Alcorn, D., Emslie, K.R., Ross, B.D., Ryan, G.B. & Tange, J.D. (1981). Selective distal nephron damage during isolated kidney perfusion. Kidney Int. 19, 638-647.

Arthus, M-F., Bergeron, M. & Scriver, C.R. (1982). Topology of membrane exposure in the renal cortex slice. Studies of glutathione and maltose cleavage. Biochim. Biophys. Acta 692, 371-376.

Bach, P.H., Ketley, C.P., Benns, S.E., Ahmed, I. & Dixit, M. (1985). The use of isolated and cultured cells in nephrotoxicity - practice, potential and problems. *In* Renal Heterogeneity and Target Cell Toxicity, ed. P.H. Bach & E.A. Lock, pp. 505-518. New York: John Wiley & Sons.

Balaban, R.S., Soltoff, S.P., Storey, J.M. & Mandel, L.J. (1980). Improved renal cortical tubule suspension: spectrophotometric study of O_2 delivery. Am J. Physiol. 238, F50-F59.

Berndt, W.O. (1976). Use of the tissue slice technique for evaluation of renal transport processes. Environ. Health Persp. 15, 73-88.

Boyer, T.D. & Rouff, S.L. (1971). Acetaminophen-induced hepatic necrosis and renal failure. J. Am. Med. Assoc. 218, 440-441.

Burg, M., Green, N., Sohraby, S., Steele, R. & Handler, J., (1982). Differentiated function in cultured epithelia derived from thick ascending limbs. Am. J. Physiol. 242, C229-C233.

Chamberlin, M.E., LeFurgey, A. & Mandel, L.J. (1984). Suspension of medullary thick ascending limb tubules from the rabbit kidney. Am J. Physiol. 247, F955-F964.

Cherian, M.G. (1985). Rat kidney epithelial cell culture for metal toxicity studies. In Vitro Cell. Devel. Biol. 21, 505-508.

Chung, S.D., Alavi, N., Livingston, D., Hiller, S. & Taub, M. (1982). Characterizatiion of primary rabbit kidney cultures that express proximal tubule functions in a hormonally defined medium. J. Cell Biol. 95, 118-126.

Cohen, L., Lapkin, R. & Kaloyanides, G.J. (1975). Effect of gentamicin on renal function in the rat. J. Pharmacol. Exp. Ther. 193, 264-273.

Cojocel, C., Maita, K., Pasino, D.A., Kuo, C-H. & Hook, J.B. (1983). Metabolic heterogeneity of the proximal and distal kidney tubules. Life Sci. 33, 855-861.

Collier, V.U., Lietman, P.S. and Mitch, W.E. (1979). Evidence for luminal uptake of gentamicin in the perfused rat kidney. J. Pharmacol. Exp. Ther. 210, 247-251.

Curthoys, N.P. & Bellemann, P. (1979). Renal cortical cells in primary monolayer culture. Exp. Cell Res. 121, 31-45.

Dworzack, D.L. & Grantham, J.J. (1975) Preparation of renal papillary collecting duct cells for study *in vitro*. Kidney Int. 8, 191-194.

Emslie, K.R., Calder, I.C., Hart, S.J. & Tange, J.D. (1981). Induction of paracetamol metabolism in the isolated perfused kidney. Xenobiot. 11, 579-587.

Endou, H., Koseki, C., Kimura, K., Yokokura, Y., Fukida, S. & Sakai, F. (1982). Use of a flow cytometer for the separation of isolated kidney cells. *In* Biochemistry of Kidney Functions, ed. F. Morel, pp. 69-78. Amsterdam: Elsevier Biomedical Press.

Eveloff, J., Haase, W. & Kinne, R. (1980). Separation of renal medullary cells: isolation of cells from the thick ascending limb of Henle's loop. J. Cell Biol. 87, 672-681.

Feldman, S., Wang, M-Y. & Kaloyanides, G.J. (1982). Aminoglycosides induce a phospholipidosis in the renal cortex of the rat: an early manifestation of nephrotoxicity. J. Pharmacol. Exp. Ther. 220, 514-520.

Gilbert, S.F. & Migeon, B.R. (1977). Renal enzymes in kidney cells selected by D-valine medium. J. Cell. Physiol. 92, 161-168.

Gstraunthaler, G., Pfaller, W. & Kotanko, P. (1985). Biochemical characterization of renal epithelial cell cultures (LLC-PK1 & MDCK). Am J. Physiol. 248, F536-F544.

Guder, W.G. & Wirthensohn, G. (1979). Metabolism of isolated kidney tubules. Interactions between lactate, glutamine and oleate metabolism. Eur. J. Biochem. 99, 577-584.

Gullans, S.R., Brazy, P.C., Dennis, V.W. & Mandel, L.J. (1984). Interactions between gluconeogenesis and sodium transport in rabbit proximal tubule. Am. J. Physiol. 246, F859-F869.

Handler, J.S., Perkins, F.M. & Johnson, J.P. (1980). Studies of renal cell function using cell culture techniques. Am. J. Physiol. 238, F1-F9.

Hassall, C.D., Gandolfi, A.J. & Brendel, K. (1983). correlation of the in vivo and in vitro renal toxicity of S-(1,2-dichlorovinyl)-L-cysteine. Drug Chem. Toxicol. 6, 507-520.

Hassall, C.D., Gandolfi, A.J., Duhamel, R.C. & Brendel, K. (1984). The formation and biotransformation of cysteine conjugates of halogenated ethylenes by rabbit renal tubules. Chem.-Biol. Interact. 49, 283-297.

Heidrich, H-G. & Dew, M.E. (1977). Homogeneous cell populations from rabbit kidney cortex. J. Cell Biol. 74, 780-788.

Hirsch, G.H. (1976). Differential effects of nephrotoxic agents on renal transport and metabolism by use of in vitro techniques. Environ. Health Persp. 15, 89-99.

Hook, J.B. & Hewitt, W.R. (1986). Toxic responses of the kidney. In Casarett & Doull's Toxicology. The Basic Science of Poisons, 3rd edition, ed. C.D. Klaassen, M.O. Amdur, J. Doull, pp. 310-329. New York: MacMillan.

Hori, R., Yamamoto, K., Saito, H., Kohno, M. & Inui, K-I. (1984). Effect of aminoglycoside antibiotics on cellular functions of kidney epithelial cell line (LLC-PK1): a model system for amonoglycoside nephrotoxicity. J. Pharmacol. Exp. Ther. 230, 742-748.

Huang, K.C. & Lin, D.S.T. (1965). Kinetic studies on transport of PAH and other organic acids in isolated renal tubules. Am. J. Physiol. 208, 391-396.

Jones, D.P., Sundby, G-B., Ormstad, K. & Orrenius, S. (1979). Use of isolated kidney cells for study of drug metabolism. Biochem. Pharmacol. 28, 929-935.

Kacew, S. & Hirsch, G.H. (1981). Evaluation of nephrotoxicity of various compounds by means of in vitro techniques & comparison to in vivo methods. In Toxicology of the Kidney, ed. J.B. Hook, pp. 77-98. New York: Raven Press.

Kluwe, W.M. (1981). Renal function tests as indicators of kidney injury in subacute toxicity studies. Toxicol. Appl. Pharmacol. 57, 414-424.

Knauss, T.C., Weinberg, J.M. & Humes, H.D. (1983). Alterations in renal cortical phospholipid content induced by gentamicin: time course, specificity, and subcellular localization. Am. J. Physiol. 244, F535-F546.

Kreisberg, J.I., Pitts, A.M. & Pretlow, T.G. (1977). Separation of proximal tubule cells from suspensions of rat kidney cells in density gradients of Ficoll in tissue culture medium. Am. J. Pathol. 86, 591-602.

Kreisberg, J.I., Hoover, R.L. & Karnovsky, M.J. (1978). Isolation and characterization of rat glomerular epithelial cells *in vitro*. Kidney Inter. 14, 21-30.

Kyle, G.M., Luthra, R., Bruckner, J.V., MacKenzie, W.F. & Acosta, D. (1983). Assessment of functional, morphological and enzymatic tests for acute nephrotoxicity induced by mercuric chloride. J. Toxicol. Environ. Health 12, 99-117.

Maack, T. (1980). Physiological evaluation of the isolated perfused rat kidney. Am. J. Physiol. 238, F71-F78.

McMurtry, R.J., Snodgrass, W.R. & Mitchell, J.R. (1978). Renal necrosis, glutathione depletion and covalent binding after acetaminophen. Toxicol. Appl. Pharmacol. 46, 87-100.

Meezan, E., Brendel, K., Ulreich, J. & Carlson, E.C. (1973). Properties of a pure metabolically active glomerular preparation from rat kidneys. I. isolation. J. Pharmacol. Exp. Ther. 187, 332-341.

Miyajima, H., Hewitt, W.R., Cote, M.G. & Plaa, G.L. (1983). Relationships between histological and functional indices of acute chemically induced nephrotoxicity. Fund. Appl. Toxicol. 3, 543-551.

Newton, J.F. & Hook, J.B. (1981). The isolated perfused kidney. Meth. Enz. 77, 94-105.

Newton, J.F., Braselton, W.E., Kuo, C-H., Kluwe, W.M., Gemborys, M.W., Mudge, G.H. & Hook, J.B. (1982). Metabolism of acetaminophen by the isolated perfused kidney. J. Pharmacol. Exp. Ther. 221, 76-79.

Newton, J.F., Yoshimoto, M., Bernstein, J., Rush, G.F. & Hook, J.B. (1983). Acetaminophen nephrotoxicity in the rat. I. Strain differences in nephrotoxicity and metabolism. Toxicol. Appl. Pharmacol. 69, 291-306.

Ojakian, G.K., & Herzlinger, D.A. (1984). Analysis of epithelial cell surface polarity with monoclonal antibodies. Fed. Proc. 43, 2208-2216.

Phillips, R., Yamauchi, M., Cote, M.G. & Plaa, G.L. (1977). Assessment of mercuric chloride-induced nephrotoxicity by p-aminohippuric acid uptake and the activity of four gluconeogenic enzymes in rat renal cortex. Toxicol. Appl. Pharmacol. 41, 407-422.

Pohl, L.R. (1979). Biochemical toxicology of chloroform. In Reviews of Biochemical Toxicology, ed. E. Hodgson, J. Bend & R.M. Philpot, pp. 79-107. New York: Elsevier North-Holland.

Rapp. N.S., Zenser, T.V., Brown, W.W. & Davis B.B. (1980). Metabolism of benzidine by a prostaglandin-mediated process in renal inner medullary slices. J. Pharmacol. Exp. Ther. 215, 401-406.

Rasmussen, H. (1975). Isolated mammalian renal tubules. Meth. Enz. 39, 11-20.

Sakhrani, L.M. & Fine, L.G. (1983). Renal tubular cells in culture. Min. Elec. Metab. 9, 276-281.

Sato, M. & Dunn, M.J. (1984). Interactions of vasopressin, prostaglandinis, and cAMP in rat renal papillary collecting tubule cells in culture. Am J. Physiol. 247, F423-F433.

Scholer, D.W. & Edelman, I.S. (1979). Isolation of rat kidney cortical tubules enriched in proximal and distal segments. Am. J. Physiol. 237, F350-F359.

Schwertz, D.W., Kreisberg, J.I. & Venkatachalam, M.A. (1986). Gentamicin-induced alterations in pig kidney epithelial (LLC-PK1) cells in culture. J. Pharmacol. Exp. Ther. 236, 254-262.

Sirica, A.E. & Pitot, H.C. (1980). Drug Metabolism and effects of carcinogens in cultured hepatic cells. Pharmacol. Rev. 31, 205-228.

Smith, J.H., Maita, K., Sleight, S.D. & Hook, J.B. (1983). Mechanism of chloroform nephrotoxicity. I. Time course of chloroform toxicity in male and female mice. Toxicol. Appl. Pharmacol. 70, 467-479.

Smith, J.H. & Hook, J.B. (1983). Mechanism of chloroform nephrotoxicity. II. In vitro evidence for renal metabolism of chloroform in mice. Toxicol. Appl. Pharmacol. 70, 480-485.

Smith, M.A., Acosta, D. & Bruckner, J.V. (in press, 1986). Development of a primary culture system of rat kidney cortical cells to evaluate nephrotoxicity of xenobiotics. Food Chem. Toxicol.

Smith, W.L. & Garcia-Perez, A. (1985). Immunodissection: use of monoclonal antibodies to isolate specific types of renal cells. Am. J. Physiol. 248, F1-F7.

Sumpio, B.E., Chaudry, I.H., & Baue, A.E. (1985). Reduction of the drug-induced nephrotoxicity by ATP-$MgCl_2$. 1. Effects on the cis-diamminedichloroplatinum-treated isolated perfused kidneys. J. Surg. Res. 38, 429-437.

Taub, M. & Sato, G. (1980). Growth of functional primary cultures of kidney epithelial cells in defined medium. J. Cell. Physiol. 105, 369-378.

Trifillis, A.L., Regec, A.L. & Trump, B.F. (1985). Isolation culture and characterization of human renal tubular cells. J. Urol. 133, 324-329.

Vinay, P., Gougoux, A. & Lemieux, G. (1981). Isolation of a pure suspension of rat proximal tubules. Am. J. Physiol. 241, F403-F411.

Wilson, P.D., Dillingham, M.A., Breckon, R. & Anderson, R.J., (1985). Defined human renal tubular epithelia in culture: growth, characterization, and hormonal response. Am. J. Physiol. 248, F436-F443.

Zenser, T.V., Mattammal, M.B. & David B.B. (1979). Cooxidation of benzidine by renal medullary prostaglandin cyclooxygenase. J. Pharmacol. Exp. Ther. 211, 460-464.

Preparation	Viability	Advantages	Disadvantages	References
Isolated perfused kidney	4 hours	-intact vasculature -drug metabolism studies -whole kidney function	-difficulty in preparation -distal reabsorptive defect -expensive	-Newton & Hook, 1983
Renal slices	4-6 hours	-ease of preparation -multiple species comparison	-heterogeneous tubule population, lack specificity for detecting distal injury	-Hirsch, 1976 -Berndt, 1976
Renal tubule suspensions	2-3 hours	-specific nephron segments	-loss of basement membrane	-Balaban et al., 1980 -Meezan et al., 1973 -Scholer & Edelman, 1979 -Vinay et al., 1981 -Cojocel et al., 1983 -Chamberlin et al., 1984
Renal cell suspensions	6-8 hours	-regional specificity	-loss of epithelial cell polarity	-Kreisberg et al., 1977 -Heidrich & Dew, 1977 -Dworzack & Grantham, 1975 -Eveloff et al., 1980 -Endou et al., 1982 -Smith & Garcia-Perez, 1985
Renal cells in culture	One-several weeks	-regional specificity -maintain cell-cell interactions and polarity	-difficult -dedifferentiation	-Handler et al., 1980 -Burg et al., 1982 -Chung et al., 1982 -Curthoys & Belleman, 1979 -Kreisberg, et al., 1978 -Sato & Dunn, 1984 -Wilson et al., 1985 -Trifillis et al, 1985

OTOTOXICITY

E.S. Harpur
MRC Mechanisms of Drug Toxicity Research Group, Pharmaceutical Sciences Institute, Aston University, Birmingham B4 7ET

INTRODUCTION

Drugs or chemicals which can damage the inner ear are termed ototoxic. The inner ear, surrounded by the temporal bone, comprises the cochlea, or organ of hearing, and the vestibular structures, the organs of balance (Figure 1). The various cavities of the inner ear are divided by membranous partitions, creating several compartments which are filled with one of two fluids: perilymph, resembling other extracellular fluids in composition, or endolymph, the only extracellular fluid in the body with an electrolyte content similar to intracellular fluid, i.e. with a high potassium, low sodium concentration. The elements of the vestibular system are the three *cristae ampullares* within the semi-circular canals and the two *maculae* of the utricle and the saccule. In each of these five structures are located the sensory cells, the vestibular hair cells (HCs), so called because a tuft of stereocilia projects from the surface of each cell. The cells are responsive to movements of the head and send information to the vestibular nuclei in the brainstem via the vestibular primary afferent neurones with which they synapse. The cochlea is not a simple curved structure as depicted in Figure 1 but rather has a helical form making several turns from base to apex (the actual number of turns varies between species) around a central bony spindle which contains the nerve supply to the sensory structures. Movement of the middle ear ossicles, including the stapes, causes displacement of the basilar membrane which separates the *scala tympani* from the *scala vestibuli*. The transduction of sound takes place in the HCs of the organ of Corti which is located on the basilar membrane. The cochlear HCs are arranged in orderly rows, a single row of inner HCs and three to five rows of outer HCs depending on the species. The HCs are activated by displacement of the stereocilia which project from their endolymphatic surfaces. The organ of Corti is innervated by both afferent and efferent neurones.

Many ototoxic substances damage both cochlear and vestibular structures, although to different extents; some are very selective for one or other sensory system. Thus any system which is to be used as a test of ototoxic potential should ideally take account of the

Figure 1. Schematic drawing of the mammalian inner ear.

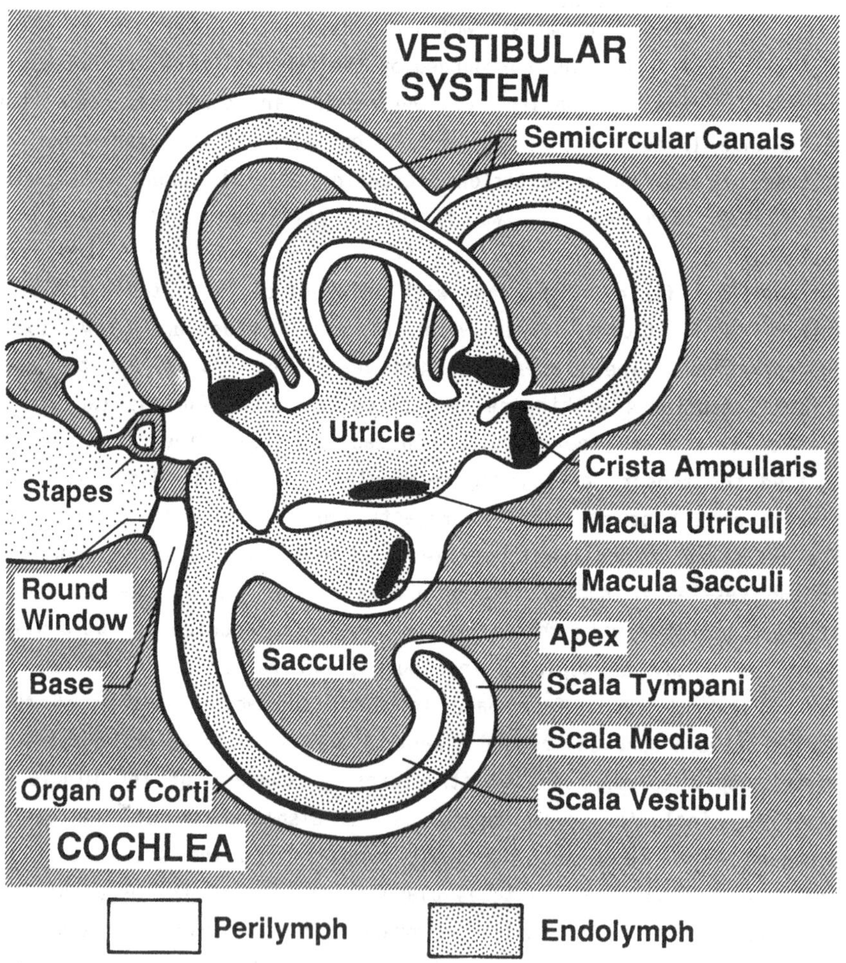

possibility that either cochlear or vestibular tissues may be the target. Although a variety of chemicals, if placed in the middle ear cavity, may be directly absorbed into the fluids of the inner ear resulting in an ototoxic response, the vast majority of reports of ototoxicity both in animals and in man concern effects which occur following systemic absorption of chemicals (see Harpur 1986, for review). Thus ototoxicity, a property of a small but growing number of chemicals, is an example of a highly selective organ-directed toxicity. The best known and most widely studied ototoxic substances are drugs, such as the aminoglycoside antibiotics and the 'loop' diuretics.

The application of histopathological methods in studies of ototoxicity has provided conclusive evidence that the primary lesion is in the peripheral end-organs. However, the end-organs are notably heterogeneous comprising several distinct tissues which include the HCs, their neural innervation and various populations of supporting cells and secretory cells. The HCs are the principal target for ototoxic drugs in both cochlear and vestibular tissues. There is also reasonable evidence to suggest that the HCs are the first target except in the case of the 'loop' diuretics, which exert their primary actions on the highly vascular secretory tissue in the lateral wall of the cochlea, known as the *stria vascularis*. Permanent hearing loss or vestibular dysfunction caused by ototoxic drugs is invariably associated with HC death. Thus, it would seem reasonable, at least in the first instance, to develop *in vitro* systems which would permit assessment of the direct toxic potential of drugs on cochlear and vestibular HCs.

Studies of the direct effects of drugs on cochlear and vestibular HCs have been carried out infrequently. Isolated systems which have been used include the lateral line organ of the fish (Wersäll & Flock 1964) or the frog (Kroese & van den Bercken 1980 and 1982) and the semicircular canal of the frog (Harada 1970; Gallais 1979; Bernard 1980 and 1983). The perfused cochlea of the anaesthetised guinea pig has also been used (Nuttall *et al.*, 1977; Konishi 1979). With only one exception these studies have examined, using electrophysiological methods, the acute effects of aminoglycoside antibiotics on HC function; Harada (1970) investigated the actions of quinine. In most cases the objective was to elucidate the mechanisms by which the drugs affected HC function although Gallais (1979) set out to compare the action of several aminoglycosides with that of a non-ototoxic antibiotic, penicillin G.

The first successful attempts at _in vitro_ organ culture of the embryonic inner ear involved the use of the avian otocyst (Fell 1928; Friedmann 1956). This preparation can achieve mature differentiation of the sensory structures _in vitro_ and has been applied to the study of ototoxic antibiotics (Friedmann & Bird 1961). While the system did appear to discriminate between ototoxic antibiotics, the aminoglycosides, and non-ototoxic antibiotics, the penicillins, only very high concentrations of aminoglycosides (about 1.0 mM) proved toxic. The apparent insensitivity of this preparation was unexplained and must place in question its value as a test system for ototoxic drugs.

It is only in the past 15 years that cultured mammalian otocysts have been widely studied. This followed the demonstration by Van de Water & Ruben (1971) that the explanted embryonic inner ear of the mouse continued to develop _in vitro_ in a manner similar to its _in vivo_ development. In the past few years there have been a few investigations of the value of cultured mouse otocyst for the study of ototoxicity _in vitro_.

In the remainder of this chapter current knowledge of the development of mammalian otocysts in culture and their use in ototoxicological investigations will be summarised.

PRACTICAL ASPECTS

Choice of Species

Most studies of inner ear tissues in culture have been conducted with a view to delineating their development during the late embryonic and early neonatal stages, i.e. during the successive phases of morphogenesis, differentiation and functional maturation. The mammalian species most frequently studied is the mouse which was originally selected (Van de Water & Ruben 1971) because many types of congenital malformations of the inner ear, with a well-defined genetic basis, had been identified in the mouse; some of these lead to lesions which resemble those occurring in the human. Furthermore Sher (1971), and several other workers before him, had described in detail the _in vivo_ development of the inner ear of the normal mouse from the 11th day of gestation to the 10th day after birth. This provided a reference by which the progress of mouse otocysts grown _in vitro_ could be measured

(Sher 1971).

A potential disadvantage in the use of the mouse otocyst in *in vitro* ototoxicological studies is the lack of information about the effects of ototoxic substances on the inner ear of the mouse *in vivo*. In contrast to the mouse, which has rarely been used in ototoxicological studies, a vast amount of information has been accumulated about the effects of ototoxic drugs on the cochlea of the guinea pig and, to a lesser extent, its vestibular structures. Recently, a few studies of the development *in vitro* of inner ear tissues from the guinea pig have been done but the use of this species presents particular problems. Most studies, with either species, have used late embryonic material but some recent attempts have been made to explant inner ear tissue from neonatal animals. This gives rise to some special difficulties which are discussed below.

Organ Culture of the Mouse Otocyst

In Table 1 are summarised the experimental details from a number of pioneering studies of culture of the mouse otocyst *in vitro*. The strain of mouse used was the CBA/CBA in all studies except that of Van de Water (1976) who used the CBA/C57 hybrid. In their initial study Van de Water & Ruben (1971) used a variety of media and examined the tissues histologically after growth *in vitro* for various intervals of time. The greatest survival of healthy cultures (90%), each showing some degree of morphogenesis and differentiation, occurred in the medium shown in Table 1. Subsequently these workers (Van de Water *et al*. 1973; Van de Water & Ruben 1974, Van de Water 1976) refined the organ culture system (Table 1). Van de Water *et al*. (1973) were able to maintain healthy specimens *in vitro* for 10 or more days. In a number of other studies the experimental conditions of Van de Water (1976) have been used with only slight modifications other than the ommission of penicillin (Table 1) with the consequent need for sterile technique (Anniko *et al*. 1979; Nordemar 1983).

Both the surgical procedure and the organ culture system were described in detail by Van de Water (1976). Gravid females were killed and the uterus removed intact and placed in a dish containing pre-warmed organ culture medium. The otocysts were dissected away from the rhombencephalon and placed in Falcon plastic organ culture dishes (No. 3010; 60 x 15 mm) and oriented with their medial surfaces in contact with the plastic surface of the dish. The outer chamber of the culture dish was moistened with sterile, pyrogen-free, distilled water and the inner dish was filled with 0.15 ml of culture medium. A gas tight closure between the culture dish and its top was affected with sterile, unbleached vaseline.

Although culture of the mouse otocyst earlier than about the 11th gestational day is not successful, possibly because the early development of the otocyst requires the influence of the rhombencephalon (Nordemar, 1983), it can be cultured from the 11th gestational day onwards (Van de Water, 1976). At about 11th-12th day of gestation the mouse otocyst has a cystic form but is not differentiated into cochlear and vestibular structures. Between days 12 and 15 there is active proliferation to form the structures of the cochlea and the vestibular system. By the 15th day most of the cells in the cochlea have passed their terminal mitoses whereas the terminal mitotic activity of the cells in the vestibular system ranges between days 14 and 18 (Ruben 1967). By day 16 morphogenesis is reaching its final stage and cyto-differentiation is in full progress.

Some aspects of the development of otocysts _in vitro_ have particular relevance to their use in toxicological investigations. For example, significant differences in the development of otocysts have been found depending on the gestational day on which they were explanted. Otocysts explanted on either the 12th or 13th gestational day readily formed sensory epithelia of vestibular character and morphological development of the semi-circular canals and a cochlear duct were seen (Van de Water _et al_. 1973). However, this kind of advanced morphological development occurred in only about 10% of the 12th gestational day explants. The 13th gestational day otocyst was much more likely to form sensory epithelia resembling the organ of Corti than the 12th day explant. Also, the 13th gestational day otocyst required a shorter period (5-6 days) of _in vitro_ development to produce differentiated sensory epithelia compared with the 12th gestational day otocyst (7-10 days). Both of these factors can probably be explained by the different degrees of development of cochlear and vestibular tissues achieved _in vivo_ prior to explantation on particular gestational days (Ruben 1967; Sher 1971). Van de Water (1976) found that only when explantation was delayed until the 13th gestational day did the gross development of the inner ear _in vitro_ progress in a manner similar to the pattern *in vivo*. Although the *in vitro* morphogenesis and cyto-differentiation of the *cristae ampullares* of inner ears explanted on the 13th gestational day is similar to the normal development *in vivo*, a delay of about 1/2 to 1 days in the gross development can be expected *in vitro* (Anniko *et al*. 1979). Furthermore, while individual HCs develop and differentiate similarly *in vitro* and *in vivo* the *cristae* frequently fail to obtain full maturation of their gross morphology *in vitro*. The corresponding maturation of the mouse cochlea, which occurs mainly post-partum *in vivo*, is not reproduced so well *in vitro* - abberant coiling and cytodifferentiation of both the organ of Corti and the stria vascularis occur *in vitro* (Anniko 1981).

Anniko *et al*. (1978) and Nordemar (1983) extended the *in vitro* culture technique to study the late stages of embryological development and the early post-natal period of development of the mouse otocyst. Otocysts were explanted on the 16th day of gestation (Table 1) and either cultured whole or bisected between the saccule and the cochlear duct, thus providing two explants, one containing vestibular structures and one containing the cochlea (Anniko *et al*. 1978).

Following 6 days in culture the explants were prepared for histological examination in the light microscope (Anniko *et al*. 1978). This time corresponds to 1 day postpartum. At the time of explantation the 16th day inner ears had already undergone most of their morphogenetic development. Subsequently, the only gross morphological changes were a lengthening, and increased arcing, of the semicircular canals. Indeed, Anniko *et al*. (1981) showed that when mouse otocysts were explanted on the 16th gestational day and maintained in culture there was negligible growth, as measured by protein content, compared with that occurring *in vivo*. However, after 6 days *in vitro* differentiation of all the vestibular sensory structures and the base to apex pattern of differentiation of the cochlear duct had occurred (Anniko *et al*. 1978). Nordemar (1983) confirmed, using electronmicroscopy, that the differentiation of HCs in the cristae was almost identical *in vivo* and *in vitro* but innervation of the HCs was delayed in the *in vitro* ears.

The influence of the presence of neural tissue (statoacoustic ganglion) and mesenchyme on the development of the otocyst *in vitro* has been studied. From some specimens Van de Water (1976) removed the statoacoustic ganglion complex at the time of explant and, using light microscopy, demonstrated that normal development of the sensory epithelia occurred in the absence of this complex. It was subsequently confirmed by Anniko _et al._ (1979) that the statoacoustic ganglion complex did not have a trophic effect on the ultrastructural differentiation of the sensory cells.

During microdissection of the otocyst epithelium the amount of surrounding mesenchyme which is removed is dependent on the technical skill of the person explanting the otocyst and will, inevitably, be variable between specimens. If insufficient mesenchyme is removed, chondrogenesis and the development of inner ear structures are impaired (Van de Water 1983). Although these effects are most marked in otocysts explanted at early stages of embryonic development they are still apparent at gestational days 12 and 13 and are manifest as impaired morphogenesis, particularly of the cochlea. However, if too much mesenchyme surrounds the otocyst its development _in vitro_ may also be impaired (Anniko & Nordemar, 1981). Li & McPhee (1979) showed that an imbalance in the amount of mesenchyme surrounding the otocyst can cause problems. Thus, an asymmetric reduction in the ventral mesenchyme resulted in failure of cochlear development despite normal development of vestibular sensory structures. Anniko (1981) pointed out that poor development of the inner ear in culture, due to a deficiency of mesenchyme, could be misinterpreted, for example, as a toxic effect of a drug present in the culture medium. Variability in the amount of mesenchyme surrounding the otocyst will also influence the penetration of any drug which is present in the culture medium. This has obvious relevance to the use of the preparation in ototoxicological studies.

A further problem which may arise during the dissection of the otocyst is that the 'hook' region - the primordial cochlea - may easily be damaged, allowing the culture medium to enter the lumen of the otocyst. Damage to this structure does not interfere with the development and maturation of the vestibular part of the labyrinth but results in either malformation or aplasia of the cochlea (Anniko 1981).

Organ Culture of the Inner Ear of the Embryonic Guinea Pig

The gestation period in the guinea pig, approximately 60 days, is much longer than that of the mouse or rat, approximately 21 days. Furthermore, whereas maturation of the mouse cochlea occurs postpartum, the inner ear of the guinea pig is both morphologically and physiologically mature at birth. The adult composition of endolymph is achieved in the fetal guinea pig about 10 days before birth (Anniko *et al.* 1982a) and about the same time the compound action potential can first be recorded in the fetal cochlea (Pujol & Holding 1973).

Anniko & Wersäll (1979) reported considerable difficulties when explanting the inner ears of fetal guinea pigs on the 30th gestational day. However, Davis & Hawrisiak (1981) achieved successful *in vitro* culture of inner ears removed from fetal guinea pigs aged between 21 and 54 gestational days. The method of Van de Water & Ruben (1974, see Table 1) was used with little modification. Early otocysts and later cartilaginous inner ears were cultured either intact or after division into dorsal (vestibular) and ventral (cochlear) portions as described by Anniko *et al.* (1978). In all cases there was considerable growth of the explants *in vitro*. The older, differentiated ears (38 - 54 gestational day explants) showed least progressive development. In early otocysts there was growth and differentiation of both cochlear and vestibular structures but the 26th - 27th gestational day explants showed the most development, paralleling the normal *in vivo* development over 12 days in culture. However, growth *in vitro* was accompanied by central tissue necrosis which was less in the divided explants in which access of the nutrient medium to the deep tissues was improved. Davis & Hawrisiak (1981) also reported difficulty in maintaining sterility and found it desirable to add antibiotics to the medium. They used penicillin (200 u/ml) and streptomycin (100 μg/ml) which would be an obvious disadvantage if this preparation were to be used in ototoxicological studies. Davis & Hawrisiak concluded that because of the above problems and further disadvantages, such as the long gestation period, the relatively slow rate of differentiation *in vivo* and *in vitro* and the small litter size, the guinea pig was less suitable than the mouse for studies of inner ear development.

Whereas Davis & Hawrisiak (1981) focused their attention on cochlear development, Anniko & Sobin (1983) used both light and electronmicroscopy to study the development of the *cristae ampullares* in otocysts explanted from fetal guinea pigs. Using a similar technique to that used earlier for the mouse otocyst (Anniko *et al.* 1979, see Table 1) they explanted inner ears on the 30th and 40th gestational days and cultured them for 1-10 days after division into cochlear and vestibular portions. Sterile procedures were used and neither antibiotics nor antimycotics were added to the culture medium. They found that the guinea pig inner ear could be maintained in culture at least until the 46th gestational day. The vestibular organs, which were close to the plane of division, were well maintained in culture and characteristic cytodifferentiation of vestibular HCs was seen. Anniko & Sobin (1983) concluded that the *in vitro* development of the embryonic inner ear of the guinea pig parallels the *in vivo* development from approximately the 25th to 45th gestational days. However, they also felt that since the vestibular organs of the mouse achieved a mature development in a much shorter time than the guinea pig and were easier to handle in large numbers they were preferable for the study of the development of the mammalian inner ear.

Organ Culture of Postnatal Inner Ear Tissue

Recently, studies have been made of the growth *in vitro* of inner ear tissues explanted from either neonatal or mature animals. The species studied have included the guinea pig (Yamashita & Vosteen 1975), the dog (Okano *et al*. 1975) and the mouse (Anniko *et al*. 1978). Both the mouse and the guinea pig were included in some studies (Anniko 1979; Anniko & Wersäll 1979; Anniko 1980). The objectives of such studies have included the delineation of the innervation of the sensory epithelia, which occurs mainly postpartum in the mouse, and of the fate of fully differentiated secretory and sensory cells. The latter objective is of particular relevance if postnatal tissues are to be used in ototoxicological studies. Data from several studies suggest that both nerve fibres and sensory cells rapidly degenerate *in vitro* when explanted postnatally. Although the sensory cells may survive for several days, their highly differentiated ultrastructure is lost within a very short time in culture. The instability of fully differentiated HCs in culture is probably due to the lack of provision of an environment resembling endolymph - which matures shortly before birth in the guinea pig (Anniko *et al*. 1982a) and shortly after birth in the mouse (Anniko & Wroblewski 1981).

A further limitation to the use of postnatal otic tissue in culture is evident from the work of Anniko *et al*. (1981). They measured the activity of adenylate cyclase and the turnover of some phospholipids during embryonic development of the mouse inner ear *in vivo* or after explantation of the otocyst at the 16th gestational day and growth in culture until a time corresponding to the postnatal period. The activity of adenylate cyclase was similar, whether the otocyst developed *in vivo* or *in vitro*, until the postnatal period when the activity in the cultured otocysts became substantially elevated compared with the activity in tissues maturing *in vivo*. This disproportionate increase in the activity of adenylate cyclase *in vitro* suggested the absence of an essential control mechanism. At this time there were also quantitative differences in phospholipid turnover between tissues developing *in vivo* and *in vitro*. Anniko *et al*. (1981) concluded that the usefulness of organ culture as a model of inner ear development was limited to the prenatal period.

EXPERIMENTAL EXAMPLES

Use of organ culture in ototoxicological investigations

Anniko & Nordemar (1981) studied the effects of two ototoxic drugs, gentamicin and ethacrynic acid, on the 13th gestational day inner ear of the CBA/CBA mouse. Explantation of the otocyst at this stage permits a study of its early morphological development. The culture technique was very similar to that of Van de Water (1976) outlined in a preceding section (see Table 1), except for the omission of antibiotics and antimycotics from the medium in which control specimens were cultured. After 1-9 days in culture, the otocysts were examined morphologically (photographically documented) and histologically, using both light and electron microscopy. Each drug was present in the culture medium at a concentration of 1, 10 or 100 μg/ml.

The approach adopted by Anniko & Nordemar (1981) to overcome two of the problems highlighted under 'Practical Aspects' - variability in the amount of mesenchyme affecting the penetration of drugs under test and the possibility of accidental damage to the hook region of the otocyst - was a compromise. In about two thirds of their explants, both controls and drug-exposed specimens, Anniko & Nordemar either incised or excised the cochlear hook to allow access of the culture medium to the lumen of the otocyst. This surgical intervention precluded study of the development of the cochlea so that the effects of gentamicin and ethacrynic acid on only the vestibular part of the inner ear were assessed. Ethacrynic acid was highly toxic to the otocyst *in vitro*: even at the lowest concentration tested (1 μg/ml) development of the otocyst was arrested. This toxic effect of ethacrynic acid appeared to be non-specific and irreversible, since specimens exposed to the drug for 3 days and then cultured in normal medium for 2-7 days were incapable of growth or differentiation. There was evidence that ethacrynic acid was exerting an antimitotic effect.

When otocysts were cultured in medium containing gentamicin, there was development of vestibular sensory structures (the *cristae ampullares* and *macula utricli*) but impaired morphogenesis, sometimes severe, was seen. A direct inflow of gentamicin-containing medium into the otocyst lumen (excised cochlear hook) caused greater morphological changes than were seen in intact otocysts (see also Anniko 1981).

Although histogenesis did proceed and differentiation of HCs and supporting cells did occur, in some specimens degenerating epithelial cells and cell debris extruded into the otocyst lumen were observed. At the intermediate dose of gentamicin (10 μg/ml) ultrastructural abnormalities, characteristic of aminoglycoside exposure, were observed mainly in the HCs. At the lowest dose of gentamicin (1 μg/ml) these changes were not seen and at the highest dose (100 μg/ml) they were observed not only in the HCs but also in the supporting cells and even in the mesenchymal cells.

A study of the effects of gentamicin on the late stages of development of the inner ear was conducted by Nordemar & Anniko (1983) using the explanted 16th gestational day inner ear of the CBA/CBA mouse. As the gross morphology of the labyrinth has developed by the 16th gestational day it is comparatively easy to dissect the inner ear from surrounding temporal bone, without damage (Anniko 1981). The explanted inner ear can either be cultured intact, surrounded by its cartilaginous capsule (Nordemar & Anniko 1983) or in two parts after surgical division of the vestibular from the cochlear portion of the labyrinth (Anniko 1981). The latter action was taken to provide standardized conditions by allowing influx of medium containing gentamicin. Nordemar & Anniko (1983) used a very similar culture technique to that described earlier (Anniko *et al*. 1979, see Table 1). Gentamicin was added to the culture medium to provide a concentration of 1, 10, 100 or 1000 μg/ml.

As a consequence of the poor development of the cochlea *in vitro* (see 'Practical Aspects') studies of the toxic effects of gentamicin on the late developing otocyst have been confined mainly to vestibular structures although Anniko (1981) has performed a pilot study on the cochlear portion of the otocyst.

Thus Nordemar & Anniko (1983) focused their attention on the effects of gentamicin on the cristae ampullares. They observed a dose-related toxicity, which was selective for the HCs and very similar to the characteristic pattern of damage caused by aminoglycoside exposure in vivo. The selectivity for the HCs was seen particularly at the lower concentrations of gentamicin (1 and 10 μg/ml). Initially (1 day), only minor ultrastructural changes were seen in some HCs but this damage became more severe with time. After 5 days in culture HCs exposed to 1 μg/ml of gentamicin showed advanced pathologies and at 10 μg/ml some were completely destroyed. Surrounding supporting cells appeared normal or showed only minor pathological changes. At the higher concentrations of gentamicin (100 and 1000 μg/ml), even after one day's exposure, there was a general degeneration of the epithelium. However, even in these specimens the supporting cells were less affected than the HCs.

Marked variability between specimens in the degree of toxic damage caused particularly by the intermediate concentrations of gentamicin was noted by Nordemar & Anniko (1983). This is reminiscent of the variability in cochlear damage which is seen after in vivo exposure when the animals are killed soon after the drug administration has ended (Harpur & Bridges 1979). In the group of explants exposed to 10 μg/ml of gentamicin some cristae were unaffected while others showed advanced degeneration. These variations were seen particularly between different explants; variations in the extent of morphological damage between cristae in the same explant were minimal. Thus, even for semiquantification of the ototoxic effects of gentamicin, Nordemar & Anniko (1983) felt that a mimimum of 5-7 organ cultures are required in each group.

Impaired development of the neural innervation of the vestibular HCs exposed to gentamicin was also seen (Nordemar & Anniko 1983). This was manifest as a delay in the appearance of nerve endings and synaptic bodies which appeared only after 5 days in culture and then only occasionally. In a pilot study Anniko (1981) evaluated damage to the cochlear portion of the inner ear after exposure in vitro to gentamicin. After exposure to 10 μg/ml of gentamicin for 3 to 4 days ultrastructural changes were seen in cochlear HCs. However, after exposure to much higher concentrations of gentamicin, 100 to 1000 μg/ml, no severely damaged HCs were seen using light microscopy. Thus the clear dose response relationship seen in the vestibular system (Nordemar & Anniko 1983) was not apparent in the cochlea. However, the study of Anniko (1981) was very limited and the results should be interpreted with caution.

In summary, it is apparent that the explanted 13th gestational day inner ear of the mouse is particularly sensitive to the toxic effects of drugs to which it is exposed in culture. Even low concentrations of gentamicin produced uncharacteristic abnormalities of cochlear development. Thus, this must be considered a model for the teratogenic effects of drugs on the otocyst rather than a model of ototoxicity (Anniko & Nordemar, 1981). By contrast the vestibular HCs of the explanted 16th gestational day inner ear of the mouse are selectively vulnerable to the toxic effects of gentamicin in a manner similar to that which has been observed *in vivo*. This 16th gestational day explant may also prove of value in determining the ototoxic effects of drugs on the developing cochlea but further studies are required to evaluate this.

Although the 16th gestational day inner ear explant is sensitive to the ototoxic effects of gentamicin in a manner similar to the inner ear *in vivo* it still remains to be shown that this is an appropriate general model of ototoxicity rather than a model of the effects of ototoxic substances on the developing ear. The study of Anniko *et al*. (1982b) makes some contribution to answering this question. Anniko *et al*. studied the ototoxic potential of two aminoglycosides, gentamicin and netilmicin, in three systems: 1) the 'standard' *in vivo* animal model involving chronic parenteral administration to the guinea pig, 2) acute (1-2 h) perfusion of the perilymphatic spaces of the cochlea of the anaesthetised guinea pig and 3) organ culture of the inner ear of the embryonic mouse. In the last model the inner ear of the CBA/CBA mouse embryo was explanted on the 16th gestational day and the explants were cultured for 5 days in the manner already described.

Netilmicin has been shown, in a diverse range of animal models and in human use, to have a low ototoxic potential (see Harpur, 1986, for review). It has also been shown consistently to be less ototoxic than gentamicin. This was confirmed by Anniko *et al.* (1982b) who administered the two drugs at doses ranging from 50 to 100 mg/kg for periods of between 18 and 30 days and evaluated the toxicity of the compounds by assessment of HC damage. Gentamicin caused profound loss of cochlear HCs at all doses and extensive damage to vestibular HCs, most severe in the central part of the *cristae ampullares*. In contrast, even at the highest dose of netilmicin, the HCs in both the cochlea and vestibular system appeared normal. In the perilymphatic perfusion model, the index of toxicity was a decline in the electrical response of the cochlea to a sound stimulus presented at a fixed intensity. Netilmicin and gentamicin reduced this electrical response significantly but the equipotent concentration of netilmicin in the perfusate was threefold higher than that of gentamicin.

In the organ culture model the toxicity of the compounds was assessed by a semiquantitative scoring of the HC damage and loss in the *cristae* and *maculae* of the vestibular system. Netilmicin had very little effect on HC morphology except at very high concentrations (1000 μg/ml) whereas with gentamicin HC damage was evident at the light microscopic level even when the concentration of the drug was only 1 μg/ml.

Thus in all three experimental models essentially the same result was obtained; netilmicin was less toxic than gentamicin. Furthermore, the ultrastructural changes observed in the HCs in the *in vitro* system were similar to those seen in the adult animals. Anniko *et al.* (1982b) thought that this validated the embryonic model for drug testing.

DISCUSSION

Only a few studies have examined the effects of ototoxic drugs, mainly the aminoglycoside antibiotics, on the mammalian inner ear in culture. The results of these studies are greatly influenced by the stage of development of the inner ear at the time of drug exposure. The use of the 13th gestational day otocyst permits a study of drug effects on morphogenesis and thus this must be considered a model for study of teratogenic effects on the inner ear (Anniko & Nordemar 1981). Reports of teratogenic damage to the ear are rare and usually occur as but one manifestation of multiple defects (d'Avignon & Barr 1964). However, ototoxic drugs do cross the placenta and gain access to fetal inner ear tissues in sufficient concentrations to cause selective damage, characteristic of that seen in adult animals (see Harpur 1986, for review). Indeed, there is evidence from in vivo studies to suggest that the cochlea may be most vulnerable to aminoglycoside-induced ototoxicity during the final stages of its maturation (Osako et al. 1979; Marot et al. 1980).

The 16th gestational day inner ear may provide a sensitive model for assessing the toxic effects of drugs on sensory cells in the inner ear. Concentrations of aminoglycoside antibiotics which are likely to be achieved in vivo in the fluids of both adult and fetal inner ears cause selective damage to the HCs of the cultured otocyst (Nordemar & Anniko 1983). In contrast, aminoglycosides are not toxic to a variety of other cells in culture even at much higher concentrations (Schafer et al. 1972; Fox & Brummett 1979). This strongly suggests that the effects observed on the cultured otocyst are truly ototoxic. However, it should be borne in mind that even with this model (the 16th gestational day otocyst) the drug is exposed to cells which are actively differentiating, rather than structurally or functionally mature. Thus, it still must be considered whether this only examines the ototoxic effects of drugs on the immature ear or whether it also models the ototoxic effects of drugs on mature sensory cells. There is some evidence for biochemical similarities, e.g. in polyphosphoinositide turnover, between fetal and adult otic tissues from mice (Anniko & Schacht 1981). This could be important, at least in the case of the aminoglycoside antibiotics, since inhibition of polyphosphoinositide turnover has been implicated as the mechanism of ototoxic action of these drugs (Schacht 1976). The study of Anniko et al. (1982b) which demonstrated that the comparative toxicities of gentamicin and netilmicin were the same on the 16th gestational day explant of the mouse inner ear and on the mature inner ear of the guinea pig, suggests that the in vitro system may be a relevant general model for the detection of ototoxicity. The observation by Anniko et al. (1982b) that netilmicin produced little or no damage to the cultured otocyst is particularly encouraging, although many more studies are necessary to demonstrate that drugs which do not damage the inner ear in vivo are also free of such effects in the in vitro system. The finding that ethacrynic acid was highly toxic to the mouse otocyst in vitro (Anniko & Nordemar 1981) is not consistent with knowledge of the effects of this drug on the inner ear in vivo.

Ethacrynic acid is reversibly toxic to the cochlea by virtue of its actions on the secretory tissues and it has only rarely been associated with HC death after prolonged administration (Crifo 1973). Fox & Brummett (1979), however, showed that ethacrynic acid was markedly cytotoxic to mouse lymphoma cells _in vitro_. The lack of correlation between the marked cytotoxicity of ethacrynic acid _in vitro_ and its low toxicity for HCs _in vivo_ may be explained by failure of the drug to penetrate to the HCs _in vivo_. These findings suggest that the otocyst in culture will be susceptible to toxic effects of some drugs which may be unrelated to their ototoxic potential.

Some further limitations to the current use of the cultured otocyst should be mentioned. Because of difficulties in reproducing _in vitro_ the development of the organ of Corti, studies to date have been largely confined to effects of drugs on vestibular structures. Furthermore, the studies have been only semi-quantitative, relying mainly on morphological assessment, using light microscopy. The difficulties in quantification of the drug effects are largely created by variability in the responses of individual explants to drug exposure. Nordemar & Anniko (1983) found that even for semiquantification of the ototoxic effects of gentamicin at least 5-7 organ cultures were required in each group. Even if this problem were overcome, quantification of HC loss in vestibular sensory epithelia would still present problems (Aran _et al._ 1982) because the lack of a regular arrangements of HCs, such as is found in the organ of Corti, means that only remaining HCs can be counted.

In conclusion, it can be said that considerable strides have been made in the last decade in the use of organ culture of the mammalian inner ear and the techniques offer considerable promise for application to assessment of ototoxicity. However, until further studies are conducted this latter use of inner ear organ culture must be regarded as experimental.

ACKNOWLEDGEMENT

The author thanks Janet Bramble for typing the manuscript.

REFERENCES

Anniko, M. (1979). Extracorporeal preservation. Organ culture of the post-natal mammalian inner ear. Acta Otolaryngol., 88, 211-9.

Anniko, M. (1980). The post-natal mammalian labyrinthine secretory epithelium in vitro. Acta Otolaryngol., 90, 237-43.

Anniko, M. (1981). Effects of gentamicin on the development of the embryonic inner ear in organ culture. In Aminoglycoside Ototoxicity, eds. S.A. Lerner, G.J.Matz & J.E. Hawkins, Jr., pp 215-27. Boston, Little Brown and Co.

Anniko, M. & Nordemar, H. (1981). Ototoxicity or teratogenicity. An analysis of drug-induced effects on the early development of the mammalian otocyst. Arch. Otorhinolaryngol., 232, 43-55.

Anniko, M., Nordemar, H., Spangberg, M.-L. & Schacht, J. (1981). Biochemical studies on the embryonic development of the mammalian inner ear in organ culture. Arch. Otorhinolaryngol., 230, 237-43.

Anniko, M., Nordemar, H. & Van de Water, T.R. (1979). Embryogenesis of the inner ear. I. Development and differentiation of the mammalian crista ampullaris in vivo and in vitro. Arch. Otorhinolaryngol., 224, 285-99.

Anniko, M. & Schacht, J. (1981). Phosphoinositides in the developing inner ear with references to brain, kidney and liver of the mouse. Int. J. Biochem., 13, 951-3.

Anniko, M. & Sobin, A. (1983). Organ culture of the crista ampullaris of the embryonic guinea pig. Arch. Otolaryngol., 109, 262-4.

Anniko, M., Sobin, A. & Wroblewski, R. (1982a). X-ray microanalysis of inner ear fluids in the embryonic and newborn guinea pig. Arch. Otorhinolaryngol., 234, 125-30.

Anniko, M., Takada, A. & Schacht, J. (1982b). Comparative ototoxicities of gentamicin and netilmicin in three model systems. Am. J. Otolaryngol., 3, 422-33.

Anniko, M. & Van de Water, T.R. (1978). Organ culture of the postnatal mouse crista ampullaris. Part I. Arch. Otorhinolaryngol., 220, 129-32.

Anniko, M., Van de Water, T.R. & Nordemar, H. (1978). Organ culture of the 16th gestational day mouse labyrinth. A model suggestion for pre- and post-partum development. Acta Otolaryngol., 86, 52-5.

Anniko, M. & Wersall, J. (1979). The inner ear and the in vitro system. Arch. Otorhinolaryngol., 224, 25-30.

Anniko, M. & Wroblewski, R. (1981). Elemental composition of the developing inner ear. Ann. Otol. Rhinol. Laryngol., 90, 25-32.

Aran, J.-M., Erre, J.-P., Guilhaume, A. & Aurousseau, C. (1982). The comparative ototoxicities of gentamicin, tobramycin and dibekacin in the guinea-pig. A functional and morphological cochlear and vestibular study. Acta Otolaryngol., Suppl. 390, 1-30.

d'Avignon, M. & Barr, B. (1964). Ear abnormalities and cranial nerve palsies in thalidomide children. Arch.Otolaryngol., 80, 136-40.

Bernard, C. (1980) Electrical activity of isolated semicircular canals in the frog. Action of streptomycin. Pflugers. Arch., 388, 93-9.

Bernard, C. (1983). Action of streptomycin and calcium on the apical membrane of hair cells of the frog isolated semicircular canal. Acta Otolaryngol., 96, 21-30.

Crifo, S. (1973). Ototoxicity of sodium ethacrynate in the guinea pig. Arch. Otorhinolaryngol., 206, 27-38.

Davis, G.L. & Hawrisiak, M.M. (1981). In vitro cultivation of the fetal guinea pig inner ear. Ann.Otol.Rhinol.Laryngol., 90, 246-50.

Fell, H.B. (1928). Development in vitro of the isolated otocyst of the embryonic fowl. Arch. exp. Zellforsch., 7, 69-81.

Fox, K.E. & Brummett, R.E. (1979). The relationship between the cytotoxicity of kanamycin and ethacrynic acid for mammalian cells in vitro and their ototoxicity in vivo. Acta Otolaryngol. 87, 72-8.

Friedmann, I. (1956). In vitro culture of the isolated otocyst of the embryonic fowl. Ann. Otol. Rhinol. Laryngol., 65, 98-103.

Friedmann, I. & Bird, E.S. (1961). The effect of ototoxic antibiotics and of penicillin on the sensory areas of the isolated fowl embryo otocyst in organ cultures: An electron-microscope study. J. Pathol. Bacteriol., 81, 81-90.

Gallais, A. (1979). Comparative study of the influence of aminoglycoside antibiotics on the activity of the horizontal semicircular canal in the frog. Acta Otolaryngol., 88, 88-96.

Harada, Y. (1970). The influence of quinine on the ampullar receptors of the isolated posterior semicircular canal of the frog. Acta Otolaryngol., 69, 200-5.

Harpur, E.S. (1986). Disorders of the ear. In Iatrogenic Diseases, Third Edition, eds. P.F. D'Arcy & J.P. Griffin, pp 713-49. Oxford: Oxford University Press.

Harpur, E.S. & Bridges, J.B. (1979). An evaluation of the use of scanning and transmission electronmicroscopy in a study of the gentamicin-damaged guinea-pig organ of Corti. J. Laryngol. Otol., 93, 7-23.

Konishi, T. (1979). Effects of local application of ototoxic antibiotics on cochlear potentials in guinea pigs. Acta Otolaryngol., 88, 41-6.

Kroese, A.B.A. & van den Bercken, J. (1980). Dual action of ototoxic antibiotics on sensory hair cells. Nature, 283, 395-7.

Kroese, A.B.A. & van den Bercken, J. (1982). Effects of ototoxic antibiotics on sensory cell functioning. Hearing Res., 6, 183-97.

Li, C.W. & McPhee, J. (1979). Influences on the coiling of the cochlea. Ann. Otol. Rhinol. Laryngol., 88, 280-7.

Marot, M., Uziel, A. & Romand, R. (1980). Ototoxicity of kanamycin in developing rats: relationship with the onset of the auditory function. Hearing Res., 2, 111-3.

Neumann, R. E. & Tytell, A.A. (1960). Serumless medium for cultivation of cells of normal and malignant origin. Proc. Soc. Exp. Biol. Med., 104, 252-6.

Nordemar, H. (1983). Embryogenesis of the inner ear. II. The late differentiation of the mammalian crista ampullaris in vivo and in vitro. Acta Otolaryngol., 96, 1-8.

Nordemar, H. & Anniko, M. (1983). Organ culture of the late embryonic inner ear as a model for ototoxicity studies. Acta Otolaryngol., 96, 457-66.

Nuttall, A.L. Marques, D.M. & Lawrence, M. (1977). Effects of perilymphatic perfusion with neomycin on the cochlear micro phonic potential in the guinea pig. Acta Otolaryngol., 83, 393-400.

Okano, Y., Yamashita, T. & Iwai, H. (1975). In vitro morphological study of cochlear epithelium. Arch. Otorhinolaryngol., 209, 151-8.

Osako, S., Tokimoto, T. & Matsuura, S. (1979). Effects of kanamycin on the auditory evoked responses during postnatal development of the hearing of the rat. Acta Otolaryngol., 88, 359-68.

Pujol, R. & Hilding, D. (1973). Anatomy and physiology of the onset of auditory function. Acta Otolaryngol., 76, 1-10.

Ruben, R.J. (1967). Development of the inner ear of the mouse: A radioautographic study of terminal mitoses. Acta Otolaryngol., Suppl. 220, 1-44.

Schacht, J. (1976). Biochemistry of neomycin ototoxicity. J. Acoust. Soc. Am., 59, 940-4.

Schafer, T.W., Pascale, A., Shimonaski, G. & Came, P.E. (1972). Evaluation of gentamicin for use in virology and tissue culture. Appl. Microbiol., 23, 565-70.

Sher, A.E. (1971). The embryonic and postnatal development of the inner ear of the mouse. Acta Otolaryngol., Suppl. 285, 1-77.

Van de Water, T. R. (1976). Effects of removal of the statoacoustic ganglion complex upon the growing otocyst. Ann. Otol. Rhinol. Laryngol., 85, Suppl. 33, 1-32.

Van de Water, T.R. (1983). Embryogenesis of the inner ear: "in vitro studies". In Development of Auditory and Vestibular Systems, ed. R. Romand, pp 337-74. New York: Academic Press.

Van de Water, T.R., Heywood, P. & Ruben, R.J. (1973). Development of sensory structures in organ cultures of the twelfth and thirteenth gestation day mouse embryo inner ears. Ann. Otol. Rhinol. Laryngol., 82, Suppl.4, 1-18.

Van de Water, T.R. & Ruben, R.J. (1971). Organ culture of the mammalian inner ear. Acta Otolaryngol., 71, 303-12.

Van de Water, T.R. & Ruben, R.J. (1974). Growth of the inner ear in organ culture. Ann. Otol. Rhinol. Laryngol., 83, Suppl. 14, 1-16.

Wersäll, J. & Flock, A. (1964). Suppression and restoration of the microphonic output from the lateral line organ after local application of streptomycin. Life Sci., 3, 1151-5.

Yamashita, T. & Vosteen, K.H. (1975). Tissue culture of the organ of Corti and the isolated hair cells from the newborn guinea pig. Acta Otolaryngol., Suppl. 330, 77-90.

Table 1. Experimental details for culture of mouse otocyst.

Reference	Gestational day on which otocyst was explanted	Dissection fluid	Culture medium	Supplements	Atmosphere*/ temp	Interval (days) at which culture medium was changed
Van de Water and Ruben (1971)	12		Medium 199 with Hank's BSS	30% FCS 0.25% lactalbumin hydrolysate 0.01 mmol sodium pyruvate 10% chick or mouse embryo extract	Air/37.5°C	4
Van de Water et al (1973)	12,13	Hank's BSS		20% FCS 10% chick or mouse embryo extract	Air/37.5°C	?
Van de Water and Ruben (1974)	12,13		Serumfree medium, Neumann & Tyrell (1960)	20% FCS 100 u/ml penicillin	Air/34.5°C	4
Van de Water (1976)	11,12,13	Culture medium		20% FCS 1% glutamine 100 u/ml penicillin	Air/34.5°C	2

Table 1 continued/

Reference	Gestational day on which otocyst was explanted	Dissection fluid	Culture medium	Supplements	Atmosphere*/ temp	Interval (days) at which culture medium was changed
Anniko et al (1978)	16	Dulbecco's PBS		10% FCS 1% glutamine 1% sodium pyruvate	Air/35°C	3
Anniko et al (1979)	13	Hank's BSS	Serumfree medium, Neumann & Tyrell (1960)	10% FCS 1% glutamine	Air/35°C	3
Anniko et al (1981)	16	?		15% FCS 1% glutamine	Air + 5%CO_2/ 37°C	3
Nordemar (1983)	16	Dulbecco's PBS		15% FCS 1% glutamine	Air + 5%CO_2/ 35°C	2

* Where not specified the atmosphere was assumed to have been air.

? Indicates no information given.

BSS Balanced salt solution.

PBS Phosphate buffered saline.

FCS Fetal calf serum.

CULTURED CELL MODELS FOR STUDYING PROBLEMS IN CARDIAC TOXICOLOGY

Nicholas Sperelakis and Ghassan Bkaily*

Department of Physiology and Biophysics
University of Cincinnati
College of Medicine
Cincinnati, OH 45267-0576
and
*Department of Biophysics, Faculty of Medicine,
University of Sherbrooke
Sherbrooke, Quebec, Canada, J1H-5N4

Outline

A. Introduction
1. Advantages of Cultured Heart Cells
2. Some Pitfalls of Using Cultured Heart Cells
3. Types of Tissues Cultured, and Types of Cultures
4. Cell Division

B. Practical Aspects
1. Cell Dissociation
2. Monolayers
3. Spherical Reaggregates
4. Cells Dissociated From Adult Hearts
5. Organ-Cultured Hearts

C. Experimental Examples
1. Developmental Changes in Membrane Electrical Properties
   a. General Changes
   b. Appearance of Fast Na^+ Channels
   c. Increase in K^+ Permeability
   d. Increase in (Na,K)-ATPase Activity, and Decrease in Cyclic AMP Level
2. Arrested Development in Organ-Cultured Young Hearts
3. Properties of Cultured Heart Cells
   a. Spherical Reaggregate Cultures Prepared From Young Hearts
   b. Reversion of Monolayer Cultures Prepared From Old Hearts
   c. Retention of Highly Differentiated Membrane Electrical Properties in Spherical Reaggregate Cultures
4. Cultured Newborn Rat Heart Cells
5. Properties of Ca^{2+} Slow Channels

A. INTRODUCTION

The first account of cultured heart cells was given by Burrows (1912), who concluded that the independent pulsatory activity of single cells was direct confirmation of the myogenic theory of heart muscle. On the basis of studies on cultured heart cells, Lewis (1928) rejected the concept of a branching syncytium in favor of cellular independence. Action potentials were obtained by impalement of cultured heart cells with microelectrodes (Crill *et al.*, 1959; Fange *et al.*, 1952; Mettler *et al.*, 1952; Sperelakis and Lehmkuhl, 1965), and details of this methodology was given by Sperelakis (1972a). The cultured cells possess pharmacological receptors virtually identical to those of cells in the original myocardium from which they were derived. That is, use of trypsin for cell dispersal does not permanently damage the cell membrane or its receptors.

Cultured cells in monolayer networks and sheets revert back to the young embryonic state. Such reverted cells are useful for studying certain properties, such as on the mechanism of the changes in type of cation channels and in K^+ permeability and on the electrogenesis of pacemaker potentials. Reverted ventricular myocardial cells may make a good model for studying the properties of cardiac nodal cells. In contrast, the cells in spherical reaggregate and strand preparations tend to retain their highly differentiated electrical properties [see book edited by Lieberman and Sano (1976) for results from several laboratories]. The reaggregates are also easier to impale with one or two microelectrodes than are the monolayers.

We will present here principally the results from our own laboratories, but the reader is referred to the book edited by Lieberman and Sano (1976) for results from other laboratories and to review articles by several investigators (Bkaily *et al.*, 1984a; Farmer *et al.*, 1983; Mitra and Morad, 1985; Schanne and Bkaily, 1981). The present chapter is an updated and expanded version of recent articles written by Sperelakis (1978, 1982, 1984).

1. Advantages of Cultured Heart Cells

The use of cultured heart cells affords unique advantages over intact myocardium for answering certain questions (Table 1). For example, the following types of studies can be performed on monolayer cells. The problem of diffusion lag in the interstitial fluid space is reduced or eliminated in monolayer culture, thus facilitating ion flux studies in a simple two-compartment system (Langer *et al.*,

1969; McCall, 1978; Seraydarian*et al.*, 1970). By using hearts of various embryonic ages for preparing the cultures, some fundamental questions of development can be answered. Cultured heart cells can be prepared that either retain highly differentiated electrical properties or have reverted ("partially dedifferentiated") electrical properties resembling young embryonic hearts. Simultaneous recording of transmembrane potentials and contractions can be made on single cells by using microelectrode and photoelectric techniques. Since cardiac muscle can be reduced to a one or two-dimensional system in monolayer culture, studies of electrotonic spread of current and cell-to-cell interactions are facilitated. The electrogenesis of various components of the action potential and pacemaker potentials can be studied in isolated single cells where propagation from, or interaction with, contiguous cells is eliminated. Voltage clamp experiments can be done on isolated single cells in which there should be adequate voltage control over the entire cell membrane, and in which the membrane current densities can be measured. Patch clamp experiments can be done on single cells in culture to examine the properties of single ion channels. Monolayer cultures of heart cells have even been used for studying the injurious effects of defibrillation current stimulation (Jones *et al.*, 1976).

Since the cells are denervated, the effects of denervation can be studied, and the direct effect of various chemicals and pharmacological agents on the myocardial cells can be determined without complications caused by neural and systemic influences. Since co-cultures of nerve and heart cells can be made, such cultures allow study of the process of nerve-muscle interactions. It is possible to produce nearly pure muscle cultures almost completely free of fibroblasts. Thus, biochemical assays can be done solely on myocardial cells, which is not possible in the intact myocardium because of the various cell types present. Microelectrophoretic injection of various substances can be done while observing electrical and mechanical effects on the injected cell. The cultured cells can be maintained in various experimental media to attempt to change the composition of the cell membranes and ascertain the concomitant changes in membrane transport and electrical properties. Cultured heart cells can be grown in chemically defined media (Halle and Wollenberger, 1971). Finally, the effects of prolonged exposure to various toxicological agents and drugs (at various concentrations) on the myocardial cells can be determined. The reader is referred to an article by Sperelakis (1981) that summarizes the effects of numerous toxic agents on heart cells. In summary, the use of cultured heart cells affords the unique opportunity to answer certain types of questions that are not readily answerable using intact cardiac muscle.

TABLE 1
Some Advantages of Cultured Heart Cells (Monolayers) for Studying Cardiovascular Toxicology

1. Long-term exposure to substances in vitro.
2. Denervated — direct effects of substances.
3. No blood flow — direct effects of substances.
4. Pure muscle cell population for biochemical assays.
5. Direct observation of living and contracting cells under microscope.
6. Excellent fixation for electron microscopy.
7. Excellent for ion flux studies. (simple 2-compartment system)
8. Retains functional receptors for neurotransmitters, hormones, and autacoids.
9. Membrane electrical properties (resting potentials, action potentials) similar to cells in intact hearts.
10. Excellent for whole-cell voltage clamp to measure the macroscopic currents, and for patch clamp to measure the single-channel currents.

2. Some Pitfalls of Using Cultured Heart Cells

Some pitfalls of working with cultured heart cells include the following. The state of electrical differentiation of the cells must be determined; i.e., it cannot be assumed that the cells will have highly differentiated electrical properties. The myofibrils may not be in a highly differentiated state, even if the cells are highly differentiated electrically; however, light microscopic examination often is sufficient to reveal if a tight parallel packing of myofibrils is present. The rate of spontaneous contractions of reverted cells is often highly variable from one hour to the next even in the same region of the culture, and there is variability from one culture to another; this problem makes studies on the effects of chemical agents on the rate of spontaneous contractions sometimes difficult to interpret. In some cases, the cells become electromechanically uncoupled, i.e., they fire action potentials but do not visibly contract. This uncoupling often occurs when the cultures are first opened and placed in an experimental chamber for electrophysiological studies. Such uncoupling can lead to erroneous conclusions, e.g., effect of a drug on automaticity, unless the cells are also impaled with microelectrodes for recording the electrical activity.

Conclusions pertaining to the effect of agents on contraction of the cells are equivocal unless experiments are also done while the cells are electrically stimulated ("paced"), because the effect of the agent could be on the pacemaker properties of the cell membrane or on the action potential generation. Cultured heart cell monolayers are difficult to impale satisfactorily with microelectrodes; this problem demands that arbitrary criteria be imposed for ascertaining adequacy of impalements. However, patch clamp techniques permit recording the action potentials and corresponding currents in single cultured cells.

With present technology, it is not possible to record the contractions of the cells quantitatively, e.g., force development. Under some conditions, such as harsh treatment during cell separation, some of the pharmacological receptors may be inactivated transiently; hence negative effects of some chemical agents must be viewed with caution. In certain types of studies, such as biochemical assays of entire cultures, contaminant cells, such as fibroblasts, will be analyzed along with the myocardial cells; therefore, the experimenter must know the degree of contamination. For example, fibroblasts are known to respond to beta-adrenergic agonists with an increase in cyclic AMP level like myocardial cells do. The metabolism of the cultured cells may shift from more aerobic to more anaerobic, and from a preponderance of tricarboxylic acid cycle towards the hexose monophosphate shunt pathway, with accompanying changes in the appropriate enzyme activities. The cells in culture may be in different states of cell division, depending on numerous factors such as the degree of confluency of the monolayers and on various factors in the serum used in the culture medium. Different batches of serum can introduce variables in the functional status of the cultured cells.

Although, there are numerous problems and potential pitfalls concerning interpretation of data collected on cultured heart cells, if reasonable precautions are taken, however, the cultured heart cells can yield important new information not readily obtainable from intact cardiac muscle preparations.

3. Types of Tissues Cultured, and Types of Cultures

Many types of animal and plant cells have been cultured, and cell lines of many of these cell types are also available. Muscle cells of all types have been cultured, including skeletal, cardiac, and smooth muscles. Smooth muscle cultures that have been made include: intestinal, vas deferens, oviduct, iris, amnion, and vascular (aortic, mesenteric, umbilical). Co-cultures of nerve and muscle have been prepared, with functional neuromuscular contacts. Co-cultures of vascular smooth muscle cells (VSM) and vascular endothelial cells can also be prepared. With respect to heart cell cultures, most preparations have been made from chick, mouse, rat, and guinea pig. Usually embryonic or early postnatal tissues are used, although adult heart cells have also been cultured.

"Tissue culture" can be divided into several subcategories: (a) In organ culture, an entire isolated organ, such as a heart or endocrine gland, is placed intact into culture medium and kept alive and functional. (b) In explant culture, a slice or a minced fragment of a tissue is placed into culture medium and maintained. In many cases, cells "grow" out of the explant by a process of repeated cell division and cell migration. (c) In cell culture, the tissue is minced and then dissociated into its individual component cells by some means (usually in Ca^{++}-free, Mg^{++}-free solution containing a proteolytic enzyme, with continual stirring). The dispersed cells are plated in culture medium and allowed to grow (i.e., divide) and to reassociate in some fashion.

The cells that grow out from the explants or the enzyme-dispersed cells adhere to the substrate (bottom of the culture dish, usually glass or plastic) and form monolayers. Cells that exhibit contact inhibition stop dividing when the monolayer cells form a confluent sheet one cell thick. In some cases, the cells form multilayers in some regions of the culture dish, in which the cells pile on top of one another to form a multilayer of cells. Monolayers and multilayers of cardiac muscle cells which contract spontaneously, often pull loose from the substrate and form three-dimensional assemblies of reaggregated cells, which sometimes are spherical in shape. The formation of such reaggregates can be expedited by growing the cells on a substrate to which they adhere poorly, such as cellophane (Halbert *et al.*, 1971). Spherical reaggregates can also be formed by spinning the enzyme-dissociated cells in a gyrotatory shaker (Moscona, 1961). For certain types of studies, enzyme-dispersed cells also can be maintained in suspension by constant shaking, which prevents them from adhering to the substrate.

For special electrophysiological experiments, the dissociated cells can be made to form long strands or thin bundles of aligned cells. For example, the cells can be plated into vessels containing glass fiber threads, to which they adhere and form a coat of cells along the entire thread (Lieberman *et al.*, 1972a, b). Unfortunately, the coating of cells often is not uniform, and there may be bare regions of thread. An alternative method ("etched substrate") is to plate the cells in a vessel whose bottom has been coated with a material to which the cells will not adhere, but in which a thin scratch has been made to expose surface favorable to cell adhesion, thus allowing the cells to align themselves in the scratch (Lieberman *et al.*, 1972b).

The above discussion has been on primary cultures of cells taken directly from a tissue. For some types of studies, secondary or tertiary cultures of "passed" cells may be used. Confluent monolayers of primary cultured cells can be shaken in the presence of low concentrations of proteolytic enzyme (e.g., trypsin) to free them from the substrate and to dissociate them again. These freed cells are then divided ("split") and plated into new culture vessels to produce "secondary" cultures. When these cells become confluent (usually within 1 to 2 weeks), the process is repeated to produce "tertiary" cultures, and so on. Some cell types retain their original characteristics for up to six such "passages" without significant "dedifferentiation" toward a stem-cell line. In those cases in which the cultured cells retain their original characteristics for a number of passages (e.g., six), these are known as a cell strain (but they have a finite life span in vitro). If this process is repeated indefinitely over many months, the cultures become known as a "cell line", presumably of cells all having a common parentage; the characteristics (both phenotype and genotype) of these cell lines may be quite different from those of the original cells. A clone of cells is made by repeated divisions of a single cell so that all daughter cells derive from a single parent cell; for example, if skeletal myoblasts are plated in very dilute solution, each myoblast forms a clone surrounding it.

Gradations in loss of some functional characteristics are seen in cells cultured for long periods. Other cell types may begin to dedifferentiate or to "revert" towards a more embryonic condition as a function of time while in primary culture. Fortunately, heart cells in primary culture can be made to retain a highly differentiated state for at least 6 weeks. All of the data on cultured heart cells and cultured VSM cells discussed below are on such primary cultures.

4. Cell Division

It is generally believed that cultured heart cells do undergo mitosis (DeHaan, 1967; Kasten, 1972; Kelly and Chacko, 1976; Mark and Strasser, 1966). However, it was reported that cardiac myocytes (from 9-day-old chick embryos) in culture, identified by PAS-positive reaction, did not proliferate, whereas the non-muscle cells did (Bogenmann and Eppenberger, 1980); although more than 50% of the myocytes synthesized DNA (incorporation of ^{3}H-thymidine and autoradiography), they merely shifted from a diploid to a tetraploid state. In addition, there is no general agreement on whether or not the mitotic state affects the state of differentiation. Some investigators suggest that dividing cells are not in a highly differentiated state. Some reports indicate that mitosis proceeds without loss of myofibrils, whereas other reports (Karsten *et al.*, 1973) indicate that contraction ceases transiently during cell division. Discussion of this problem of mitosis and differentiation is given in a review by Rumyantsev (1977). Mitosis and organogenetic movements continue when the cells are depolarized in high K^+ (Pappano and Sperelakis, 1969c; Manasek and Monroe, 1972).

It is not clear whether contact inhibition of cell division occurs among heart cells in vitro. Multilayer regions can be found in cultures prepared at high plating density, indicating that cells can overgrow one another. The density of cells plated may influence their viability and function through secretion of factors into the medium ("conditioned medium") (Gordon and Brice, 1974). Cell mobility of embryonic chick ventricular cells, as measured by intermixing of radiolabeled and unlabeled cells, was high for young (6-day-old) cells but steadily declined during development (Gershman *et al.*, 1979). Addition of dibutyryl cyclic AMP (1.2 mM) plus theophylline (1.0 mM) greatly decreased the mobility, particularly of the younger cells. The authors concluded that the cyclic AMP level was one regulatory factor in cell movements and that contact inhibition was operative.

B. PRACTICAL ASPECTS

1. Cell Dissociation

The main focus of this chapter is on primary cell cultures produced from enzyme-dissociated cells. Embryonic or early postnatal tissue is generally used for preparing cell cultures because the myocardial cells are more easily freed from the tissue. For cultured chick heart cells, fertilized chicken eggs can be obtained from a local hatchery on a weekly basis and incubated in an egg incubator at 37° C with daily rotation. The eggs are opened when the embryos are between 3 and 20 days old (hatching occurs at 21 days), and the hearts removed. The hearts from approximately 12 embryos are pooled together (in chilled Ringer solution) to make one preparation. The hearts are washed free of blood in Ringer solution (5° C), and the atria dissected and discarded (except when atrial cultures are desired). The ventricles are then minced with a small scissors. Cell separation is carried out by stirring (with a magnetic stirring bar) in a Ca^{++}-free, Mg^{++}-free Ringer solution (37° C) containing glucose (100 mg%) and 0.05% trypsin. Other proteolytic enzymes may also be used to separate the cells, such as collagenase (with or without hyaluronidase); in general, there seems to be no important difference in the properties of the cultured cells regardless of which enzyme is used to separate the cells from the intercellular matrix.

For vascular smooth muscle cell cultures, elastase or collagenase (with and without hyaluronidase) is most often used. The activity of collagenase increases with increasing Ca^{2+} concentration. It is important that the concentration of trypsin not be too high or that the exposure period not be too long. Numerous studies have shown the damaging action of trypsin on the cell membrane (Hodges*et al.*, 1973) and on intracellular proteins (Maizel*et al.*, 1974), and the metabolism of cultured cells may be affected by this damage, particularly during the first 24 to 48 hr in culture (Phillips, 1967). However, trypsin-dissociated cells quickly recover adhesiveness to one another (Steinberg*et al.*, 1973). The use of a Ca^{++} -free, Mg^{++} -free solution (contaminant Ca^{++} and Mg^{++} present only, e.g., about 10^{-6} M) facilitates the separation of the cells; in fact, some tissues, e.g., epithelia, dissociate in Ca^{2+}-free, Mg^{2+}-free solution alone without the need of a proteolytic enzyme. Mechanical shearing forces facilitate cell separation, as for example, by the vigorous stirring of the dissociation solution. Other methods of producing mechanical shearing forces have also been used in various laboratories.

During the dissociation process, at intervals of 5-15 min, the cloudy cell-containing supernatant is decanted into chilled culture medium (containing normal Ca^{++} and Mg^{++}). The combination of cold and serum rapidly inactivates the trypsin, thus the exposure of the already-freed cells to trypsin is minimized. Fresh dissociation solution is added to the undissociated tissue, and the process is repeated from five to seven times. The first one or two removals are discarded because they contain a large fraction of nonmuscle cells, and the remaining ones are pooled together. The cells are washed by light centrifugation (50 to 200 g for 5-10 min) into a pellet. Then the supernatant is aspirated or decanted, replaced with fresh culture medium, and the cells resuspended. Washing is often repeated for a second or third time to completely remove the dissociating enzymes. Embryonic heart cells usually become rounded immediately after cell separation, but this does not mean that they are severely damaged, as in the case of adult heart cells.

The usual composition of the culture medium is 10% or 15% serum (fetal calf or horse), 40% nutrient solution (such as Puck's N-16 or Medium 199), and 45-50% balanced salt solution (Hank-Ringer). The chemical composition of the various synthetic media, such as Medium 199, Puck's N-16, NCTC-135, basal medium Eagle (BME), modified Eagle medium (MEM), Dulbecco's modified Eagle medium (DMEM), Hanks Minimum Essential Medium (HMEM), L-15, etc., are usually given in the catalogs of the companies that supply the media. In general, these media contain various amino acids, glucose, vitamins, inorganic salts, and a variety of other components. Some media are claimed to promote the growth and well-being of specific types of cells. The type of serum used may be important as well, and it is thought that fetal serum contains a higher concentration of a factor that promotes cell division. Some investigators also add chick embryo extract (CEE), bought commercially or prepared in their own laboratory, to the culture medium to promote cell growth and viability. In order to facilitate the sealing of a patch clamp microelectrode, a low serum concentration (2-5%) is sometimes used to prevent the cells from becoming too thin.

Antibiotics, such as penicillin plus streptomycin (50 units/ml) or gentamicin, may be added to the medium. But if careful sterile procedures are used throughout, antibiotics and fungicides (e.g., Fungizone) may be avoided. All solutions used are sterilied by passing through filters with pore diameters of approximately 0.2 μm. All glassware and dissecting instruments are sterilized by autoclaving; plasticware used for culture vessels is purchased already sterilized and wrapped; and all dissections and procedures are carried out in a laminar-flow hood (presterilized with ultraviolet rays).

The washed pellet of cells is diluted with sufficient culture medium to give a concentration of approximately 0.5 to 1.0 x 10^6 cells/ml for plating into the culture vessels or for gyrotation. The optimal plating density can be determined by serial dilution and assaying for some selected parameter, e.g., rate of cell proliferation. Some workers pass the cell suspension through a small-pore nylon mesh to disrupt any large multicellular aggregations before plating.

In some cases, the dissociation solution is modified to contain elevated K^+ (10-25 mM) and ATP (5 mM), because this modification may facilitate the production of highly electrically differentiated cells (McLean and Sperelakis, 1974). The addition of insulin to the culture medium also appears to promote a state of high electrical differentiation, including high tetrodotoxin (TTX) sensitivity (LeDouarin *et al*., 1974; Suignard, 1979). A very simple method (Bkaily *et al*., 1986a, b, c) to separate single cells, from chick embryo heart and rabbit aortic smooth muscle preparations, consists of using a solution of HMEM (Gibco) containing 0.1% trypsin and 1.8 mM Ca^{2+}. This solution (without trypsin; with 5% serum) can be used for culturing the cells, and helps protect the cells against enzyme damage.

It is also possible to culture adult tissues (Jacobson, 1977; Jacobson *et al*., 1983; Farmer *et al*., 1983; Bkaily *et al*., 1984a; Mitra and Morad, 1985).

2. Monolayers

For producing monolayer cultures, the cells are plated into the desired type of culture vessels (e.g., modified Carrell flasks with removable lids (Bellco), plastic Petri dishes, or plastic Falcon flasks). A glass coverslip can be placed in the culture vessel so that the coverslip with adhering cells can be removed and placed into another chamber for experimentation. A volume of 1 - 3 ml of cell suspension is added per culture vessel. The cells settle to the bottom of the culture dish over a period of 12 to 48 hr if left undisturbed, and become attached to the substrate. They divide and make contact with one another to form various monolayer patterns, such as loose random networks, strands, rosettes, and confluent sheets. Confluent sheets are usually produced when the cells are plated at higher densities. Usually the myocardial cells in suspension contract spontaneously, each with its own independent rhythm. Shortly after the monolayer cells make morphological contact with one another (within 10 - 50 min), they contract synchronously, indicating that they have formed functional junctions. One or more cells acts as a pacemaker to drive the others. At low plating densities, regions of isolated single cells are often found. Such isolated single cells are suitable for whole-cell voltage clamp. Monolayer cells can be impaled with one or two microelectrodes to examine their electrophysiological properties or the patch electrode technique can be used (Bkaily *et al*., 1986a, c; Sperelakis, 1972a; Sperelakis and McLean, 1978a).

Since fibroblasts and endothelioid cells adhere to the substrate much faster than do myocardial cells, if the plated cells are allowed to settle for only 30 to 90 min and then poured off carefully, many of the fibroblasts will remain stuck to the dish and can thus be discarded. If this procedure of differential adhesion is serially repeated for 3 - 6 times, a myocardial-enriched, fibroblast-depleted culture can be thus produced (Horres *et al*., 1979). In addition, an inhibitor of fibroblasts can be added to the culture medium. Such "pure" cultures are not necessary for most electrophysiological studies, but could facilitate interpretation of biochemical types of experiments. But even without such procedures, the percentage of beating myocardial cells in a monolayer culture is often 70% to 90%; thus the proportion of nonmuscle cells may be quite low.

The cultures may be "fed" once or twice a week with fresh culture medium, if desired, but primary cultures of heart cells survive quite well for several weeks without such feeding. In fact, some types of cells prefer "conditioned medium" (medium in which other cells are growing or have grown). For example, it has been reported that the ratio of the number of cells to the volume of the medium has a critical value below which the cells will not proliferate because they are unable to "condition the medium" adequately (Earle *et al*., 1951). Since the volume of culture medium (e.g., 3 ml) is relatively large compared to the volume of cells (wet weight of approximately 1-3 mg), there is almost no acidosis produced (pH indicator added to the culture medium or medium pH checked with a pH meter) after 1 - 3 weeks in culture.

The cultures survive very well even if the culture vessels are sealed to the incubator atmosphere (compressed air and 5% CO_2, filtered and washed). Presumably the amount of oxygen available in the culture vessel (e.g., about 8 ml air in a Carrell flask) is sufficient to last the cells for several weeks. The oxygen tension may be important in determining the rate of cell proliferation (Hollenberg, 1971) and relative activity of glycolytic versus oxidative metabolism. Cultured chick heart cells, while primarily dependent on glucose for energy metabolism, retain a capacity to utilize fatty acids, whereas cultured mammalian fetal heart cells lack this ability (Rosenthal and Warshaw, 1973). Mammalian fetal heart cells in culture seem to adapt to low environmental oxygen tension by diminished synthesis of contractile proteins and a shift in lactic dehydrogenase isozyme pattern, without a decrease in cellular energy stores (Karsten *et al*., 1973). Some laboratories place a group of open culture vessels in a large closed plastic box, which can be "flushed" daily with any desired gas mixture.

Wentzel *et al*. (1970) showed that the spontaneous beating of cultured neonatal rat heart cells (confluent monolayers and multilayers) was maintained for a longer time if the plating concentration was high (e.g., 0.5 x 10^6 cells/ml) than when it was low (e.g., 1.3 x 10^3 cells/ml). In addition, the higher the proportion of muscle cells to nonmuscle cells in the culture, the longer the period that beating was maintained. The addition of nicotine (0.016 to 0.6 mM) to the culture medium also prolonged the beating period. Similarly, it was found that high carbon monoxide (75% of atmosphere for periods up to 26 days) not only inhibited the overgrowth of muscle cells by endothelioid cells, but also prevented the usual time-dependent reduction in spontaneous beating rate (Brenner and Wenzel, 1972).

3. Spherical Reaggregates

In addition to the monolayer preparations and fiberglass strands described above, the cells can also be reaggregated into small spheres of about 100 to 500 μm in diameter by either of two methods. (1) The cells can be plated into glass culture dishes containing cellophane squares on the bottom. Since the cells do not adhere very well to cellophane, they pull free and form small (0.1 to 0.5 μm) spherical reaggregates spontaneously (Halbert *et al*., 1971; McLean and Sperelakis, 1976; Nathan *et al*., 1976). (2) Alternatively, the cells can be placed into Ehrlenmeyer flasks and rotated on a gyrotatory shaker for about 48 hr (Mettler *et al*., 1952). The cells make contact with one another in the vortex of the solution and stick together. The longer the gyrotation period, the larger the spherical reaggregates become. Rotation for 24 to 48 hr produces reaggregates varying between 50 μm to 400 μm in diameter. Larger reaggregates are not desirable because of a tendency for the cells in the core to become hypoxic and necrotic. After the rotation period, the spherical reaggregates can be transferred to a regular culture vessel and cultured for up to 6 weeks. The reaggregates will stick lightly to the substrate (or tightly in some cases with outgrowth). The entire reaggregate contracts synchronously.

The spherical reaggregates are transferred to a heated (37° C) bath containing fresh culture medium or Ringer solution for microelectrode impalements. There are several advantages of spherical reaggregates over monolayers, the most notable of which is the much easier microelectrode impalements due to the three-dimensional packing of cells and to isolation from vibrations (shock-mounting). An advantage of spherical reaggregates ("mini-heart") over an intact heart is that the contractions are more feeble, so that it is often possible to remain in the same cell for a prolonged period. In addition, since there are no blood vessels in the reaggregates, the effect of a drug under investigation cannot be on the rate of perfusion.

Reaggregates that are composed of highly electrically-differentiated cells usually do not contract spontaneously, but do contract in response to electrical stimulation. Reaggregates that are composed of reverted cells generally contract spontaneously at a rate of approximately 1 sec^{-1}. The properties of the cells do not seem to change very much, if at all, during incubation periods of 5-30 days. The number of TTX-sensitive reaggregates can be increased if Ca^{2+} is replaced by Sr^{2+} or Ba^{2+} during the trypsin dispersion (Bkaily *et al.*, unpublished results).

Scanning electron microscopy has been done on heart reaggregates at various stages of formation by Shimada *et al.* (1974; 1976). They showed that a thin fibroblastic coat eventually completely covers the reaggregate. Fibroblasts from within the center of the reaggregate worked their way out to the surface.

4. Cells Dissociated From Adult Hearts

Isolated adult myocytes can be prepared by enzymatic perfusion of adult hearts (Altschuld *et al.*, 1980; Berry *et al.*, 1970; Carlson *et al.*, 1978; Nag *et al.*, 1977; Pretlow *et al.*, 1972; Vahouny *et al.*, 1970, 1979) or by mechanical disaggregation (Bloom *et al.*, 1974). The methods used are similar to those developed to disperse and culture heart cells from embryonic and neonatal animals (for review see Kuzuya *et al.*, 1983; Sperelakis, 1982). For preparing isolated adult cardiomycytes, the species that have been used include rat, mouse, dog, rabbit, guinea pig, human, bovine, and cat (Altschuld *et al.*, 1980; Berry *et al.*, 1970; Bkaily *et al.*, 1984a; Carlson *et al.*, 1978; Nag *et al.*, 1977; Pretlow *et al.*, 1972; Vahouny *et al.*, 1970, 1979).

Numerous investigators have obtained isolated adult mammalian cardiomyocytes by a variety of techniques. In 1970, Berry *et al.* obtained morphologically intact myocytes by perfusing hearts with collagenase and hyaluronidase. Vahouny *et al.* (1970) used trypsin and collagenase in their incubation medium to obtain isolated cardiac cells. Powell and colleagues (1976) isolated cardiomyocytes by perfusing hearts with collagenase and albumin. In general, isolated cardiomyocytes are prepared by perfusing or incubating whole adult hearts or fragments with a Ca^{2+}-free solution. This solution washes out residual blood and weakens the intercellular cement. Tissues are then treated with solutions of varying Ca^{2+} concentrations that contain multiple enzymes to remove the glycocalyx. Finally, the cells are dispersed by one of a variety of mechanical procedures (for review see Bkaily *et al.*, 1984a; Farmer *et al.*, 1983; Mitra and Morad, 1985).

Type I and type II collagenase are used by most investigators preparing isolated cardiomyocytes. This crude collagenase requires Ca^{2+} for activation, and is inhibited by cysteine and EDTA. Therefore, many investigators add some Ca^{2+} to the medium (e.g., 1 μM) to activate the collagenase. However, ventricular myocytes obtained by these methods are often rounded cells that have been damaged. Some cells, although rod-shaped, exhibit the calcium paradox. Other cells beat spontaneously, indicative of damage during dispersion. The rod-shaped cells generally do not survive more than a few hours. Although these isolated cells usually have a resting potential (RP) of only about -30 to -50 mV, normal resting potentials can be obtained by exposing the cells to high concentrations of calcium (5-10 mM) (Powell *et al.*, 1981) or by incubating them for a period in a high K^+ medium (Isenberg and Klockner, 1982).

Clark *et al.* (1978) reported a procedure for dissociating cells from adult rat hearts without causing major cell damage. These investigators used a combination of collagenase (0.5 %) and hyaluronidase (0.2 %), followed by a solution containing EDTA (0.5 mM), taurine (30 mM), and dimethylsulphoxide (DMSO, 10 % v/v). They reported that the DMSO protected the cells against degeneration during the isolation, and permitted physiological levels of $[Ca]_o$ to stimulate rhythmic contractions without inducing cell damage. The ultrastructure of the isolated cells was normal. The cells remained intact for up to 1 hr if stored at 0 to 4° C; longer storage periods produced some degeneration of the cells. Other investigators also have succeeded in preparing isolated cardiac cells by enzymatic digestion that tolerate external $[Ca]_o$ in the millimolar range (Farmer *et al.*, 1977; Glick *et al.*, 1974; Powell *et al.*, 1978; Powell and Twist, 1976; Rajs *et al.*, 1978). However, these isolated fibers usually beat spontaneously.

Isenberg and Klockner (1980) demonstrated that the RPs and action potentials (APs) of isolated rat heart myocytes [dissociated by collagenase (1 mg/ml) and hyaluronidase (1 mg/ml) in a Ca^{++}-free solution] were similar to those of cells in intact rat hearts. The "calcium paradox" (cells going into contracture, becoming spherical, and dying) was avoided by incubating the cells in high K^+ (> 100 mM) and substrate-enriched solutions before stepwise elevation of $[Ca]_o$ to 3.6 mM. Voltage clamp experiments were also done on these myocytes (using a single microelectrode method), and the inward slow current (I_{si}) was measured.

Lee *et al.* (1979), using the dispersal method of adult rat hearts described by Powell and Twist and drawing the isolated single cells (cylinders, approximately 15-25 μm diameter by 100 μm length) into a suction pipette (about 20 μm diameter), reported that the cells had high RPs (-70 to -90 mV), pacemaker potentials, and fast-rising TTX-sensitive APs. Using internal perfusion of the cells and with blockade of I_K (by Cs^+), I_{Ca} (by Co^{++} or Ca^{++}-free), and I_{Cl} (Cl-free solution), they were able to measure the fast inward Na^+ current (I_{Na}) in voltage clamp experiments. Because the surface area of the cell could be measured accurately, the current densities were obtained.

Bkaily *et al.* (1984a) used a modified bristle method (Jacobson, 1977; Jacobson *et al.*, 1983) for mechanical dispersion of adult single heart cells with enzyme-free medium containing Sr^{2+} or Ba^{2+} as a replacement for Ca^{2+}, and obtained healthy rod-shaped Ca^{2+}-tolerant single adult cells. These myocytes did not contract spontaneously, had a normal RP, and were TTX sensitive. The yield was improved by the following modification (Bkaily *et al.*, 1984a): A Ca^{2+}-free medium containing 0.1% trypsin and 1.8 mM Sr^{2+} was used for perfusion of the whole heart, which was stimulated electrically during the enzymatic perfusion. When the contraction of the heart became greatly weakened, the perfusing solution was replaced by trypsin-free medium. After a few minutes, the ventricle was minced, and the bristle dispersion was begun. This method gave a large number of dispersed cells. Recently, a uniform enzymatic method for dissociation of myocytes from adult hearts was described by Mitra and Morad (1985).

Brown *et al.* (1981) used one-electrode and two-electrode suction pipettes to record the fast Na^+ current. Patlak and Ortiz (1985) found three types of Na^+ channels: fast, slow, and ultraslow. Several types of K^+ channels were reported in single myocytes, such as inward rectifier, outward rectifier, ATP-dependent, Ca^{2+}-dependent, Na^+-dependent, 4-AP sensitive, and acetylcholine-activated K^+ currents. Single adult myocytes retain insulin receptors and a strong Na/K pump.

5. Organ-Cultured Hearts

It is also advantageous in some cases to organ-culture hearts in order to answer some specific questions. For example, young embryonic hearts can be removed from the fetus before innervation reaches the heart and placed in organ culture for the purpose of answering such questions as: (a) what is the effect of innervation on the properties of the cells? and (b) will the heart continue to differentiate in vitro? Thus, one variable is the develomental stage of the hearts when placed in culture. As might be expected, the younger the embryonic age of the heart (which also means the smaller the heart), the better they survive in culture. Organ-cultured hearts have been prepared primarily from embryonic chicks (McLean *et al.*, 1976; Renaud and Sperelakis, 1976; Renaud *et al.*, 1978; Shigenobu and Sperelakis, 1974, 1975; Sperelakis *et al.*, 1974; Sperelakis and Shigenobu, 1974), and from fetal mice (DeLuca *et al.*, 1974; Ingwall *et al.*, 1975; Kaufman *et al.*, 1977; Roeske *et al.*, 1977; Wildenthal, 1971 a, b, 1973). Most of the studies on embryonic chick hearts concern their electrophysiological properties. In contrast, most of the studies on the fetal mouse hearts concern metabolic studies, e.g., on the adenine nucleotides, and the effects of hypoxia, ischemia, substrates, hormones, and temperature on survival and function of the hearts.

The methods for culturing various types of mature organs have been described (Trowell, 1959). The methods used for making organ-cultured hearts, either completely immersed in culture medium or at an interface between culture medium and moist air, have been described in detail (Renaud and Sperelakis, 1976; Shigenobu and Sperelakis, 1974; Sperelakis *et al.*, 1974; Sperelakis and Shigenobu, 1974). Likewise, the methods used for producing blood-perfused hearts grafted onto the chorioallantoic membrane of a host embryonic chick have been published (Renaud and Sperelakis, 1976).

C. EXPERIMENTAL EXAMPLES

1. DEVELOPMENTAL CHANGES IN MEMBRANE ELECTRICAL PROPERTIES

a. General Changes

The anterior half of the flat 16-20 hr-old chick embryo blastoderm contains bilateral "precardiac" areas (mesoderm) whose cells are destined to form the heart (Rosenquist and DeHaan, 1966). Twin tubular primordia are formed bilaterally from the precardiac mesoderm and fuse to form a single tubular heart (Patten, 1956). The tubular heart begins contracting spontaneously at 30-40 hr (9 - 19 somite stage) (Romanoff, 1960). The blood pressure is very low (1-2 mm Hg), and propagation of the peristaltic contraction wave is very slow (approx 1 cm/sec in 3-day hearts) (Romanoff, 1960). Chambers first appear in the heart on about day 5, and circulation to the chorioallantoic membane is established, so that metabolism of the embryo becomes aerobic at that time. The nerves arrive at the heart on about day 5 (Romanoff, 1960), but they do not become functional with respect to neurotransmitter release until considerably later (Enemar*et al*., 1965; Pappano, 1976). The heart rate of the chick embryo increases from approximately 50 beats/min on day 1.5 to 220 beats/min on day 8.

Electron microscopy of young chick hearts shows that there are only few and short myofibrils (Fig. 1). The sarcomeres are not complete, and the myofibrils run in all directions, including perpendicular to one another. There is an abundance of ribosomes and rough endoplasmic reticulum, and large pools of glycogen are found in the cells. As development progresses, the number of myofibrils increases and they become aligned. By day 18, the ultrastructure of the myocardial cells is similar to that of cells in adult hearts.

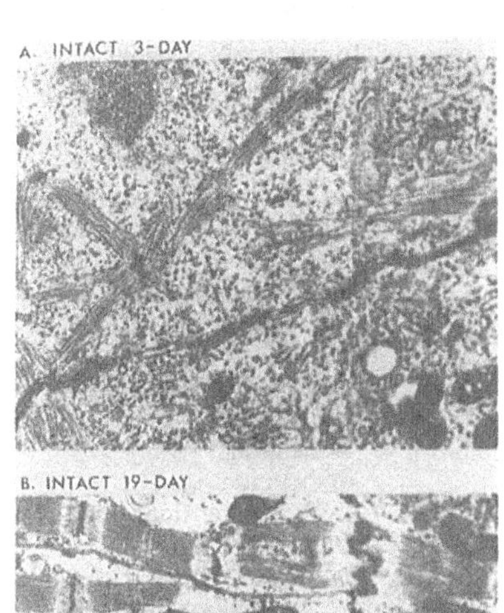

FIG. 1. Cell ultrastructure of young (three days in ovo) and old (19 days in ovo) embryonic chick hearts in situ. **A:** Three-day ventricular cell demonstrating paucity and nonalignment of myofibrils. Ribosomes are abundant in the cytoplasm. The contiguous cells are held in close apposition by desmosomes. **B:** 19-day ventricular cells with abundant and aligned myofibrils. A convoluted intercalated disc appears between contiguous cells. Taken from Sperelakis *et al*., 1976; Sperelakis and McLean, 1978a, b.

b. Appearance of Fast Na^+ Channels

In order to determine the state of membrane differentiation of the cultured cells, comparison should be made with the properties of intact chick hearts at different stages of development in situ. The electrical properties of the heart undergo sequential changes during development (Bernard, 1976; Ishima, 1968; Schneider and Sperelakis, 1975; Shigenobu and Sperelakis, 1971; Sperelakis *et al.*, 1967). The myocardial cells in young (2-3 days in ovo) hearts possess slowly-rising (10-30 V/sec) action potentials (APs) preceded by pacemaker potentials (Fig. 2A). The upstroke is generated by Na^+ influx through slow Na^+ channels, which are insensitive to TTX (Fig. 2B). Kinetically-fast Na^+ channels that are sensitive to TTX make their initial appearance on about day 4, and increase in density until about day 18. The maximal rate of rise of the AP ($+\dot{V}_{max}$) increases progressively from day 3 through day 18, when the adult $\dot{V}_{max}$ of approximately 150 V/sec is attained (Fig. 2E). From day 5 to day 7, fast Na^+ channels coexist with a large complement of slow channels. TTX reduces $+\dot{V}_{max}$ to the value observed in 2-day hearts, i.e., 10-20 V/sec, but the APs persist (Fig. 2 C-D). After day 8, the APs are completely abolished by TTX (Fig. 2F), and depolarization to less then -50 mV now abolishes excitability. This indicates that the AP-generating channels consist predominantly of fast Na^+ channels, most of the slow Na^+ channels having been lost (functionally) so that insufficient numbers remain to support regenerative excitation. Addition of some positive inotropic agents increases the number of available Ca^{++} slow channels in the membrane, and leads to regain of excitability in cells whose fast Na^+ channels have been inactivated (Schneider and Sperelakis, 1975; Shigenobu and Sperelakis, 1972).

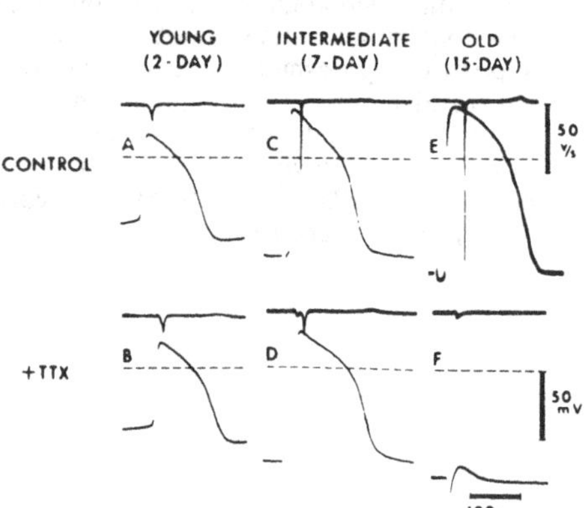

FIG. 2. Development of sensitivity to TTX of intact embryonic chick hearts with increasing embryonic age. **A-B:** Intracelluar recordings from a 20-day-old heart before **(A)** and 20 min after **(B)** the addition of TTX (20 μg/ml). **C-D:** Recordings from a 7-day-old heart before **(C)** and 2 min after **(D)** the addition of TTX (2 μg/ml). (Note depression of the rate of rise in **D.**) **E-F:** From a 15-day-old heart prior to **(E)** and 2 min after **(F)** the addition of TTX (1 μg/ml). The upper traces give dV/dt; this trace has been shifted relative to the V-t trace to prevent obscuring dV/dt. The horizontal broken line in each panel represents zero potential. (Modified from Sperelakis and Shigenobu, 1974.)

c. Increase in K^+ Permeability

Young embryonic chick hearts have a low K^+ permeability (P_K) (Sperelakis, 1980; Sperelakis and Shigenobu, 1972). This accounts for the low resting potential (RP) of about -45 mV and for the high incidence of automaticity in the ventricular area of the tubular heart. The incidence of pacemaker potentials in cells in young hearts is very high, and this incidence decreases during development, roughly in parallel with the increase in P_K (Sperelakis and McLean, 1978b; Sperelakis and Shigenobu, 1972). As deduced from RP versus log $[K]_o$ curves for hearts of different ages, the low RP in young hearts is caused by a high P_{Na}/P_K ratio of approximately 0.2. The $[K]_i$ level is about 130 mM in 3-day-old hearts compared to 150 mM in 15-day-old hearts; hence, the K^+ equilibrium potential (E_K) is about -91 mV (at a $[K]_o$ of 4 mM) in 3-day hearts. The P_{Na}/P_K ratio decreases to about 0.1 by day 5, and is between 0.05 and 0.01 by day 15. The increase in RP parallels the change in the P_{Na}/P_K ratio. Because the input resistance of the cells is high in young hearts (about 13 MΩ), a low P_K is primarily responsible for the high P_{Na}/P_K ratio. Carmeliet *et al.* (1976 a,b) have also shown from ^{42}K flux measurements that P_K is several-fold lower in 6-day hearts than in 19-day hearts.

d. Increase in (Na,K)-ATPase Activity and Decrease in Cyclic AMP Level

The (Na,K)-ATPase specific activity is low in young chick hearts and increases progressively during development, reaching the final adult value by about day 18 (Sperelakis, 1972b). Although the Na-K pump capability is thus low in young hearts, it is sufficient to maintain a relatively high $[K]_i$. The Na-K pump is aided in the task by the low P_K; that is, in young hearts, the pump capability is low but the ion leak is correspondingly low.

The cyclic AMP level is very high in young hearts, and it decreases during development. The drop is rapid at first and then more slowly, declining to the final adult level by about day 16 (McLean *et al.*, 1975; Renaud *et al.*, 1978). Since elevation of cyclic AMP leads to an increase in the number of available slow Ca^{++} channels (Schneider and Sperelakis, 1975; Shigenobu and Sperelakis, 1972), the decrease in cyclic AMP level during development could be related to the concomitant decrease in density of available slow channels (in the absence of positive inotropic agents). It has been proposed that a protein constituent of the slow channel must be phosphorylated by activation of cyclic AMP-dependent protein kinase in order for the channel to be available for voltage activation (see section C-5).

2. ARRESTED DEVELOPMENT IN ORGAN-CULTURED YOUNG HEARTS

Organ culture of embryonic hearts <u>in vitro</u> provides a powerful means of analyzing the changes that occur during normal development <u>in situ</u>. When 3-

day-old chick embryonic hearts are placed intact into organ culture for 10-14 days, these muscle cells do not continue to differentiate electrically or morphologically (Sperelakis *et al.*, 1974; Sperelakis and Shigenobu, 1974). The impaled cells have low RPs and slow-rising TTX-insensitive APs (Fig. 3). That is, their properties are identical to those of fresh noncultured 3-day-old hearts. They do not gain fast Na^+ channels and retain their slow Na^+ channels, as indicated by the fact that Mn^{++} (1 mM) does not block the APs but D600 (verapamil analog) does (Fig. 3). The cells are arrested in the stage of differentiation attained at the time of explanation. The same was true of young hearts grafted onto the chorioallantoic membrane of a host chick and thereby blood perfused (Renaud and Sperelakis, 1976) (Fig. 3). Therefore, something in the in situ environment of the heart in the developing embryo must control the appearance of the fast Na^+ channels. A possible trophic influence of the innervation is not known.

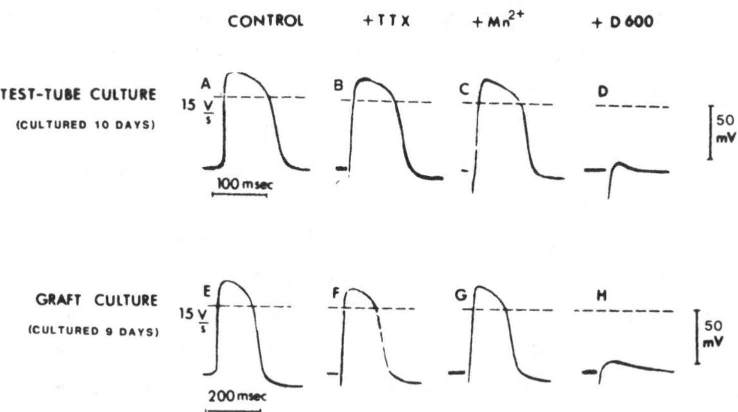

FIG. 3. Lack of gain of fast Na^+ channels in organ-cultured young (3-day-old) embryonic chick hearts. **A-D:** Tissue in test-tube culture for 10 days. **E-H:** Tissue in graft culture for 9 days. As shown in **A** and **E**, the control action potentials had slow rates of rise of about 15 V/sec. Addition of tetrodotoxin (TTX: 2 μg/ml) had little or no effect on the rate of rise of the action potential **(B,F)**. Addition of Mn^{++} (1 mM), a known blocker of Ca^{++} current, did not affect the action potentials **(C,G)**. However, D600 (10^{-6}M), a known blocker of slow channels, did abolish the action potentials **(D,H)**. Note the different time scale in **E-H** compared to **A-D**, and that the action potential durations were longer in the graft cultures compared to the test-tube cultures, for the same pacing frequency and temperature. (Modified from Renaud and Sperelakis, 1976.)

In contrast, the sensitivity to ACh continues to differentiate in organ culture. Dong *et al.* (1986) showed that, whereas fresh non-cultured 3-day-old embryonic chick hearts (atrial portion) are essentially insensitive to ACh, the sensitivity to

ACh increases markedly during organ culture for 14 days. It is not known whether the number of muscarinic responses increases and/or the N_i coupling protein increases.

When organ-cultured young hearts were incubated with RNA-enriched extracts obtained from adult chicken hearts, fast Na^+ channels appeared de novo, the RPs increased, automaticity ceased, and the APs were rapidly rising and completely sensitive to TTX (McLean *et al.*, 1976) (Fig. 4C-D). There was a lag period of about 6 days before the effects became demonstrable. These findings indicate that further differentiation can be induced in vitro. The induction was prevented by cycloheximide, an inhibitor of protein synthesis, thus suggesting that synthesis of new protein is required for the appearance of the fast Na^+ channels. In agreement with these findings, it has been recently demonstrated that mRNA injected into frog oocytes can induce ion channels (Gundersen *et al.*, 1984).

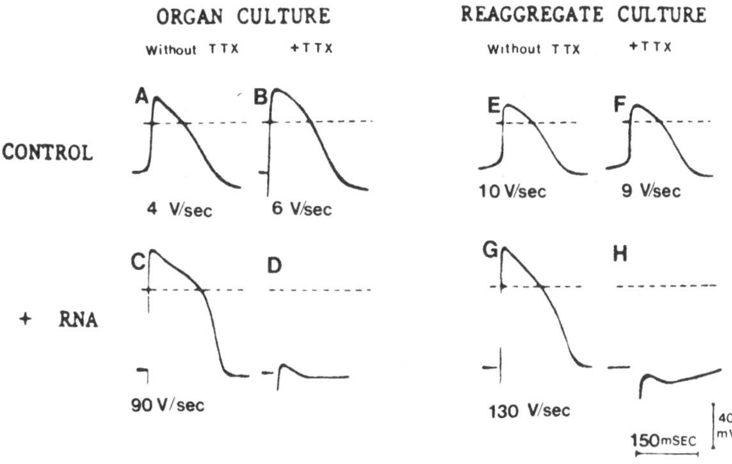

FIG. 4. Arrest of development of young (3-day) embryonic myocardial cells in organ-cultured intact hearts **(A-B)** and in cultured reaggregates **(E-F)**, and induction of further differentiation by culturing with RNA-enriched extracts from adult hearts **(C-D, G-H)**. **A-B:** Records from one cell in a 3-day-old intact heart organ cultured for 10 days before **(A)** and after **(B)** addition of TTX (1 μg/ml), and showing the arrest of development. **C-D:** Records from one cell in an organ-cultured 3-day-old heart treated with RNA showing a fast rate of rise (90 V/sec) **(C)** and complete blockade by TTX **(D)**. **E-F:** Records from one cell in a spherical reaggregate before **(E)** and after **(F)** TTX (1 μg/ml), illustrating the failure of membrane differentiation, including lack of fast Na^+ channels. **G-H:** Records from one cell in a spherical reaggregate culture treated with RNA showing a fast rate of rise (130 V/sec) and a high resting potential (-75 mV) **(G)**; TTX (0.1 μg/ml) rapidly abolished the action potential **(H)**. Electric field stimulation applied in **B, C, D, G, H.** (Modified from McLean *et al.*, 1976.)

Survival of old embryonic hearts (nonperfused) is much more difficult unless the hearts are minced into small fragments (Renaud and Sperelakis, 1976; Sperelakis and Shigenobu, 1974). In the latter case, the cells in the heart fragments tend to retain their highly differentiated electrical properties, including relatively large stable RPs with moderately fast-rising TTX-sensitive APs upon electrical stimulation (Renaud and Sperelakis, 1976). When whole hearts were cultured, survival was for a shorter period (e.g., up to 6 days). Whole fetal mouse hearts in organ culture also survive for similar periods (Wildenthal, 1971a).

3. PROPERTIES OF CULTURED HEART CELLS

a. Spherical Reaggregate Cultures Prepared From Young Hearts

When spherical reaggregate cultures were prepared from 3-day-old embryonic hearts and cultured for 10 days, no evidence for differentiation was obtained (McLean *et al.*, 1976; Pelleg and Sperelakis, unpublished observations). The impaled cells had low RPs, pacemaker potentials, and slowly-rising (about 10 V/sec) APs that were not sensitive to TTX (Fig. 4 E-F). In contrast, DeHaan and coworkers (1976) reported that reaggregates of 4-day-old cells exhibited increasing rates of rise of the APs over several days in culture (cf. Nathan and DeHaan, 1978). Since day 4 is on the edge of the intermediate period, it is possible that genes coding for the production of fast Na^+ channel protein had been activated prior to culturing.

When the spherical reaggregate cultures prepared from 3-day-old embryonic hearts were incubated with mRNA-enriched extracts obtained from adult chicken hearts, the cells proceeded to differentiate after a lag period of several days, as in the case of organ-cultured young hearts. There were large stable RPs and rapidly rising TTX-sensitive APs (McLean*et al.*, 1976) (Fig. 4G-H).

b. Reversion of Monolayer Cultures Prepared from Old Hearts

When ventricular myocardial cells from 14- to 20-day-old embryonic chick hearts are dispersed in trypsin and placed into standard monolayer cell culture, the cells lose many of their myofibrils within a short time. After several days in culture, there are only few and incomplete myofibrils. Thus, the ultrastructure rapidly reverts to that characteristic of the young embryonic state. However, the cells tend to regain more myofibrils after long periods in culture (Mark and Strasser, 1966). It has also been found that the ultrastructure closely resembles the adult ultrastructure if the cultured cells are placed into media containing low serum concentrations (which presumably inhibits cell division and favors differentiation) (Jones*et al.*, 1976). In addition, it has been found that even isolated single heart cells in culture may contain a dense packing of myofibrils (S.

Chacko, personal communication). Collagenase-dissociated cells exhibit less myofibrillar disruption than trypsin-dissociated cells (Jongsma *et al*., 1976). Numerous enzyme and metabolic changes also occur in cultured heart cells rapidly after culture (Harary *et al*., 1964; Sperelakis, 1972a; Warshaw and Rosenthal, 1972).

When monolayer cells, derived from old embryonic hearts and cultured for 3-14 days, are impaled with microelectrodes, it is found that the RPs are low and the APs are slowly rising ($+\dot{V}_{max}$ of 3-15 V/sec), and the overshoot is small (Fig. 5C). Hyperpolarizing current pulses increase AP amplitude, but $+\dot{V}_{max}$ is increased only a relatively small amount. With depolarizing pulses, spike amplitude and $+\dot{V}_{max}$ decrease and go to zero at an E_m of about -20 mV. There is loss of TTX sensitivity (Sperelakis and Lehmkuhl, 1965; Rosen and Fuhrman, 1971; McDonald *et al*., 1972; Renaud, 1973) (Fig. 5D). The APs closely resemble those found in young embryonic hearts (compare Fig. 5C with Fig. 2A), and not those found in old embryonic hearts from which the cells were derived (compare Fig. 5C-D with Fig. 5A-B or with Fig. 2E-F). Thus, the ventricular cells taken from 14- to 20-day embryonic hearts revert to the early embryonic state (or partially dedifferentiate) with respect to the AP-generating mechanism: fast Na^+ channels are functionally lost and slow Na^+ channels are gained. This reversion can occur rapidly, often being complete within 24 hr (McLean and Sperelakis, 1974).

The inward current during the AP is carried mainly by Na^+ ion because the overshoot is a function of log $[Na]_o$, with a slope approaching the theoretical 60 mV/decade (Pappano and Sperelakis, 1969b). $+\dot{V}_{max}$ is also dependent on $[Na]_o$ (Sperelakis and Lehmkuhl, 1968). A small inward Ca^{++} current participates in the electrogenesis of the rising phase and overshoot of the AP. In fact, in cells whose excitability is abolished in zero Na^+, elevation of $[Ca]_o$ to 10 mM, or addition of Sr^{++} or Ba^{++} (2-10 mM) leads to rapid appearance of APs. Thus, purely divalent cation spikes can be produced in cultured heart cells. The divalent cations presumably pass through either slow Ca^{++} channels or the slow Na^+ channels.

Shortly after separation from the ventricle, many of the myocardial cells in suspension beat spontaneously at independent rhythms (Sperelakis and Lehmkuhl, 1964). This indicates that the normally nonpacemaker ventricular cells of old embryonic hearts rapidly gain automaticity upon cell separation. This suggests that a marked decrease in P_K occurs, because to exhibit automaticity, cells must have a low g_K and a low g_{Cl}. When the cells are cultured for a few days, the RPs are low and many cells exhibit pacemaker potentials (Fig. 5C). The input resistance increases to nearly double (10 MΩ) that of cells in intact hearts (Sperelakis, 1979b). These facts are consistent with a low P_K. A plot of resting potential versus log $[K]_o$ suggests that the extrapolated $[K]_i$ is 90-100 mM in the reverted cells, corresponding to an E_K (at a $[K]_o$ of 4 mM) of -82 mV. This value is considerably greater than the measured average RP of about -55 mV, hence indicating that the P_{Na}/P_K ratio is high (presumably because P_K is low). Thus, P_K also tends to revert back toward the young embryonic state in cultured monolayers. In fact, in some isolated single cells in culture, P_K is so low that the cells are depolarized beyond the level that APs can be produced (beyond the inactivation potential for the slow channels); therefore, these cells do not contract spontaneously (Pappano and Sperelakis, 1969a). However, if these cells are impaled with one or two microelectrodes, it is found that the membrane resistance is very high and that spontaneous APs and contractions appear upon application of hyperpolarizing current pulses (Fig. 6J-L). These cells exhibit a prominent hyperpolarization when $[K]_o$ is raised to 10-15 mM.

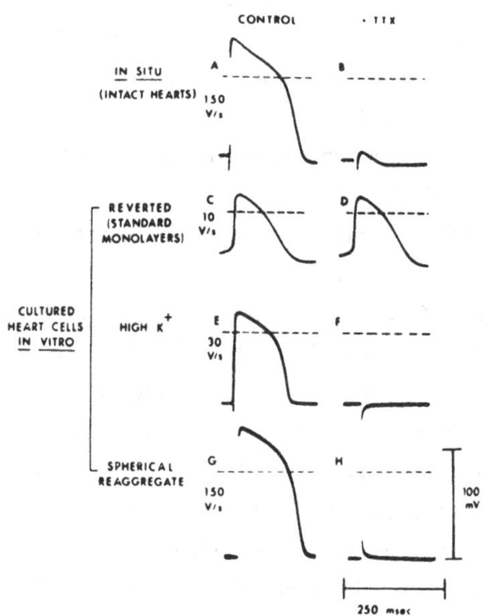

FIG. 5. Comparison of electrophysiological properties of intact old (16-day) embryonic chick hearts in situ (A-B) with those of trypsin-dispersed old ventricular myocardial cells in cultures prepared by three different methods (C-H). A-B: Intact heart; control action potential (A) was rapidly rising (150 V/sec), had a high stable resting potential (about -80 mV), and was completely abolished by tetrodotoxin (TTX; 0.1 μg/ml) (B). C-D: Standard reverted monolayers; control action potential was slowly rising (10 V/sec), was preceded by a pacemaker potential, the resting potential was low (about -50 mV) (C), and TTX did not alter the action potential (D). E-F: Partially reverted cells cultured as monolayers in media containing elevated K^+ concentration (25 mM); control action potential had a rate of rise of 30 V/sec (E), lacked a pacemaker potential, had a moderately high resting potential (-60 mV), and was completely abolished by TTX (F). G-H: Highly differentiated cells in spherical reaggreagate culture; control action potentials were rapidly rising (150 V/sec), the resting potentials were high (-80 mV) (G), and TTX abolished the action potentials (H). (Modified from McLean & Sperelakis, 1974, 1976; Sperelakis & Shigenobu, 1974.)

Some of the monolayer cells behave as nonpacemaker cells (Sperelakis and Lehmkuhl, 1964). Application of depolarizing or hyperpolarizing current pulses does not alter the frequency of firing in these cells (Fig. 6A-B). Sufficient hyperpolarization causes failure of the APs; but unlike the true pacemaker cells, small driving junctional potentials continue at unaltered frequency during the pulse (Fig. 6C). The junctional potentials probably represent the interaction with contiguous firing cells (Sperelakis, 1979b). In contrast, true pacemaker cells respond to small depolarizing current pulses by an increase in firing rate, and to small hyperpolarizing pulses by a decrease in firing frequency (Fig. 6D-F). There is an absence of junctional potentials when firing is abolished in true pacemaker cells (Fig. 6F). Quiescent cells can be induced to exhibit trains of APs during application of long-duration depolarizing pulses (Fig. 6G), and anodal-break excitation can be elicited by brief hyperpolarizing pulses (Fig. 6I).

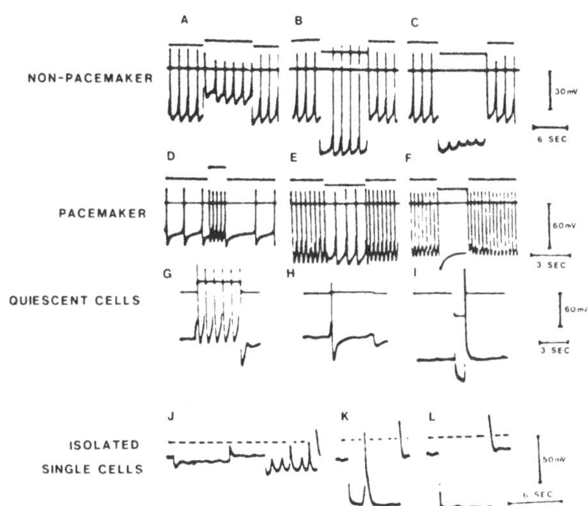

FIG. 6. Effect of polarizing current on non-pacemaker and pacemaker reverted heart cells in monolayer culture. **A–C:** Non-pacemaker cell; frequency of firing unaltered by current pulses of 0.6 **(A)** and 1.4 nA **(B)**; at 1.5 nA, action potentials were prevented, but driving junctional potentials remained at unaltered frequency **(C)**. **D–F:** Three different pacemaker cells; depolarizing current pulse of 1.2 nA markedly increases rate of firing **(D)**, whereas hyperpolarizing pulses slow the frequency **(E**, 0.6 nA) or cause cessation of firing **(F**, 1.2 nA). **G–I:** Quiescent cells can be induced to fire during depolarizing current pulses (1.4 nA in **G** and 0.2 nA in **H**), or at the termination of hyperpolarizing current pulses **(I**, 2 nA). **J–L:** Recordings from an isolated single cell in culture that was quiescent and had a very low resting potential. Hyperpolarizing current pulses of 0.2 and 0.4 nA **(J)**, 0.8 nA **(K)**, and 0.9 nA **(L)** elicited anodal-break responses as well as spontaneous firing during the pulse **(J–K)**; the frequency of firing during the pulse was a function of the degree of hyperpolarization, indicating true pacemaker behavior. (Modified from Pappano and Sperelakis, 1969a; Sperelakis and Lehmkuhl, 1964.)

In some true pacemaker cells, application of a hyperpolarizing current pulse, large enough to shut off the train but too small to elicit anodal-break excitation, turns off the train (Fig. 7A). Subsequent application of a hyperpolarizing pulse sufficiently large to elicit anodal-break excitation (or a brief depolarizing pulse sufficient to trigger a single AP) turns the train back on (Fig. 7B). This suggests that, in this form of automaticity, each AP is responsible for triggering the next one. In some cases, the train turns off and on paroxysmally (Fig. 7C). In such cases, it can be seen that a depolarizing afterpotential or delayed after-depolarization (DAD) follows the hyperpolarizing afterpotential. DADs have been described in adult ventricular and Purkinje cells, and are precipitated by ouabain or other methods of producing Ca^{++} overload of the SR. The DADs give rise to triggered automaticity and consequent ectopic foci for arrhythmias. The DADs are generated by Ca^{++} release from the SR, which activates a Ca^{++}-activated mixed Na-K channel, the transient inward current (I_{ti}) channel.

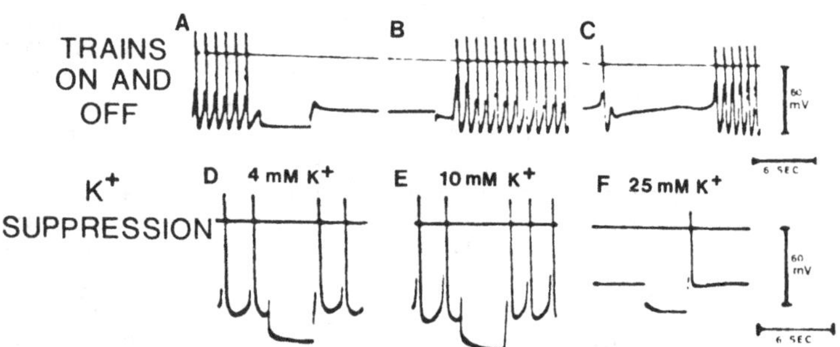

FIG. 7. Impalement of one cell in a monolayer culture with one microelectrode. **A–C:** Trains of spontaneous action potentials turned off **(A)** and on **(B)** by small hyperpolarizing pulses. Automatic firing was stopped by a 1.2 nA pulse too small to cause anodal-break excitation; firing reinstated by a larger pulse (1.8 nA), which produced anodal-break excitation **(B)**. **C:** Spontaneous arrest of firing and resumption of firing in a cell; note depolarizing after-potential following the hyperpolarizing after-potential. **D–F:** Recordings from one true pacemaker cell illustrating suppression of automaticity by elevation of extracellular K^+. In 4 mM **(D)** and 10 mM **(E)** K^+, automaticity was not suppressed, whereas elevation of K^+ to 25 mM caused depolarization and cessation of spontaneous action potential generation, but anodal-break excitation elicited an action potential **(F)**. Hyperpolarizing current pulses of 4.8 nA applied in each panel. (Modified from Lehmkuhl & Sperelakis, 1965; Sperelakis & Lehmkuhl, 1966.)

Automaticity is suppressed by elevation of $[K]_o$ above 15 mM (Fig. 7D-F). The g_K is a function of both P_K and $[K]_o$, and P_K is also increased in elevated $[K]_o$ (Carmeliet *et al.*, 1976a, b; DeHaan, 1970; McDonald and DeHaan, 1973). Distinction between suppression of automaticity and depolarization block of excitability is clearly demonstrated in Fig. 7F, in which automaticity of the same cell is completely suppressed, yet the cell is capable of producing an AP upon anodal-break stimulation.

Automaticity is rapidly induced by 2-5 mM Ba^{++}, presumably by its effect of decreasing P_K (Sperelakis and Lehmkuhl, 1966; Sperelakis*et al*., 1967) and perhaps also by its increasing the inward background depolarizing current through acting as a current carrier. Partial depolarization is produced, and membrane resistivity is greatly increased. If the depolarization produced is too great (beyond the inactivation potential for the slow channels), the cell becomes quiescent but will fire spontaneous APs (and contract concomitantly) during the application of hyperpolarizing current pulses. Sr^{++} (5-10 mM) also induces automaticity in quiescent cells concomitant with hyperpolarization (Sperelakis and Lehmkuhl, 1966). Depolarizing afterpotentials are produced, and the APs ride on top of large sinusoidal-like oscillations. Sr^{++} also hyperpolarizes cells partially depolarized by ouabain or local-anesthetic inhibition of the (Na,K)-ATPase.

Heart cells partially depolarize when $[K]_o$ is lowered from the normal level (e.g., 4 mM) to about 1 mM. The same is true of embryonic chick hearts (Carmeliet*et al*., 1976b) and of cultured embryonic chick heart cells (Pappano and Sperelakis, 1969a). The mechanism for this effect is usually given (Sperelakis, 1979a) as a combination of: (a) inhibition of the electrogenic Na^+ pump potential, and (b) decrease in P_K and g_K as function of low $[K]_o$. Carmeliet*et al*. (1976b) reported that there was substantial dependence of P_K on $[K]_o$ in intact chick embryonic hearts. In contrast, Horres*et al*. (1979), using cultured chick embryonic (11-day-old) heart cells oriented into cylindrical strands of about 60 μm diameter, reported that ^{42}K efflux does not decrease in K^+-free media; they concluded that low $[K]_o$ does not decrease P_K. They suggested that in intact heart preparations, the observed decrease in ^{42}K efflux could result from diffusional limitations in the interstitial space. If so, this would be another example of an advantage of using cultured heart cells to investigate the properties of myocardial cells.

Cultured heart cells exhibit the phenomena of postdrive hyperpolarization and consequent (overdrive) suppression of automaticity (Pelleg*et al*., 1980). Post-drive hyperpolarization is due to stimulation of the electrogenic Na^+ pump potential because of the increased $[Na]_i$ resulting from the increased frequency of APs. The cultured monolayer cells have a lowered (Na,K)-ATPase specific activity (Sperelakis and Lee, 1971).

McLean *et al.* (1975) reported that monolayers prepared from old embryonic hearts had a basal cyclic AMP level about 50% higher than in the control intact hearts, whereas Renaud *et al.* (1978) reported that the basal cyclic AMP level in both monolayers and spherical reaggregates was somewhat lower than in the control hearts. However, a large increase in cyclic AMP level after addition of isoproterenol occurred consistently in both studies, and confirms that functional beta-adrenergic receptors are present in the cultured cells. Clo *et al.* (1980) reported that the cAMP level was influenced by the serum concentration. The basal cyclic AMP level of monolayer cultures of chick embryonic (8-10 days old) heart cells was 20.0 pmol/mg protein when equilibrated in low serum (0.5%) for 24 hr, but the level was lowered to 14.5 pmol/mg after the cells were exposed to 20% horse serum for 15 hr.

It was found that separating cells and culturing them in media containing elevated K^+ (12-60 mM) helped the cells to retain more highly differentiated electrical properties (McLean and Sperelakis, 1974). The RPs were higher (about -60 mV) and automaticity was absent in most cells, indicating that P_K was not as greatly reverted. Although the APs were only moderately faster rising ($+\dot{V}_{max}$ of about 30-40 V/sec), they were completely abolished by TTX (Fig. 5E-F). Thus, it appears that some fast Na^+ channels are retained and the number of slow Na^+ channels is not greatly increased under these conditions. Addition of ATP (5 mM) to the medium seemed to have a slight beneficial effect, especially in combination with elevated K^+, for retention or regain of differentiated membrane properties. Therefore, cell separation and culture in high K^+ media acted to prevent complete reversion to the young embryonic state. It has been reported that TTX sensitivity of cultured heart cells depends on cell associations (Sachs *et al.*, 1973). Single cells in monolayer culture of chick embryo heart (13-20-days-old), dispersed in HMEM containing 0.1% trypsin, showed a RP of -85 mV, $+\dot{V}_{max}$ of about 150 V/s, and TTX sensitivity (Bkaily *et al.*, 1986a).

Chenoval *et al.* (1972) were the first to suggest that fibroblasts may produce changes in the apparent electrical properties of myoblasts in culture. Lompre *et al.* (1979) reported that cells isolated from 6-day-old embryonic chick hearts were automatic, had low maximal diastolic potential ($-E_{max}$), and had low $+\dot{V}_{max}$ of the APs at 4 hr and 24 hr after dissociation. After 48 hr, very few cells remained spontaneously active, and the RP and $+\dot{V}_{max}$ recovered to values close to those of cells in intact hearts. With longer culture periods, many fibroblasts were present, and the myocardial cells now had automaticity, low $+\dot{V}_{max}$, and little or no TTX sensitivity. These reverted parameters were attributed to the proliferation of the fibroblasts, because in pure myoblast cultures, the cells were nonautomatic and developed fast-rising TTX-sensitive APs when stimulated. A possible influence of fibroblasts on the state of differentiation of rat heart cell reaggregates was also suggested by Jourdon and Sperelakis (1980). The technique of differential adhesion for removing fibroblasts was first applied to heart cell cultures by Blondel *et al*. (1971). It was suggested that two cultured heart cells not in physical contact with one another may be synchronized (in beating) by a third large nonmuscle cell (e.g., endothelioid) (Goshima, 1970, 1971; Goshima and Tonomura, 1969; Hyde *et al*., 1969; Mark *et al*., 1967).

The importance of fibroblastic contamination in some types of studies, e.g., ^{45}Ca fluxes, on cultured heart cells (from neonatal rats) is emphasized by the fact that pure fibroblast cultures had similar ^{45}Ca washout curves and kinetics as nearly pure myoblast cultures, and La^{3+} exerted similar effects on the ^{45}Ca uptakes and washouts (Langer and Frank, 1972).

c. Retention of Highly Differentiated Membrane Electrical Properties in Spherical Reaggregate Cultures

Many cells in spherical reaggregates and in cylindrical strands retain fully differentiated electrophysiological properties identical to those of the intact old embryonic hearts in situ (Fig. 5) (McLean and Sperelakis, 1976). Such cells had high RPs of about -80 mV, and pacemaker potentials were absent; this indicates that P_K was high. The plot of E_m versus log $[K]_o$ indicated a P_{Na}/P_K ratio of about 0.02, and a $[K]_i$ of about 130 mM (Fig. 8B). The input resistance averaged approximately 5 MΩ (Fig. 8D). The APs had fast rates of rise (100-200 V/sec), and they were completely blocked by TTX (Fig. 5H). $+\dot{V}_{max}$ diminished as the cells were progressively depolarized by elevation of $[K]_o$, and all excitability was abolished at an E_m of about -50 mV (Fig. 8A). In addition, a short chronaxie of about 0.5 msec was found (Fig. 8C), indicative of high excitability comparable to that of adult cardiac muscle.

Not all cells were highly differentiated. Some cells in the same reaggregate, or cells in another reaggregate in the same culture vessel, had partially or completely reverted. That is, there was a wide spectrum of degrees of reversion. Aging the cultures for several weeks sometimes improved the incidence of highly differentiated cells.

The retention of pharmacological receptors can be assayed by the induction of Ca^{++} slow channels in the sarcolemma. To facilitate the detection of slow channels, the fast Na^+ channels were blocked by using TTX (Fig. 9). Then, addition of agents such as catecholamines and methylxanthines, which rapidly increase the number of slow channels available for activation upon stimulation, cause the appearance of slowly-rising overshooting APs (the "slow APs") (Fig. 9C). The slow APs are accompanied by contractions. Both Ca^{++} and Na^{+} inward currents participate in the slow AP (Shigenobu and Sperelakis, 1972; Schneider and Sperelakis, 1975). The slow APs are blocked by agents that block slow Ca^{++} current, including Mn^{2+}, La^{3+}, and verapamil. The effect of isoproterenol is blocked by beta-adrenergic blocking agents (Fig. 9G-H), thus indicating the presence of functional beta-adrenergic receptors. Angiotensin-II also induced slow APs, and its action is blocked by specific angiotensin receptor blocking agents (Fig. 9K-L) (Freer *et al*., 1976). Finally, histamine also induces slow APs, and its action is blocked by histamine H_2-receptor blocking agents (Fig. 9O-P) (Josephson *et al*., 1976). Thus, the cells possess functional receptors for a variety of agents.

Hermsmeyer and Robinson (1977) reported that ventricular cells, isolated from 13-day-old chick embryos and cultured (monolayers) for 3-5 days in vitro, were highly sensitive to norepinephrine (ED_{50} of 0.80 nM) and acetylcholine (ED_{50} of 0.37 nM) with respect to the frequency of spontaneous beating. Pulse (transient) application of the autonomic agents caused approximately two orders of magnitude more sensitivity compared to a constant concentration.

It was reported that cultured 14-day-old embryonic chick heart cells possess two classes of receptors for insulin (Santora *et al*., 1979). The affinity constants were 5.0 nM^{-1} and 0.026 nM^{-1} for the high and low affinity sites, respectively; the binding capacities were 600 and 9,000 molecules/cell, respectively. Occupancy of the lower affinity class of insulin receptors correlated quantitatively with insulin stimulation of amino acid (2-aminoisobutyric acid) transport in the cells.

Although it was found that, in a given reaggregate, the sarcolemmal electrical properties of most cells were highly differentiated, the ultrastructure of the cells in that same reaggregate exhibited the characteristic appearance of an immature cardiomyoblast. There were only few and incomplete myofibrils, and they were not aligned. The morphology was similar to that of 3-day-old intact hearts. Cultured strand reaggregates described by Lieberman *et al*. (1972b) exhibited a highly differentiated morphology, including aligned myofibrils and well-developed intercalated disks. Jones *et al*. (1976) reported highly differentiated morphology and electrophysiology in multilayer cultures of chick heart cells incubated in media with reduced serum concentrations.

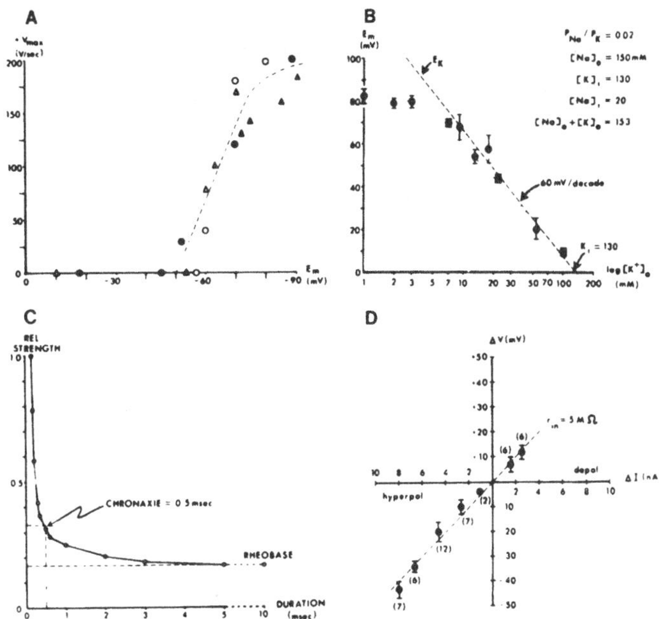

FIG. 8. Summary of some electrophysiological properties of highly differentiated (electrically) cells in spherical reaggregate cultures. **A:** Plot of $+V_{max}$ versus membrane potential (E_m) from aggregates in four separate cultures (different symbols) with complete inactivation of the fast Na^+ channels at about -50 mV. Resting potential varied by elevation of $[K]_o$. Each point represents the mean of four to seven values obtained from different reaggregates within a culture. **B:** Plot of E_m versus the log of external K^+ concentration ($[K]_o$) (equimolar substitution of K^+ for Na^+) extrapolates to an internal $[K]_i$ of 130 mM. The slope of the points in high $[K]_o$ is about 60 mV/decade; the straight line gives the K^+ equilibrium potential (E_K) calculated from the Nernst equation. The dotted line was calculated from the Goldman constant-field equation for a P_{Na}/P_K ratio of 0.02 and for the ion concentrations given in the figure. **C:** Strength-duration curve obtained from an impaled cell having a chronaxie of 0.5 msec. **D:** Voltage/current relation gave an average input resistance of about 5MΩ; data obtained from cells in several different aggregates (150 to 300 μm in diameter). (Modified from McLean and Sperelakis, 1976.)

Evidence was obtained from double microelectrode impalements that cell-to-cell propagation occurs throughout the spherical reaggregates (50-400 μm in diameter). However, no evidence of low-resistance connections between cells could be obtained in reaggregates containing the most highly differentiated cells (McLean and Sperelakis, 1980). In reaggregates containing reverted cells (with pacemaker potentials), moderate to strong electrotonic interaction between the two microelectrodes was obtained in about 50% of the cell pairs. DeHaan and

Fozzard (1975) reported strong electrotonic interactions between all cells in reaggregates, and Lieberman (1973) reported strong interaction in strand preparations. Jongsma and van Rijn (1972) also reported strong electrotonic interaction in monolayers of rat heart cells, whereas Lehmkuhl and Sperelakis (1965) reported weak or absent electrotonic interaction in monolayers of chick heart cells, except in the case where long and thick strands were impaled. Thus, cultured heart cells exhibit different degrees of electrotonic coupling depending on the condition. It has been reported that nonmyocardial cells, such as fibroblasts, may become electrically coupled to myocardial cells in culture (Goshima, 1976).

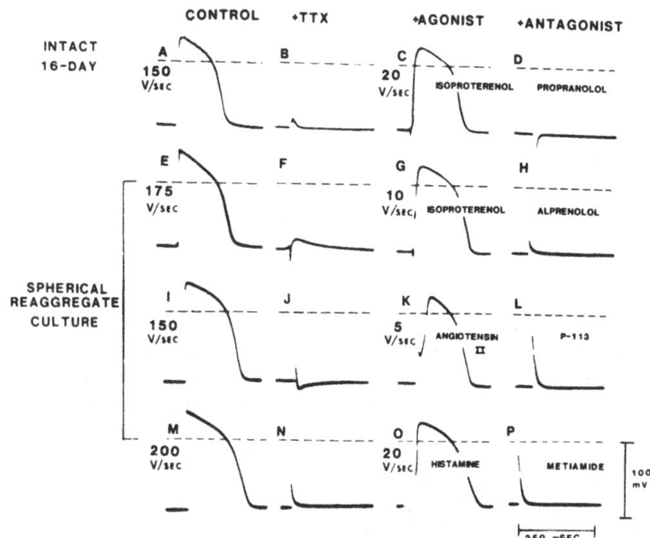

FIG. 9. Demonstration of functional receptors for positive inotropic agents in intact old (16-day) embryonic chick hearts **(A-D)** and in cultured spherical reaggregates of trypsin-dispersed ventricular cells **(E-P)**. Following blockade of the fast Na^+ channels by tetrodotoxin, positive inotropic agents induce slow responses which are blocked by specific antagonists. **A-D:** Records from a ventricular cell in an intact 16-day-old heart. The control, rapidly-rising (150 V/sec) action potential **(A)** was abolished by tetrodotoxin (TTX; 0.1 µg/ml) **(B)**. Addition of isoproterenol (10^{-6}M) induced a slowly-rising (20 V/sec) overshooting electrical response **(C)** which was blocked by propranolol (10^{-5}M) **(D)**. **E-H:** Records from one cell in a cultured spherical reaggregate showing control action potential **(E)** abolished by TTX (0.1 µg/ml) **(F)**; isoproterenol (3×10^{-5}M) induced a slow response **(G)** which was blocked by the specific beta-adrenergic receptor antagonist, alprenolol (10^{-7}M). **I-L:** Records from one cell in another reaggregate showing control action potential **(I)** and its blockade by TTX **(J)**; a slow response was induced by angiotensin II (10^{-6}M) **(K)** and was blocked by its competitive antagonist, P-113 (10^{-5}M) **(L)**. **M-P:** Records from one cell in another reaggregate showing control action potential **(M)** and its blocked by TTX **(N)**; histamine (10^{-5}M) induced a slow response **(O)** which was abolished by the H_2 antagonist, metiamide (10^{-5}M) **(P)**. (Modified from Freer *et al.*, 1976; Josephson *et al*, 1976; Shigenobu and Sperelakis, 1972; Sperelakis, 1978.)

Small spherical reaggregates of cultured chick embryonic heart cells have been successfully used for voltage clamp analysis, including measurement of the fast inward current (Ebihara *et al.*, 1980; Nathan and DeHaan, 1979). Shrier and Clay (1980) used a two-microelectrode voltage clamp to study the pacemaker current (Ip) from cultured reaggregates (ventricular cells) of 7, 12, and 17-day-old chick embryos. The reversal potential for Ip indicated that it was a pure K^+ current. The intensity of Ip decreased during development, paralleling the decline in automaticity.

4. CULTURED NEWBORN RAT HEART CELLS

A number of electrophysiological studies have been made on cultured rat heart cells, both monolayer and reaggregate cultures, prepared from neonatal rats (e.g., 2-6 days old). The rat cultures, like the chick cultures, exhibit different states of electrical differentiation, depending on the preparation methods, on whether the cells are as monolayers or reaggregates, and perhaps on the number of fibroblasts present. For example, some monolayer cultures exhibit fast-rising APs (Athias *et al.*, 1979), whereas others do not (Schanne *et al.*, 1977). Reaggregate cultures exhibited highly differentiated electrical properties similar to those of the intact rat hearts (Jongsma *et al.*, 1978). Jourdon and Sperelakis (1980) found that reaggregate cultures of neonatal rat ventricular cells cultured under standard conditions had a low RP and a low $+\dot{V}_{max}$. TTX only slightly decreased $+\dot{V}_{max}$, whereas verapamil completely blocked the APs. Thus, the inward current seemed to be predominantly a slow current. However, in reaggregates produced by reducing the amount of fibroblasts, by using the differential attachment technique, the AP parameters were similar to intact noncultured hearts. Thus, it appears that removal of fibroblasts allows highly differentiated electrical properties to be maintained in reaggregate cell culture.

McCall (1976a), using confluent monolayer cultures of trypsin-dispersed neonatal rat ventricular cells, found that the contraction frequency and Na^+ influx of the cells were unaffected by TTX but were markedly reduced by verapamil (10^{-8}-10^{-5}M) in a dose-dependent manner. The contraction frequency was not affected by $\Delta [Ca]_o$ between 0.3 and 3.0 mM, but declined as $[Na]_o$ was lowered (to 40 mM), thus showing a relationship between automaticity and Na^+ influx. McCall demonstrated that local anesthetics, such as procainamide, produced a prompt dose-dependent reduction in Na^+ influx and in the frequency of spontaneous contractions. These effects were readily reversible. Since a close correlation was found between the verapamil-sensitive part of the Na^+ influx and contraction frequency, McCall concluded that automaticity was dependent on the verapamil-sensitive Na^+ influx. McCall (1976b) did related studies with quinidine.

An electro-optical method was used to ascertain the beating responses of cultured rat heart cells (monolayers) to halothane (Strong *et al.*, 1975). Halothane (2-5 vol %) exerted negative chronotropic and negative inotropic effects in a dose-dependent manner. Inhibition of glycolysis (by 2-deoxyglucose) increased the sensitivity to halothane. Halothane also was found to decrease the rate of ATP production.

5. PROPERTIES OF Ca^{++} SLOW CHANNELS

Histamine and beta-adrenergic agonists, subsequent to binding to their specific receptors, stimulate adenylate cyclase with resultant elevation of cyclic AMP levels. These positive inotropic agents also induce the slow APs, presumably by making more Ca^{2+} slow channels available in the membrane and/or increases their mean open time. Therefore, it was postulated that a protein constituent of the slow channels is phosphorylated by means of a cyclic AMP-dependent protein kinase (Schneider and Sperelakis, 1975; Shigenobu and Sperelakis, 1972; Sperelakis and Schneider, 1976). The phosphorylated slow channel is presumably the form more available for voltage activation. Cyclic AMP and its dibutyryl derivative also induced the slow APs, but only after a long lag period (15-30 min), as would be expected from slow elevation of intracellular cAMP level. The GTP analog (5'-guanylimidodiphosphate [GPP(NH)P) (10^{-5} - 10^{-3} M), an agent known to activate adenylate cyclase directly, induced slow APs in cultured reaggregates of chick heart cells within 5-20 min (Josephson & Sperelakis, 1978). Prostaglandin $F_{1\alpha}$, which is known to increase cyclic AMP levels in many tissues, induced slow APs in K^+-depolarized cultured chick heart cells within 5 min. Intracellular injection of the catalytic subunit of the cAMP-dependent protein kinase induced and enhanced the slow APs (Bkaily and Sperelakis, 1984) and potentiated I_{si} (Brum *et al.*, 1983). Intracellular injection (by the liposome method) of an inhibitor of the cAMP-dependent protein kinase into cultured chick heart cells depressed and abolished the slow APs (Bkaily and Sperelakis, 1984). The effect of the inhibitor was rapidly reversed by injection of the catalytic subunit of the cAMP-dependent protein kinase. Thus, the intracellular level of cyclic AMP controls the availability of the Ca^{++} slow channels in the myocardial sarcolemma by phosphorylation.

Fluoride ion, in low concentrations (< 1 mM), induces the slow APs and acts as a positive inotropic agent, but does not elevate cyclic AMP (Vogel *et al.*, 1977). Fluoride ion may act by inhibiting the phosphatase that dephosphorylates the slow channel protein, thereby resulting in a larger fraction of phosphorylated channels.

Injection of cyclic GMP into cultured chick heart cells by the liposome method (Bkaily and Sperelakis, 1985) or by pressure injection (Wahler and Sperelakis, 1985) depressed and abolished the slow APs. Nitroprusside (which elevates cyclic GMP by direct stimulation of guanylate cyclase) depressed the slow APs of cultured chick heart cells, and prostaglandin $F_{2\alpha}$, which is known to increase cyclic GMP levels, abolished the naturally-occurring slow APs of cultured chick heart cells (Bkaily and Sperelakis, unpublished observations). Therefore, cyclic GMP regulates the functioning of the myocardial Ca^{2+} slow channels in a manner that is antagonistic to that of cyclic AMP. The effect of cyclic GMP may be mediated through phosphorylation of a protein that regulates the functioning of the slow channels. It is possible that the slow channel protein, or an associated regulatory protein, has a site that when phosphorylated, inhibits the slow channel.

Acetylcholine (ACh) increases g_K, and thereby hyperpolarizes SA nodal cells (therefore depressing automaticity) and shortens the duration of the AP in atrial myocardial cells. This would also tend to suppress slow APs in atrial cells by increasing the overlapping outward K^+ current, and so diminishing the net inward current. ACh also exerts a negative inotropic effect on the ventricular myocardium that has been stimulated by β-adrenergic agonists. That is, activation of the muscarinic receptor in ventricular cells reverses the stimulation of the adenylate cyclase complex produced by β-adrenergic agonists. Activation of the β-adrenergic receptor activates the regulatory (stimulatory) component (N_s or G_s coupling protein) of the adenylate cyclase complex, whereas activation of the muscarinic receptor activates an inhibitory regulatory component of the enzyme (N_i or G_i coupling protein). Josephson and Sperelakis (1982) demonstrated, in voltage clamp experiments on cultured chick ventricular cells, that ACh depresses the inward slow current, I_{si}, but did not increase the outward K^+ current. It is possible that the depression of the potentiated I_{si} is mediated by lowering of the cyclic AMP level (that was elevated by activation of the β-adrenergic receptor).

Inhibitors of calmodulin, namely trifluoperazine (TFP) and calmidazolium, inhibit the slow APs of cultured chick heart cells (Bkaily and Sperelakis, 1986; Bkaily *et al.*, 1984b). Subsequent injection of calmodulin could reverse the inhibition produced by calmidazolium. Therefore, it appears that calmodulin also plays a potentiating role in the regulation of the myocardial Ca^{2+} slow channels. It is possible that a protein associated with the slow channel is phosphorylated by the Ca^{2+}-calmodulin dependent protein kinase, and potentiates the effects of cAMP-dependent phosphorylation.

The induced slow APs are blocked by hypoxia, ischemia, and metabolic poisons, accompanied by a lowering of the cellular ATP level (Schneider and Sperelakis, 1974). Under conditions in which the slow channels are blocked, the fast Na^+ channels are unaffected, thus indicating a differential dependence on metabolic energy. The slow APs blocked by valinomycin are restored by elevation of the glucose concentration (Vogel and Sperelakis, 1978). These findings are consistent with the phosphorylation hypothesis, since ATP is required for phosphorylation. The Ca^{2+} slow channels are blocked at acid pH, nearly complete blockade occurring at pH 6.0, whereas the fast Na^+ channels are not significantly affected at this pH (Vogel and Sperelakis, 1977). In summary, these peculiar properties of the slow channels allow the myocardial cells to exert control over the Ca^{++} influx across the cell membrane and thereby the force of contraction. Such control may serve as a protective mechanism to conserve ATP under adverse conditions of transient regional ischemia (Sperelakis and Schneider, 1976).

The Ca^{2+} slow channels are not blocked by TTX, whereas they are blocked by the Ca^{2+} antagonistic drugs, e.g., verapamil, nifedipine, and diltiazem, and by Mn^{2+} and La^{3+} at low concentrations (Shigenobu *et al*., 1974). The local anesthetics, in contrast, do not distinguish between the fast and slow channels, the dose-response curves for both types of channels being virtually identical (Josephson and Sperelakis, 1976). Ouabain (10^{-6}-10^{-5}M) blocks the slow APs induced in reaggregated cell cultures by isoproterenol (Josephson and Sperelakis, 1977; Schneider and Sperelakis, 1975). This finding could partly account for the toxic effects of high concentrations of cardiac glycosides.

The bee venom toxin apamin, at a very low concentration, produced a transitory increase in $+\dot{V}_{max}$ and overshoot, followed by a progressive decrease of the amplitude and $+\dot{V}_{max}$ of the spontaneous slow Ca^{2+}-dependent APs in cultured heart cell reaggregates (Bkaily *et al*., 1985). Washout of the apamin was difficult, but addition of quinidine during the washout period allowed complete recovery of the slow APs. Use of whole-cell voltage clamp to study the effects of apamin on the slow inward Ca^{2+} current (I_{si}) of single cultured embryonic chick heart cells showed similar results. However, the inhibitory effects of apamin on I_{si} was accompanied by an increase in outward K^+ current. The effects of apamin on I_{si} and I_K were blocked by quinidine. Spider venom was also found to block specifically the Ca^{2+} current in single cultured embryonic chick heart cells (Bkaily *et al*., unpublished observations).

The effects of two antifibrillatory compounds, bretylium tosylate and its pharmacological analog bethanidine sulfate, were studied on single cultured cells of embryonic chick heart using whole-cell voltage clamp technique (Bkaily *et al.*, unpublished observations). Bethanidine and bretylium (10^{-4} M) blocked the K^+ currents. The site of action of these two compounds was extracellular. When injected intracellularly, bretylium and bethanidine blocked the fast Na^+ inward current. Extracellular bretylium or bethanidine did not decrease I_{Na}. Neither bethanidine nor bretylium blocked the Ca^{2+} slow current in these cells.

6. CULTURED VASCULAR SMOOTH MUSCLE CELLS

Cultured reaggregates of vascular smooth muscle (VSM) cells from embryonic chick that contracted spontaneously have been produced (Hermsmeyer *et al.*, 1976; McLean and Sperelakis, 1977). Single cells were trypsin-dispersed from arteries and veins (great vessels near the heart and mesenteric vessels) isolated from 10- to 20-day-old chick embryos, and induced to reaggregate into small spheres (100-400 μm in diameter) either by gyrotation or by plating on cellophane. Many of these spherical reaggregates contracted spontaneously or in response to electrical stimulation during culture periods of up to 6 weeks. When the reaggregates were allowed to adhere to a glass substrate, cells emigrated from the spheres to form aprons of monolayered cells, which continued to contract. Thick and thin myofilaments and characteristic "dense bodies" were observed in a large fraction of the cells examined by electron microscopy. This ultrastructure is rather typical for smooth muscle cells, and the muscle cells can readily be distinguished from fibroblasts (which contain extensive rough ER).

The VSM cells in these primary cultures had RPs of -40 to -60 mV and overshooting APs with maximal rates of rise usually about 4-10 V/sec (McLean and Sperelakis, 1977). Such electrophysiological properties are characteristic of smooth muscle cells. In addition, the APs were insensitive to TTX, as expected since smooth muscle cells do not possess fast Na^+ channels. The APs were preceded by pacemaker potentials, which are responsible for the spontaneous firing.

Cultured monolayers and reaggregates of VSM cells from rat aorta (Harder and Sperelakis, 1979; Zelcer and Sperelakis, 1981) and of smooth muscle cells from guinea pig vas deferens (Chamley and Campbell, 1974; McLean *et al.*, 1979) have also been prepared. Spontaneously contracting monolayer cultures of VSM cells from rat aorta, which were passed several times and maintained for up to 3 months, also have been characterized (Kimes and Brandt, 1976), and spontaneously contracting monolayer cultures of venous smooth muscle have been prepared (S. Chacko, personal communication).

Reaggregates of VSM cells from rabbit aorta fired APs (in presence of TEA) in response to electrical stimulation. The TEA-induced slow APs were sensitive to Ca^{2+} blocking agents (Fig. 10).

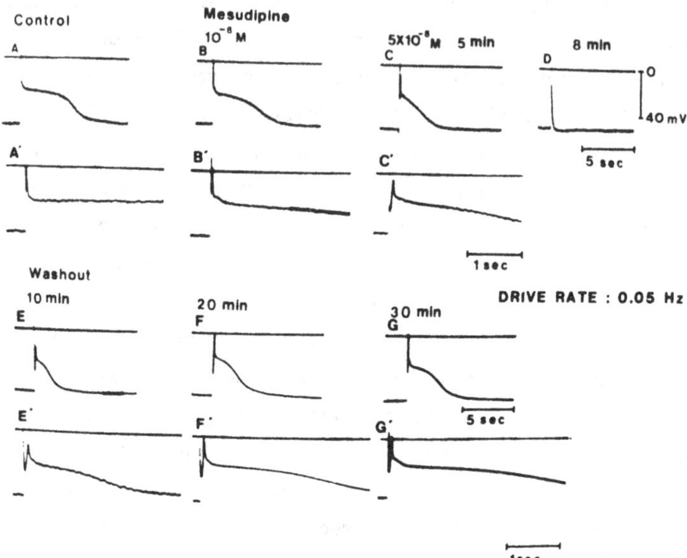

FIG. 10. Effect of mesudipine on cultured VSM cell reaggregates (A-D) and washout (E-G). **A:** Control slow AP in normal Ringer with 10 mM TEA. **B:** Addition of 10^{-8} M mesudipine depressed the AP plateau duration. **C-D:** Elevation of the mesudipine concentration to $5x10^{-8}$ M further depressed (C, 5 min) and completely blocked the slow APs (D, 8 min). **A',B',C':** The same records as A,B,C, respectively, at faster sweep speed to show the spike component of the AP. **E-G:** Washout of the drug restored excitability; degree of recovery depicted at 10 min (E), 20 min (F), and 30 min (G). **E',F',G':** The same records as E,F,G, respectively, at faster sweep speed. Drive rate was 0.05 Hz. All records are from the same impalement. Taken from Molyvdas and Sperelakis, 1984.

Therefore, these results indicate that identifiable VSM cells can be successfully maintained in primary culture as reaggregates for several weeks, and that these cells retain electrical properties similar to those of smooth muscle cells in intact adult blood vessels. Thus, this preparation provides a convenient system for electrophysiological and pharmacological studies of VSM cells. Some obvious advantages of these cultured cells include the relatively easy impalement of the reaggregates by one or two microelectrodes (probably because of the absence of tough connective tissue) and the absence of innervation. One notable disadvantage is the great difficulty in producing cultured mammalian VSM cells capable of contracting.

Since the K^+ conductance in aortic VSM cells is very large, agents that block K^+ channels increase excitability and allow APs to be generated. In patch clamp studies (cell attached configuration), using cultured single cells (monolayer) from rabbit aorta, a high-conductance K^+ channel (90 pS) was found that was sensitive to voltage and $[K]_o$ (Bkaily *et al.*, 1986c). In the whole cell voltage clamp configuration, two different K^+ currents were found in the same cell; the first K^+ current showed mostly outward rectification, whereas the second type did not show any rectification. TEA and Ba^{2+} were found to block both types of I_K. In contrast, bethanidine and apamin blocked type-one K^+ current, but increased type-two K^+ current. Apamin had effects similar to those of bethanidine, but the reversal potential for the bethanidine-stimulated current was different from the apamin-stimulated K^+ current. In addition, the apamin-sensitive I_K was sensitive to calcium blocking agents and to quinidine (Bkaily *et al.*, 1985). The increase of g_K by bethanidine and apamin suggests that these compounds may produce vasodilatation by abbreviating the Ca^{2+} entry (e.g., when g_K is very high, aortic cells do not respond to electrical stimulation).

D. DISCUSSION AND CONCLUSIONS

This chapter attempts to give a brief, and perhaps oversimplified, summary of cultured heart and VSM cells as model systems for studying the physiology, pharmacology, biochemistry, and toxicology of myocardial and VSM cells. The general techniques used are briefly described, and references are given so that the reader can study any topic in greater detail. The types of culture preparations commonly used, such as monolayers and spherical reaggregates, are given, and some of the advantages and disadvantages of working with cultured cells are summarized.

In order to provide the reader with a reference point with which to assess the functional state of the myocardial cells in culture, a brief description is given of some of the key properties of the cells that change during normal development of the heart in situ. It is demonstrated that the cells in standard monolayer cultures (primary) initially isolated from old embryonic hearts usually possess the characteristics of cells in intact young embryonic hearts; that is, they tend to revert back to the young embryonic state ("partial differentiation"). They possess little or no functional fast Na^+ channels and have a low P_K, thus resulting in a low RP, automaticity, and slow-rising TTX-insensitive APs. In contrast, cells in spherical reaggregate cultures often retain (or regain) their initial highly differentiated electrical properties: they have large stable RPs and fast-rising TTX-sensitive APs.

However, some spherical reaggregates contain cells which possess reverted properties, indicating that reaggregation, although an important factor, is not sufficient. Many factors, some unknown, appear to influence the degree of differentiation observed in cultured heart cells. These factors may include: embryonic age of the hearts, possible damage during cell separation, plating density, reaggregation, composition of the culture medium, period in culture, and presence of fibroblasts.

The cultured cells retain their pharmacological receptors. The ultrastructure of the cultured myocardial cells often reverts to the early embryonic state, even in those cases in which the cell membrane remains highly differentiated. On the other hand, cultured heart cells (monolayers) can be made which possess a tight packing of parallel and completed myofibrils.

Immature myocardial cells placed in vitro normally do not continue to differentiate, either electrically or morphologically, although the response to ACh differentiates in organ-cultured young chick hearts. However, addition of an mRNA-enriched extract from adult chicken hearts to the culture medium allows electrical differentiation to proceed after a lag period of several days, in both reaggregate cell cultures prepared from young embryonic hearts and organ-cultured intact young embryonic hearts.

Spontaneously contracting spherical reaggregate cultures of smooth muscle cells can also be made from VSM as well as from other smooth muscles, such as vas deferens. These cultured cells can be relatively easily impaled with one or two microelectrodes, and the cells retain the same electrical properties they possessed in the intact muscle. Single VSM cells in culture are a very suitable preparation for study of single ion channels and toxin or drug action using whole-cell voltage clamp or patch clamp techniques.

In conclusion, cultured heart cells and VSM cells can be used to study and to answer a wide variety of multidisciplinary questions that are difficult or impossible to answer in intact cardiac muscle or intact blood vessels.

ACKNOWLEDGEMENTS

The work on which this chapter is based was supported by grants from the U.S. Public Health Service (HL-11155 and HL-18711) to Dr. Sperelakis and from the FRSQ, CRMC and FQMC to Dr. Bkaily. Dr. Bkaily is a scholar of the Canadian Heart Association. These studies were performed in collaboration with Dr. D. Lehmkuhl, Dr. A.J. Pappano, Dr. M.J. McLean, Dr. J.-F. Renaud, Dr. K. Shigenobu, Dr. A. Pelleg, Dr. S. Vogel, Dr. I. Josephson, and Dr. J. Ousterhout.

REFERENCES

Altschuld, R.A., Gibb, L., and Kruger, F.A. (1980). Calcium tolerance of isolated rat heart cells. Fed. Proc., 39 (No. 6):1787 (Abstr.).

Athias, P., Frelin, C., Groz, B., Dumas, J.P., Klepping, J., and Padieu P. (1979). Myocardial electrophysiology: Intracellular studies on heart cell cultures from newborn rts. Pathologie Biologie (Paris), 27:13-19.

Bernard, C. (1976). Establishment of ionic permeabilities of the myocardial membrane during embryonic development of the rat. In: Development and Physiological Correlates of Cardiac Muscle, edited by M. Lieberman and T. Sano, pp. 169-184, Raven Press, New York.

Berry, M.N., Friend, D.S., and Scheuer, J. (1970). Morphology and metabolism of intact cells isolated from adult rat heart. Circ. Res., 26:679-687.

Bkaily, G., Payet, M.D., Renaud, J.-F., Sauve, R., Bacaner, M.B., and Sperelakis, N. (1986b). Bethanidine blocked I_K, increased I_{Na} and the force of contraction of heart cells. (Submitted).

Bkaily, G., Renaud, J.-F., Payet, M.D., Sauve, R., Bacaner, M.B., and Sperelakis, N. (1986c). Bethanidine, increased one type of potassium current and relaxed aortic vascular smooth muscle cells. (Submitted).

Bkaily, G., Sauve, R., Payet, M.D., and Sperelakis, N. (1986d). A high conductance single K^+ channel in cultured vascular smooth muscle cells of rabbit aorta. Submitted for publication.

Bkaily, G. and Sperelakis, N. (1984). Injection of protein kinase inhibitor into cultured heart cells blocks calcium slow channels. Am. J. Physiol. 246:H630-H634.

Bkaily, G. and Sperelakis, N (1985). Injection of guanosine 5'-cyclic monophosphate into heart cells blocks calcium slow channels. Am. J. Physiol. 248:H745-H749.

Bkaily, G. and Sperelakis, N. (1986). Calmodulin is required for a full activation of the calcium slow channels in heart cells. J. Cyclic Nucleotide and Protein Phos. Res. 11:25-34.

Bkaily, G., Sperelakis, N., and Doane, J. (1984a). A new method for preparation of isolated simple adult myocytes. Am. J. Physiol. 247:H1018-H1026.

Bkaily, G., Sperelakis, N., and Eldefrawi, M. (1984b). Effects of the calmodulin inhibitor, trifluoperazine, on membrane potentials and slow action potentials of cultured heart cells. Eur. J. Pharmacol. 105:23-31.

Bkaily, G., Sperelakis, N., Renaud, J.-F., and Payet, M.D. (1985). Apamin, a highly specific Ca^{2+} blocking agent in heart muscle. Am. J. Physiol. 248:H961-H965.

Blondel, B., Roijen, I., and Cheneval, J.P. (1971). Heart cells in culture: A simple method for increasing the proportion of myoblasts. Experientia, 27:356-358.

Bloom, S., Brady, A.J., and Langer, G.A. (1974). Calcium metabolism and active tension in mechanically disaggregated heart muscle. J. Mol. Cell. Cardiol., 6:137-147.

Bogenmann, E., and Eppenberger, H.M. (1980). DNA-synthesis and polyploidization of chicken heart muscle cells in mass cultures. J. Mol. Cell. Cardiol., 12:17-27.

Brenner, G.M., and Wenzel, D.G. (1972). Carbon monoxide and cultured rat heart cells. I. Inhibition of cell growth and maintenance of beating rate. Toxicol. Appl. Pharmacol., 23:251-262.

Brown, A.M., Lee, K.S., and Powell, T. (1981). Voltage clamp and internal perfusion of single rat heart muscle cells. J. Physiol. 318:455-477.

Brum, G., Flockerzi, V., Hofmann, F., Osterrieder, W., and Trautwein, W. (1983). Injection of catalytic subunit of cAMP-dependent protein kinase into isolated cardiac myocytes. Pflugers Arch. 398:147-154.

Burrows, M.T. (1912). Rhythmische Kontractionen der isolierten Herzmuskelzelle ausserhalb des Organismus. Munchen. Med. Wschr., 59:1473-1475.

Carlson, E.C., Grosso, D.S., Romero, S.A., Frangakis, C.J., Byus, C.V., and Bressler, R. (1978). Ultrastructural studies of metabolically active isolated adult rat heart myocytes. J. Molec. Cell. Cardiol., 10:449-459.

Carmeliet, E., Horres, C.R., Lieberman, M., and Vereecke, J.S. (1976a). Developmental aspects of potassium flux and permeability of the embryonic chick heart. J. Physiol., 254:673-692.

Carmeliet, E., Horres, C.R., Lieberman, M., and Vereecke, J.S. (1976b). Potassium permeability in the embryonic chick heart: Change with age, external K, and valinomycin. In: Developmental and Physiological Correlates of Cardiac Muscle, edited by M. Lieberman and T. Sano, pp. 103-116. Raven Press, New York.

Chamley, J.H. and Campbell, G.R. (1974). Mitosis of contractile smooth muscle cells in tissue culture. Exptl. Cell Res. 84:105-110.

Chenoval, H.P., Hyde, A., Blondel, A., and Girardier, L. (1972). Heart cells in culture: Metabolism, action potential, and transmembrane ionic movements. J. de Physiologie (Paris), 64:413-430.

Clark, M.G., Gannon, B.J., Bodkin, N., Patten, G.S., and Berry, M.N. (1978). An improved procedure for the high-yield prepartion of intact beating heart cells from the adult rat: Biochemical and morphologic study. J. Molec. Cell. Cardiol., 10:1101-1121.

Clo, C., Coccolini, M.N., Tantini, B., and Caldarera, C.M. (1980). Increased sensitivity of heart cell cultures to norepinephrine after exposure to polymine synthesis inhibitors. Life Sciences, 27:67-73.

Crill, W.E., Rumry, R.E., and Woodbury, J.W. (1959). Effects of membrane current on transmembrane potentials of cultured chick embryo heart cells. Am. J. Physiol., 197:733-735.

DeHaan, R.L. (1967). Spontaneous activity of cultured heart cells. In: Factors Influencing Myocardial Contractility, edited by R.D. Tanz, F. Kavaler, and J. Roberts, pp. 217-230. Academic Press, New York.

DeHaan, R.L. (1970). The potassium-sensitivity of isolated embryonic heart cells increases with development. Develop. Biol., 23:226-240.

DeHaan, R.L., and Fozzard, H. (1975). Membrane responses to current pulses in spheroidal aggregates of embryonic heart cells. J. Gen. Physiol., 65:207-222.

DeHaan, R.L., McDonald, T.F., and Sachs, H.G. (1976). Development of tetrodotoxin sensitivity of embryonic chick hearts in vitro. In: Developmental and Physiological Correlates of Cardiac Muscle, edited by M. Lieberman and T. Sano, pp. 155-168. Raven Press, New York.

DeLuca, M.A., Ingwall, J.S., and Bittl, J.A. (1974). Biochemical responses of myocardial cells in culture to oxygen and glucose deprivation. Biochem. Biophys. Res. Commun., 59:749-756.

Dong, L., Sperelakis, N., and Wahler, G. (1986). Development of physiological responses to acetylcholine during organ culture of young embryonic chick hearts. J. Dev. Physiol. 8:000-000.

Earle, W.R., Sanford, K.K., Evans, V.J., Waltz, H.K., and Shannon, J.E., Jr. (1951). The influence of inoculum size on proliferation in tissue culture. J. Natl. Cancer Inst., 12:133-154.

Ebihara, L., Shigeto, N., Lieberman, M., and Johnson, E.A. (1980). The initial inward current in spherical clusters of chick embryonic heart cells. J. Gen. Physiol., 75:437-456.

Enemar, A., Falck, B., and Hakanson, R. (1965). Observations on the appearance of norepinephrine in the sympathetic nervous system of the chick embryo. Dev. Biol., 11:268-283.

Fange, R., Persson, H., and Thesleff, S. (1952). Electrophysiologic and pharmacological observations on trypsin-disintegrated embryonic chick hearts culture in vitro. Acta Physiol. Scand., 38:173-183.

Farmer, B.B., Harris, R.A., Jolly, W.W., Hathaway, D.R., Katzberg, A., Watanabe, A.M., Whitlow, A.L., and Besch, H.R., Jr. (1977). Isolation and characterization of adult rat heart cells. Arch. Biochem. Biophys., 179:545-558.

Farmer, B.B., Mancina, M., Williams, E.S., and Watanabe, A.M. (1983). Isolation of calcium tolerant myocytes from adult rat hearts: Review of the literature and description of a method. Life Sci. 33:1-8.

Freer, R.J., Pappano, A.J., Peach, M.J., Bing, K.T., McLean, M.J., Vogel, S., and Sperelakis, N. (1976). Mechanism of the positive inotropic action of angiotensin II on isolated cardiac muscle. Circ. Res., 39:178-182.

Gershman, H., Weis, G., and Barstow, N. (1979). Dibutyryl cyclic AMP suppresses mobility of embryonic chick heart cells in aggregates. J. Cell Sci., 37:243-255.

Glick, M.R., Burns, S.H., and Reddy, W.J. (1974). Dispersion and isolation of beating cells from adult rat heart. Analyt. Biochem., 61:32-42.

Gordon, H.P., and Brice, M.C. (1974). Intrinsic factors influencing the maintenance of contractile embryonic heart cells in vitro. II. Biochemical analysis of heart muscle conditioned medium. Exptl. Cell Res., 85:311-318.

Goshima, K. (1970). Formation of nexuses and electronic transmission between myocardial and FL cells in monolayer culture. Exp. Cell Res., 63:124-130.

Goshima, K. (1971). Synchronized beating of myocardial cells mediated by FL cells in monolayer culture and its inhibition by trypsin-treated FL cells. Exp. Cell. Res., 65:161-169.

Goshima, K. (1976). Beating of myocardial cells in culture. In: Developmental and Physiological Correlates of Cardiac Muscle, edited by M. Lieberman and T. Sano, pp. 197-216. Raven Press, New York.

Goshima, K., and Tonomura, Y. (1969). Synchronized beating of embryonic mouse myocaridal cells mediated by FL cells in monolayer culture. Exp. Cell Res., 56:387-392.

Gundersen, C.B., Miledi, R., and Parker, I. (1984). Messenger RNA from human brain induces drug- and voltage-operated channels in Xenopus oocytes. Nature 308:421-424.

Halbert, S.P., Bruderer, R., and Lin, T.M. (1971). In vitro organization of dissociated rat cardiac cells into beating three-dimensional structure. J. Exptl. Med., 133:677-695.

Halle, W., and Wollenberger, A. (1971). Myocardial and other muscle cell cultures. In: Methods in Pharmacology, Vol. 1, edited by A. Schwartz, pp. 191-246. Appleton-Century-Crofts, New York.

Harary, J., Fujimoto, A., and Kuramitsu, H. (1964). Enzyme changes in cultured heart cells. Natl. Cancer Inst. Monographs, 13:257-271.

Harder, D.R., and Sperelakis, N. (1979). Action potential generation in reaggregates of rat aortic smooth muscle cells in primary culture. Blood Vessels, 16:186-201.

Hersmeyer, K., DeCino, P., and White, R. (1976). Spontaneous contractions of dispersed vascular muscle in cell culture. In Vitro, 12:628-634.

Hermsmeyer, K., and Robinson, R.B. (1977). High sensitivity of cultured cardiac muscle cells to autonomic agents. Am. J. Physiol., 233:C172-C179.

Hodges, G.M., Livingston, D.C., and Franks, L.M. (1973). The localization of trypsin in cultured mammalian cells. J. Cell Sci., 12:887-897.

Hollenberg, M. (1971). Effect of oxygen on growth of cultured myocardial cells. Circ. Res., 28:148-157.

Horres, C.R., Aiton, J.F., and Lieberman, M. (1979). Potassium permeability of embryonic avian heart cells in tissue culture. Am. J. Physiol., 236:C163-C170.

Hyde, A., Blondel, B., Matter, A., Cheneval, J.P., Filloux, B., Girardier, L. (1969). Homo- and heterocellular junctions in cell cultures: An electrophysiological and morphological study. Progr. Brain Res., 31:283-311.

Ingwall, J.S., DeLuca, M.A., Sybers, H.D., and Wildenthal, K. (1975). Fetal mouse hearts: A model for studying ischemia. Proc. Natl. Acad. Sci. (U.S.A.), 72:2809-2813.

Isenberg, G., and Klockner, U. (1980). Glycocalyx is not required for slow inward calcium current in isolated rat heart myocytes. Nature, 284:358-360.

Isenberg, G. and Klockner, V. (1982). Calcium tolerant ventricular myocytes prepared by preincubation in a "KB Medium". Pfluegers Arch. 335:6-18.

Ishima, Y. (1968). The effect of tetrodotoxin and sodium substitution on the action potential in the course of development of the embryonic chicken heart. Proc. Japan. Acad., 44:170-177.

Jacobson, S.L. (1977). Culture of spontaneously contracting myocardial cells from adult rats. Cell Struct. Funct. 2:1-9.

Jacobson, S.L., Kennedy, C.B., and Mealing, A.R. (1983). Evidence for functional sodium and calcium ion channels in the membrane of cultured cardiomyocytes of adult rat. Can. J. Physiol. Pharmacol. 61:1312-1316.

Jones, J.L., Proskauer, C., Jones, R.E., Paull, W.K., Williams, E.H., and Lepeschkin, E. (1976). Differentiation of myocardial cells in monolayer cell culture. Fed. Proc., 35:319, (Abstract #638).

Jongsma, H.J., Lieberman, M., DeBruijne, J., and Van Ginneken, A.C.G. (1978). Electrophysiological properties of rat heart cells in vitro and in tissue culture. In: Recent Advances in Studies on Cardiac Structure and Metabolism, Vol. II, Heart Function and Metabolism, edited by T. Kobayashi, T. Sano, and N.S. Dhalla, pp. 19-24. University Park Press, Baltimore.

Jongsma, H.J., and van Rijn, H.E. (1972). Electrotonic spread of current in monolayer cultures of neonatal rat heart cells. J. Membr. Biol., 9:341-360.

Josephson, I., Renaud, J.-F., Vogel, S., McLean, M.J., and Sperelakis, N. (1976). Mechanism of the histamine-induced positive inotropic action in cardiac muscle. Europ. J. Pharmacol., 35:393-398.

Josephson, I., and Sperelakis, N. (1976). Local anesthetic blockade of Ca^{++}-mediated action potentials in cardiac muscle. Eur. J. Pharmacol., 40:201-208.

Josephson, I., and Sperelakis, N. (1977). Ouabain blockade of inward slow current in cardiac muscle. J. Mol. Cell. Cardiol., 9:409-418.

Josephson, I., and Sperelakis, N. (1978). 5'-Guanylimidodiphosphate stimulation of slow Ca^{++} current in myocardial cells. J. Mol. Cell. Cardiol., 10:1157-1166.

Josephson, I. and Sperelakis, N. (1982). On the ionic mechanism underlying adrenergic-cholinergic antagonism in ventricular muscle. J. Gen Physiol. 79:69-86.

Jourdon, P., and Sperelakis, N. (1980). Electrical properties of cultured heart cell reaggregates from newborn rat ventricles: Comparison with intact noncultured ventricles. J. Mol. Cell. Cardiol., 12:1441-1458.

Karsten, U., Kossler, A., Janiszewski, E., and Wollenberger, A. (1973). Influence of variations in pericellular oxygen tension on individual cell-growth, muscle-characteristic proteins, and lactate dehydrogenase isoenzyme pattern in cultures of beating rat heart cells. In Vitro, 9:139-146.

Kasten, F.H. (1972). Rat myocardial cells in vitro: Mitosis and differentiated properties. In Vitro, 8:128-149.

Kelly, A.M., and Chacko, S. (1976). Myofibril organization and mitosis in cultured cardiac muscle cells. Develop. Biol., 48:421-430.

Kimes, B.W. and Brandt, B.L. (1976). Characterization of two putative smooth muscle cell lines from rat thoracic aorta. Exptl. Cell Res. 98:349-366.

Kuzuya, F., Naito, M., Asai, K.-I., Shibata, K., and Iwata, Y. (1983). Effect of the calcium blocker, lanthanum, on bovine aortic smooth muscle cells in culture. Artery 12:51-59.

Langer, G.A., and Frank, J.S. (1972). Lanthanum in heart cell culture: Effect on calcium exchange correlated with its localization. J. Cell Biol., 54:441-455.

Langer, G.A., Sato, E., and Seraydarian, M. (1969). Calcium exchange in a single layer of rat cardiac cells studied by direct counting of cellular activity of labeled calcium. Circ. Res., 24:589-597.

LeDouarin, G., Renaud, J.-F., Renaud, D., and Coraboeuf, E. (1974). Influence of insulin on sensitivity to tetrodotoxin of isolated chick embryo heart cells in culture. J. Mol. Cell. Cardiol., 6:523-529.

Lee, K.S., Weeks, T.A., Kao, R.L., Akaike, N., and Brown, A.M. (1979). Sodium current in single heart muscle cells. Nature, 278:269-271.

Lehmkuhl, D. and Sperelakis, N. (1965). Electrotonic spread of current in cultured chick heart cells. J. Cell. Comp. Physiol. 66:119-134.

Lewis, W.H. (1928). Cultivation of embryonic heart muscle. Carnegie Inst. Wash. Contrib. Embryol., No. 90, 18:1-12.

Lieberman, M. (1973). Electrophysiological studies of a synthetic strand of cardiac muscle. Physiologist, 16:551-563.

Lieberman, M., Sawanobori, T., Shigeto, N., and Johnson, E.A. (1972a). Physiologic implications of heart muscle in tissue culture. In: Developmental and Physiological Correlates of Cardiac Muscle, edited by M. Lieberman and T. Sano, pp. 139-154. Raven Press, New York.

Lieberman, M., Roggeveen, A.E., Purdy, J.E., and Johnson, E.A. (1972b). Synthetic strands of cardiac muscle: Growth and physiological implications. Science, 175:909-911.

Lieberman, M., and Sano, T., Eds. (1976). Developmental and Physiological Correlates of Cardiac Muscle, pp. 1-322. Raven Press, New York.

Lompre, A.M., Poggioli, J., and Vassort, G. (1979). Maintenance of fast Na-channels during primary culture of embryonic chick heart cells. J. Molec. Cell. Cardiol., 11:813-825.

Maizel, A., Nicolini, C., and Baserga, R. (1974). Early cardiac morphogenesis is independent of function. Devel. Biol., 27:584-588.

Manasek, F.J., and Monroe, R.G. (1972). Early cardiac morphogenesis is independent of function. Devel. Biol., 27:584-588.

Mark, G.E., Hackney, J.D., and Strasser, F.F. (1967). Morphology and contractile behavior of cultured heart cells, and their response to various oxygen concentration. In: Factors Influencing Myocardial Contractility, edited by R.D. Tanz, F. Kavaler and J. Roberts, pp. 301-315. Academic Press, New York.

Mark, G.E., and Strasser, F.F. (1966). Pacemaker activity and mitosis in cultures of newborn rat heart ventricle cells. Exptl. Cell Res., 44:217-233.

McCall, D. (1976a). Effect of quinidine and temperature on sodium uptake and contraction frequency of cultured rat myocardial cells. Circ. Res., 39:730-735.

McCall, D. (1976b). Effect of verapamil and of extracellular Ca and Na on contraction frequency of cultued heart cells. J. Gen. Physiol., 68:537-549.

McCall, D. (1978). Responses of cultured heart cells to procainamide and ligocaine. Cardiovasc. Res., 12:529-536.

McDonald, T.F., and DeHaan, R.L. (1973). Ion levels and membrane potentials in chick heart tissue and cultured cells. J. Gen. Physiol., 61:89-109.

McDonald, T.F., Sachs, H.G., and DeHaan, R.L. (1972). Development of sensitivity to tetrodotoxin in beating chick embryo hearts, single cells, and aggregates. Science, 176:1248-1250.

McLean, M.J., Lapsley, R.A., Shigenobu, K., Murad, F., and Sperelakis, N. (1975). High cyclic AMP levels in young chick embryonic hearts. Dev. Biol., 42:196-201.

McLean, M.J., Renaud, J.-F., Sperelakis, N., and Niu, M.C. (1976). mRNA induction of fast Na^+ channels in cultured cardiac myoblasts. Science, 191:297-299.

McLean, M.J., and Sperelakis, N. (1974). Rpaid loss of sensitivity to tetrodotoxin by chick ventricular myocardial cells after separation from the heart. Exptl. Cell. Res., 86:351-364.

McLean, M.J., and Sperelakis, N. (1976). Retention of fully differentiated electrophysiological propeties of chick embryonic heart cells in vitro. Dev. Biol., 50:134-141.

McLean, M.J., and Sperelakis, N. (1977). Electrophysiological recordings from spontaneously contracting reaggregates of cultured vascular smooth muscle cells from chick embryos. Exptl. Cell Res., 104:309-318.

McLean, M.J., and Sperelakis, N. (1980). Differences in degree of electrotonic interaction between highly differentiated and reverted cultured heart cell reaggregates. J. Memb. Biol., 57:37-50.

Mettler, F.A., Grundfest, H., Crain, S.M., and Murray, M.R. (1952). Spontaneous electrical activity from tissue cultures. Trans. Am. Neurol. Assoc., 77:52-53.

Mitra, R. and Morad, M. (1985). A uniform enzymatic method for dissociation of myocytes from heart and stomachs of vertebrates. Am. J. Physiol. 249:H1056-H1060.

Molyvdas, P.A. and Sperelakis, N. (1984). Effects of calcium antagonistic drugs on various heart tissues, including blockade of the slow channels and depression of postdrive hyperpolarization. In: Calcium Antagonists: Mechanism of Action on Cardiac Muscle and Vascular Smooth Muscle (N. Sperelakis and J. Calufield, eds.), Martinus Nijhoff Publishers, Boston, pp. 153-178.

Moscona, A. (1961). Rotation mediated histogentic aggregation of dissociated cells. Exptl. Cell Res., 22:455-475.

Nag, A.C., Fischman, D.A., Aumont, M.C., and Zak, R. (1977). Studies of isolated adult rat heart cells: The surface morphology and the influence of extracellular calcium ion concentration on cellular viability. Tissue and Cell, 9:419-436.

Nathan, R.D., and DeHaan, R.L. (1978). In vitro differentiation of a fast Na^+ conductance in embryonic heart cell aggregates. Proc. Natl. Acad. Sci., 75:2776-2780.

Nathan, R.D., and DeHaan, R.L. (1979). Voltage clamp analysis of embryonic heart cell aggregates. J. Gen. Physiol., 73:175-198.

Nathan, R.D., Pooler, J.P., and DeHaan, R.L. (1976). Ultraviolet-induced alterations of beat rate and electrical properties of embryonic chick heart cell aggregates. J. Gen. Physiol. 67:27-44.

Pappano, A.J. (1976). Development of autonomic neuroeffector transmission in the chick embryo heart. In: Developmental and Physiological Correlates of Cardiac Muscle, edited by M. Lieberman and T. Sano, pp. 235-248. Raven Press, New York.

Pappano, A.J., and Sperelakis, N. (1969a). Low K^+ conductance and low resting potentials of isolated single heart cells. Am. J. Physiol., 217:1076-1082.

Pappano, A.J., and Sperelakis, N. (1969b). Spike electrogenesis in cultured heart cells. Am. J. Physiol., 217:615-624.

Pappano, A.J., and Sperelakis, N. (1969c). Spontaneous contractions of cultured heart cells in high K^+ media. Exptl. Cell Res., 54:58-68.

Patlak, J.B. And Ortiz, M. (1985). Slow currents through single sodium channels of the adult rat heart. J. Gen. Physiol. 86:89-104.

Patten, B.M. (1956). The development of the sinoventricular conduction system. U. Mich. Med. Bull., 22:1-21.

Pelleg, A., Vogel, S., Belardinelli, L., and Sperelakis, N. (1980). Overdrive suppression of automaticity in cultured chick myocardial cells. Am. J. Physiol./Heart and Circulatory Physiol., 238:H24-H30.

Phillips, H.J. (1967). Some metabolic changes resulting from treating kidney tissue with trypsin. Can. J. Biochem., 45:1495-1504.

Powell, T., Steen, E.M., Twist, V.W., and Woolf, N. (1978). Surface characteristics of cells isolated from adult rat myocardium. J. Molec. Cell. Cardiol., 10:287-292.

Powell, T., Sturridge, M.S., Suvarna, S.K., Terrar, D.A., and Twist, V.W. (1981). Intact individual heart cells isolated from human ventricular tissue. Br. Med. J. 283:1013-1015.

Powell, T., and Twist, V.W. (1976). A rapid technique for the isolation and purification of adult cardiac muscle cells having respiratory control and a tolerance to calcium. Biochem. Biophys. Res. Commun., 72:327-333.

Pretlow, T.E., Glick, M.R., and Reddy, W.J. (1972). Separation of beating cardiac myocytes from suspensions of heart cells. Am. J. Pathol., 67:215-223.

Rajs, J., Sundberg, M., Sundby, G.-B., Danell, N., Tornling, G., Biberfeld, P., and Jakobsson, S.W. (1978). A rapid method for the isolation of viable cardiac myocytes from adult rat. Exptl. Cell Res., 115:183-189.

Renaud, J.-F. (1973). Etude de l'evolution en culture primaire des cardiomyoblastes embryonnaires de poulet. Thesis, University of Nantes.

Renaud, J.-F., and Sperelakis, N. (1976). Electrophysiological properties of chick embryonic hearts grafted and organ-cultured in vitro. J. Mol. Cell. Cardiol., 8:889-900.

Renaud, J.-F., Sperelakis, N., and LeDouarin, G. (1978). Increase of cyclic AMP levels induced by isoproterenol in cultured and noncultured chick embryonic hearts. J. Molec. Cell. Cardiol., 10:281-286.

Roeske, W.R., Ingwall, J.S., DeLuca, M., and Sybers, H.D. (1977). Thermally induced myocardial preservation and necrosis in deprived fetal mouse hearts. Am. J. Physiol., 232:H275-H282.

Romanoff, A. (1960). The Avian Embryo: Structure and Functional Development, pp. 1-1305. Macmillan, New York.

Rosen, J.S., and Fuhrman, F.A. (1971). Comparison of the effects of atelapidtoxin with those of tetrodotoxin, saxitoxin, and batrachotoxin on beating of cultured heart cells. Toxicology, 9:411-415.

Rosenthal, M.D., and Warshaw, J.B. (1973). Interaction of fatty acid and glucose oxidation by cultured heart cells. J. Cell Biol., 58:332-339.

Rosenquist, G., and DeHaan, R.L. (1966). Migration of precardiac cells in the chick embryo: A radio-autographic study. Contrib. Embryol. Carnegie Inst. Washington, 263:113-121.

Rumyantsev, P.P. (1977). Interrelations of the proliferation and differentiation processes during cardiac myogenesis and regeneration. Int. Rev. Cytol., 51:189-273.

Sachs, H.G., McDonald, R.F., and DeHaan, R.L. (1973). Tetrodotoxin sensitivity of cultured embryonic heart cells depends on cell interactions. J. Cell Biol., 56:255-258.

Santora, A.C., Wheeler, F.B., DeHaan, R.L., and Elsas, L.J. (1979). Relationship of insulin binding to amino acid transport by cultured 14-day embryonic chick heart cells. Endocrinology, 104:1059-1068.

Schanne, D.F. and Bkaily, G. (1981). Explanted cardiac cells: A model to study drug actions? Can. J. Physiol. 59:443-467.

Schanne, O.F., Ruiz-Ceretti, E., Rivard, C., and Chartier, D. (1977). Determinants of electrical activity in clusters of cultured cardiac cells from neonatal rats. J. Mol. Cell. Cardiol., 9:269-283.

Schneider, J.A., and Sperelakis, N. (1974). The demonstration of energy dependence of the isoproterenol-induced transcellular Ca^{++} current in isolated perfused guinea pig hearts: An explanation for mechanical failure of ischemic myocardium. J. Surg. Res., 16:389-403.

Schneider, J.A., and Sperelakis, N. (1975). Slow Ca^{++} and Na^+ current channels induced by isoproterenol and methylxanthines in isolated perfused guinea pig hearts whose fast Na^+ channels are inactivated in elevated K^+. J. Mol. Cell. Cardiol., 7:249-273.

Seraydarian, M.W., Sato, E., and Harary, I. (1970). The effect of inhibitors on the calcium exchange of heart cells in tissue culture. J. Mol. Cell. Cardiol., 1:439-444.

Shigenobu, K., and Sperelakis, N. (1971). Development of sensitivity to tetrodotoxin of chick embryonic hearts with age. J. Mol. Cell. Cardiol., 3:271-286.

Shigenobu, K., and Sperelakis, N. (1972). Ca^{++} current channels induced by catecholamines in chick embryonic hearts whose fast Na^+ channels are blocked by tetrodotoxin. Circ. Res., 31:932-952.

Shigenobu, K., and Sperelakis, N. (1974). Failure of development of fast Na^+ channels during organ culture of young embryonic chick hearts. Devel. Biol., 39:326-330.

Shigenobu, K., and Sperelakis, N. (1975). Prolongation of the action potential plateau of embryonic chick hearts organ-cultured in the presence of cyclic AMP. Jap. J. Pharmacol., 25:481-484.

Shimada, Y., and Fischman, D.A. (1976). Cardiac cell aggregation by scanning electron microscopy. In: Developmental and Physiological Correlates of Cardiac Muscle, edited by M. Lieberman and T. Sano, pp. 81-102. Raven Press, New York.

Shimada, Y., Moscona, A.A., and Fischman, D.A. (1974). Scanning electron microscopy of cell aggregation: Cardiac and mixed retina-cardiac cell suspensions. Devel. Biol., 36:428-446.

Shrier, A., and Clay, J.R. (1980). Pacemaker currents in chick embryonic heart cells change with development. Nature, 283:670-671.

Sperelakis, N. (1972a). Electrical properties of embryonic heart cells. In: Electrical Phenomena in the Heart, edited by W.C. DeMello, pp. 1-61. Academic Press, New York.

Sperelakis, N. (1972b). (Na^+,K^+)-ATPase activity of embryonic chick heart and skeletal muscles as a function of age. Biochem. Biophys. Acta, 266:230-237.

Sperelakis, N. (1978). Cultured heart reaggregate model for studying cardiac toxicology. Proceedings of the Conference on Cardiovascular Toxicology, Environ. Health Perspect. 26:243-267.

Sperelakis, N. (1979a). Origin of the cardiac resting potential. In: Handbook of Physiology, The Cardiovascular System, Vol. I. The Heart, edited by R.M. Berne and N. Sperelakis, pp. 187-267. Am. Physiol. Soc., Bethesda, Maryland.

Sperelakis, N. (1979b). Propagation mechanisms in heart. Ann. Rev. Physiol., 41:441-457.

Sperelakis, N. (1980). Changes in membrane electrical properties during development of the heart. In: The Slow Inward Current and Cardiac Arrhythmias, edited by D.P. Zipes, J.C. Bailey, and V. Elharrar, pp. 221-262. Martinus Nijhoff, The Hague.

Sperelakis, N. (1981). Effects of cardiotoxic agents on the electrical properties of myocardial cells. In: Cardiac Toxicology, Vol. 1, pp. 39-108, edited by T. Balazs, CRC Press, Boca Raton, Florida.

Sperelakis, N. (1982). Cultured heart cell reaggregate model for studying cardiac toxicology. In: Cardiovascular Toxicology, edited by E.W. VanStee, Raven Press, New York.

Sperelakis, N. (1984). Electrophysiological characterization of cultured heart cells and cultured vascular smooth muscle cell preparations for studies on cardiovascular toxicity. In: Proceedings of the 16th Annual Meeting of the Society of Toxicology of Canada, Symposium on Cardiovascular Toxicology. pp 9-47.

Sperelakis, N., Forbes, M.S., Shigenobu, K., and Coburn, S. (1974). Organ-cultured chick embryonic heart cells of various ages. Part II. Ultrastructure. J. Mol. Cell. Cardiol., 6:473-483.

Sperelakis, N., and Lee, E.C. (1971). Characterization of (Na^+,K^+)-ATPase isolated from embryonic chick hearts and cultured chick heart cells. Biochem. Biophys. Acta, 233:562-579.

Sperelakis, N., and Lehmkuhl, D. (1964). Effect of current on transmembrane potentials in cultured chick heart cells. J. Gen. Physiol., 47:895-927.

Sperelakis, N., and Lehmkuhl, D. (1965). Insensitivity of cultured chick heart cells to autonomic agents and to tetrodotoxin. Am. J. Physiol., 209:693-698.

Sperelakis, N., and Lehmkuhl, D. (1966). Ionic interconversion of pacemaker and nonpacemaker cultured chick heart cells. J. Gen. Physiol., 49:867-895.

Sperelakis, N., and Lehmkuhl, D. (1968). Ba^{++} and Sr^{++} reversal of the inhibition produced by ouabain and local anesthetics on membrane potentials of cultured heart cells. Exptl. Cell Res., 49:396-410.

Sperelakis, N., and McLean, M.J. (1978a). Electrical properties of cultured heart cells. In: Recent Advances in Studies on Cardiac Structure and Metabolism Vol. 12, edited by T. Kobayashi, Y. Ito, and G. Rona, pp. 645-666. University Park Press, Baltimore.

Sperelakis, N., and McLean, M.J. (1978b). The electrical properties of embryonic chick cardiac cells. In: Fetal and Newborn Cardiovascular Physiology, Vol. 1, Developmental Aspects, edited by L.D. Longo, pp. 191-236. Garland Press, New York.

Sperelakis, N., and Schneider, J.A. (1976). A metabolic control mechanism for calcium ion inlux that may protect the ventricular myocardial cell. Am. J. Cardiol., 37:1079-1085.

Sperelakis, N., Schneider, J.A., and Harris, E.J. (1967). Decreased K^+ conductance produced by Ba^{++} in frog sartorius fibers. J. Gen. Physiol., 50:1565-1583.

Sperelakis, N., and Shigenobu, K. (1972). Changes in membrane properties of chick embryonic hearts during development. J. Gen. Physiol., 60:430-453.

Sperelakis, N., and Shigenobu, K. (1974). Organ-cultured chick embryonic heart cells of various ages. Part I. Electrophysiology. J. Mol. Cell Cardiol., 6:449-471.

Sperelakis, N., Shigenobu, K., and McLean, M.J. (1976). Membrane cation channels: Changes in developing hearts, in cell culture, and in organ culture. In: Developmental and Physiological Correlates of Cardiac Muscle, edited by M. Lieberman and T. Sano, pp. 209-234, Raven Press, New York.

Steinberg, M.S., Armstrong, P.B., and Granger, R.E. (1973). On the recovery of adhesiveness by trypsin-dissociated cells. J. Memb. Biol., 13:97-128.

Strong, L., Hartzell, C.R., and McCarl, R.L. (1975). Halothane and the beating response and ATP turnover rate of heart cells in tissue culture. Anesthesiology, 42:123-132.

Suignard, G. (1979). Metabolisme poteique et sensibilite a la tetrodotoxine des cardiomyblastes cultives in vitro: Infouence de l'insuline. J. de Physiol. (Paris) 75:733-740.

Trowell, O.A. (1959). The culture of mature organs in a synthetic medium. Exptl. Cell Res., 16:118-147.

Vahouny, G.V., Starkweather, R., and Davis, C. (1970). Preparation of beating heart cells from adult rats. Science, 167:1616-1618.

Vahouny, G.V., Wei, R.W., Tamboli, A., and Albert, E.N. (1979). Adult canine myocytes: Isolation, morphology, and biochemical characteristics. J. Molec. Cell. Cardiol., 11:339-357.

Vogel, S., and Sperelakis, N. (1977). Blockade of myocardial slow inward current at low pH. Am. J. Physiol., 233:C99-C103.

Vogel, S., and Sperelakis, N. (1978). Valinomycin blockade of myocardial slow channels is reversed by high glucose. Am. J. Physiol., 234:H46-H51.

Vogel, S., Sperelakis, N., Josephson, I., and Brooker, G. (1977). Fluoride stimulation of slow Ca^{++} current in cardiac muscle. J. Mol. Cell. Cardiol., 9:461-475.

Wahler, G.M. and Sperelakis N. (1985). Intracellular injection of cyclic GMP depresses cardiac slow action potentials. J. Cyclic Nucleo. & Prot. Phos. Res. 10:83-95.

Warshaw, J.B., and Rosenthal, M.D. (1972). Changes in glucose oxidation during growth of embryonic heart cells in culture. J. Cell Biol., 52:283-291.

Wenzel, D.G., Wheatley, J.W., and Byrd, G.D. (1970). Effect of nicotine on cultured rat heart cells. Toxicol. Appl. Pharmacol., 17:774-785.

Wildenthal, K. (1971a). Long-term maintenance of spontaneously beating mouse hearts in organ culture. J. Appl. Physiol., 30:153-157.

Wildenthal, K. (1971b). Responses to cardioactive drugs of fetal mouse hearts maintained in organ culture. Am. J. Physiol., 221:238-241.

Wildenthal, K. (1973). Studies of fetal moust hearts in organ culture: Metabolic requirements for prolonged function in vitro and the influence of cardiac maturation on substrate utilization. J. Mol. Cell. Cardiol., 5:87-99.

Zelcer, E. and Sperelakis, N. (1981). Angiotensin induction of active responses in cultured reaggregates of rat aortic smooth muscle cells. Blood Vessels 18:263-279.

USE OF THE ISOLATED RAT HEART FOR THE DETECTION OF CARDIOTOXIC AGENTS.

A. Cockburn
Honeypot Lane, Stock, Nr. Ingatestone,
Essex, CM4 9PE

1 INTRODUCTION

The toxicological development and therapeutic utility of a number of important drugs is frequently limited by their potential for cardiotoxicity. Such side effects may develop acutely or chronically and can range from minimal electrocardiographic (ECG) changes to permanent cardiac damage, or even sudden death (Marshall and Lewis, 1973). Inevitably much time and effort has been spent investigating ways to improve the predictability of myocardial involvement. This has resulted in the proliferation of often complex animal models (Rona, 1967; Balazs et al, 1969; Osborne and Dent, 1973; Chapple et al, 1976), and highly sophisticated schemes of clinical monitoring (Lahtinen et al, 1982). The detection of cardiotoxicity nevertheless remains complicated by the large functional reserve of the heart which can mask mechanical impairment, its ability to develop resistance to further damage after certain insults (Joseph et al, 1983) and also to repair foci of myocarditis (Lehr, 1972; Bach and Cockburn, in press).

Damage to the heart generally occurs either as a consequence of direct cellular toxicity or due to remote effects on the neural, humoral and haemodynamic influences which normally control it. The latter indirect toxicity is frequently seen as a result of exaggerated pharmacological response at the high dose levels commonly used in routine toxicological studies (Herman et al, 1979).

While the toxic end point may be the same it is important to appreciate and differentiate these mechanisms when assessing the significance of cardiotoxicity. Unfortunately, the intact animal seldom provides a suitable model in which to unravel mechanisms of target organ toxicity due to the interaction of numerous organs and systems. This is especially true in the case of the heart, and was central to the decision to develop the isolated organ as a model for the detection of directly acting cardiotoxins. These can affect the functioning and structure of the heart muscle, its innervation and conducting pathways, its vasculature, the valves or any combination of these.

Classically the isolated perfused heart has been employed to investigate the physiology, pharmacology and biochemistry of the organ (Ross, 1972). The original method of Langendorff (1895) has been widely used and despite numerous modifications, survives because of its technical simplicity and robustness. The modified procedure, which utilises the rat heart, not only distinguishes functional from structural change but, used in conjunction with *in vivo* toxicological protocols, can also differentiate direct from indirect cardiotoxins. The following chapter provides details of the technique and the methods used for its validation including responses to the reference cardiotoxin isoprenaline and to ischaemia. Beyond the scope of this Chapter, the model has also been used to evaluate the cardiotoxic potential of a variety of other drugs, each of which has given a clearcut and characteristic response. Considerable potential exists for the system for closely controlled screening studies (Breed et al, 1979; Lee et al, 1985), interventions aimed at mitigating cardiotoxicity (Yates et al, 1980) and the study of toxic mechanisms (Singal et al, 1981).

2 PRACTICAL ASPECTS

The apparatus described is relatively inexpensive but supports the isolated heart in good physiological condition for a minimum of 3 hours. Many modifications have been made to the basic Langendorff apparatus and as these are fundamental to the stability and reproducibility of the model, the rationale for their incorporation is discussed. The rat heart was chosen for perfusion not only for practical reasons but also because of the extensive use of the rat in toxicology and hence the ready ability to make *in vitro*/*in vivo* comparisons.

2.1 Perfusion apparatus

The modified Langendorff system described, permits excellent perfusion of the coronary vessels and hence myocardium with the drug under investigation (Figure 1).

Fig. 1. Basis of 'Langendorff' perfusion of heart. The aortic valve closes when pressure is exerted from above (reverse flow). Medium must pass into the coronary vessels to supply heart muscle, since it cannot now enter the left ventricle. The ventricle can empty only when intraventricular pressure rises above that in the aorta, to open the aortic valve. (From Ross, B.D., Perfusion Techniques in Biochemistry, 1972, Clarendon Press).

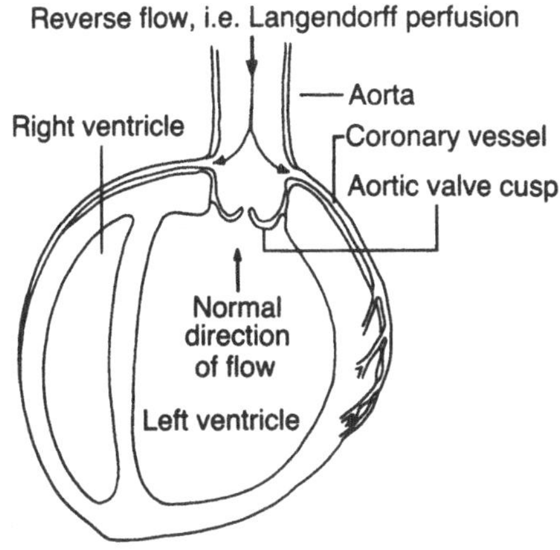

A non-recirculating system was employed (Figure 2) the essential components of which comprise an oxygenator, a constant flow peristaltic pump (Watson Marlow, MHRE22, UK), an in-line 0.45 µm pore cellulose acetate filter (Millipore (UK) Ltd.), a warming coil (Aimer Scientific Supplies, UK), and a heart chamber. Both the warming coil and perfusion chamber are water jacketed and connected via a circulating pump (Charles Austin Pumps, UK), to a water bath (Grant Camlab Ltd, UK), which maintains the temperature of the perfusate as it enters the heart at 36.5°C $\pm$ 0.5°C. The cardiac chamber is essential to maintain adequate warmth and humidity about the heart and has a short vertical port on one side to allow entry of a ventricular epicardial electrode which, apart from steadying the heart, serves with the aortic electrode for the recording of bipolar surface ECG. A small outlet in the base of the chamber enables the collection of coronary effluent for analysis.

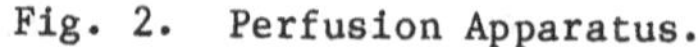

Fig. 2. Perfusion Apparatus.

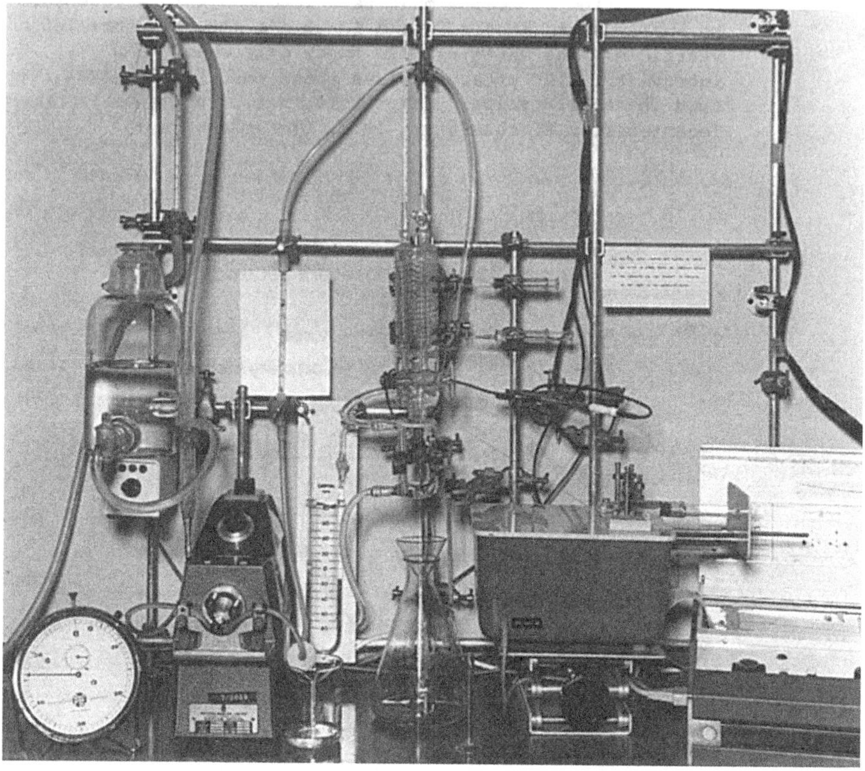

In order to prevent bubbles entering the heart, which rapidly prove fatal, two cannulae, each connected to a disposable syringe, are employed to aspirate coalesced gas bubbles from the descending portion of the warming coil immediately above the heart. A third cannula, situated immediately adjacent to the aortic cannula is used for the timed infusion of test substances. The oxygenator consists of a vessel containing perfusate into which 95% O_2:5% CO_2 is continuously bubbled at 700 ml/min through a sealed polythene tube (8 mm OD) perforated with a 21 gauge needle. The oxygen tension at the outlet of the oxygenator is about 450 mm/Hg. A variable flow peristaltic pump enables rapid alteration of flow rate, normally maintained at 4.8 ml/min. The warming coil is that described by J.B.E. Baker (1951) and incorporates an overflow bubble trap, a point at which temperature can be measured, and a side arm for the connection of a manometer to measure perfusion pressure.

2.2 Perfusion medium

Modified Krebs-Henseleit bicarbonate buffer medium, pH 7.4, (Krebs and Henseleit, 1932) containing 1300 units/l Heparin BP is used as perfusate. Twenty mg/litre ascorbic acid is added as an anti-oxidant in order to protect test substances. During preparation of the perfusion medium, the calcium and phosphate salts are not brought together in less than the final volume to prevent precipitation (Umbreit et al, 1964). The osmolality, determined by freezing point depression, is 304 mosmol/l and the oxygen tension of the perfusate on entry to the heart ranges between 200 and 350 mm/Hg.

2.3 Animals and isolation of the heart

Male Sprague Dawley rats, weighing between 200 g and 300 g and fed a normal maintenance diet and tap water *ad libitum*, are used.

To isolate the heart the donor rat is lightly anaesthetised with ether and killed by cervical dislocation. The abdominal cavity is opened at the xiphisternum and the diaphragm transected. The rib cage is gently raised and incised along each side in turn. The anterior wall of the chest is then folded back. Pericardial and any filamentous tissues are removed from the heart. The organ is lifted upwards and forwards with the fingers, and the great vessels cut with blunt tipped curved scissors approximately 5 mm distal to the base, leaving all pulmonary and most thymic tissue behind. The heart is then carefully blotted dry and any remaining connective or thymic tissue rapidly pulled away. Next the heart is transferred immediately to a pre-weighed petri-dish containing 0.9% heparinised saline (1300 units/l) chilled to +4°C. The whole procedure should not exceed 30 seconds.

2.4 Perfusion technique

In all experiments the flow of warmed oxygenated perfusion fluid through the apparatus is established some 20 minutes before excision and preparation of the heart. The aorta of the freshly isolated heart is then slipped onto the polythene perfusion cannula (1.34 mm OD), using fine curved forceps, and is held in place by the upper margin of the aorta using a modified No. 4 Blalock clamp. The latter also serves as the aortic electrode for recording epicardial ECGs. The aorta is then ligatured in place, ensuring that the tip of the cannula is above the aortic valves. The arrested heart resumes spontaneous contraction within 10 seconds.

A 30 minute period is then allowed for the heart to stabilise. During the first 5-15 minutes the beat is often irregular but subsequently normalises with a rate of 180-260 beats/min. Drug infusions are then carried out at 0.08 ml/min by means of a syringe pump over the following 100 minutes after which the heart is allowed a period of 30 minutes during which to recover. At the end of each experiment, the heart is removed, blotted dry with filter paper and weighed before fixation in 10% buffered formol saline to facilitate subsequent processing for histopathological examination, if required.

It is recommended that all experiments are carried out at the same time each day to minimise cardiac rhythmical changes. Tharp and Folk (1965) have shown that isolated rat hearts display a distinct circadian rhythm with elevated rates each evening and lower rates during the day.

2.5 Measurements of viability and stability

A number of critical parameters are measured on the freshly isolated heart to monitor the physiological viability, stability and response of the preparation. Scope exists for many other parameters to be included but the basic model was established with the minimum number for diagnostic speed and simplicity. Any hearts not responding within normal limits during the initial 30 minutes stabilisation period are rejected.

Enzyme efflux. One to 2 ml samples of coronary effluent are collected serially in plastic vials and stored at +4°C until the end of each experiment. Samples are collected at the following times after mounting the heart:-

Stabilisation period: + 1, 5, 15, 30 minutes
Infusion period : + 35, 45, 60, 80, 105, 130 minutes
Recovery period : + 145, + 160 minutes

Creatine kinase activity (CK) - (ATP:creatine phosphotransferase EC 2.7.3.2.) is measured as an index of structural damage. Activity is expressed in I.U./l at 30°C: the limit of sensitivity in the assay used, was 8 I.U./l.

Epicardial ECG and heart rate (HR) (Figure 3). Surface ECGs are differentially recorded at a sensitivity of 0.25 mV/mm, between the aortic stump and ventricular apex, using either lead III or the augmented lead AVL conformation.

Fig. 3. Photograph of the purfused heart showing location of ECG electrodes, aortic reservoir and warming jacket. (LA, LL, RL, AVL - standard ECG leads).

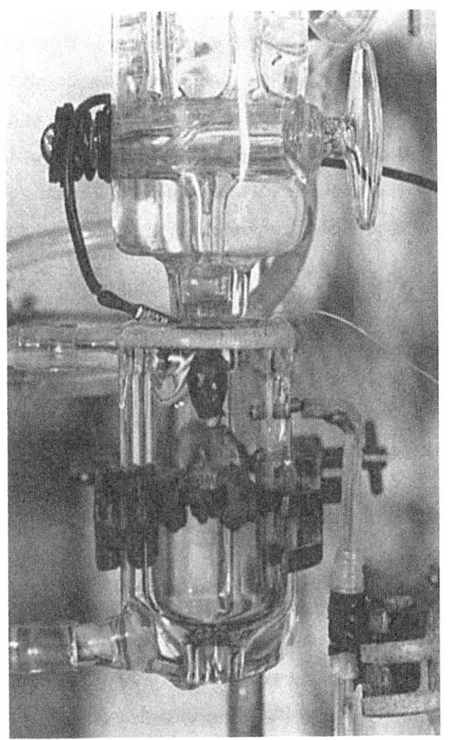

Heart rate is calculated directly from ECG paper traces recorded at 25 mm/sec.

Coronary flow rate. The flow rate of 4.8 ml/min is not altered after the stabilisation period and always remains between a maximum and minimum of 5.2 ml/min and 4.4 ml/min, respectively.

Perfusion pressure (PP). Perfusion pressure is measured using a mercury manometer connected to a side arm on the aortic cannula. This provides a sensitive index of coronary resistance.

Oedema formation. Colloid is not included in the perfusion fluid as it results in frothing during oxygenation which leads to coronary embolisation. In consequence, varying degrees of cardiac swelling occur in all studies. This is quantified by recording heart wet weight before and after each experiment.

2.6 Control data (Table 1)

After completion of the 30 minute 'stabilisation' period, perfusion fluid is infused at 0.08 ml/min over the next 100 minutes followed by a 30 minute 'recovery' period. Under these conditions, each of the parameters of viability and stability remain steady and enzyme release barely detectable for periods of up to 3 hours. The initial reduction in CK release is in accord with the results obtained by de Leiris et al, (1969) for lactate dehydrogenase and probably represents 'washing-out' of enzyme containing plasma due to coronary perfusion. Following isolation of the heart, early ECGs show marked ST segment elevation indicating hypoxia. On continued perfusion the degree of ST segment elevation decreases. Apart from the lower heart rate, bipolar ECGs from the isolated heart show striking similarities to those obtained *in vivo* from untreated male rats. Increases in the wet weight of the heart of 12-34% occur typically during the experimental period due to oedema formation.

3 EXPERIMENTAL EXAMPLES

The model was initially validated in terms of diagnostic potential, by assessing response to three diverse insults. Isoprenaline hydrochloride (ISO) was chosen as a well documented cardiotoxic agent, ischaemia to mimic coronary thrombosis, and physical injury, by lancing the apex of the heart, to cause cell disruption, e.g. as in endomyocardial biopsy or cardiac catheterisation.

3.1 Isoprenaline (Figure 4)

Infusions of 1 to 100 mg ISO were approximately equivalent to concentrations of 2 to 200 µg/ml. Higher doses caused profound arrhythmias. It has been estimated that 100 mg ISO infused into the isolated heart at the rate of 1 mg/min is equivalent to the maximum cardiac burden following 25 mg/kg by the subcutaneous route to the intact rat.

TABLE 1

CONTROL VALUES FOR INDICES OF VIABILITY AND STABILITY WITH THE ISOLATED PERFUSED RAT HEART

INDICES	PERFUSION TIME (min)											
	STABILISATION				INFUSION						RECOVERY	
	1	5	15	30	5	15	30	50	75	100	15	30
CK Release I.U./1 at 30°C	33.25 ±13.71	20.0 ±7.04	21.25 ±8.40	12.50 ±5.84	<8.0 -	<8.0 -	<8.0 -	<8.0 -	<8.0 -	<8.0 -	<8.0 -	<8.0 -
HR Beats/min	206.50 ±136.5	140.67 ±30.78	165.67 ±28.90	230.0 ±15.28	235.67 ±20.22	257.67 ±32.64	243.0 ±43.0	255.0 ±28.43	261.0 ±31.21	260.0 ±30.55	249.33 ±24.91	245.0 ±25.98
PP mm/Hg	*	12.75 ±1.11	13.25 ±0.75	13.0 ±0.71	13.0 ±0.71	13.0 ±0.71	12.75 ±0.85	12.75 ±0.85	13.0 ±0.71	12.5 ±1.04	12.5 ±1.04	12.75 ±1.11
ECG at 25 mm/sec AVL	at 30 min			HR 200	at 100 min				HR 200		at 30 min	HR 200
ECG from Untreated S.D. rat, Lead III at 50 mm/sec												HR 480

Each point represents the mean ± standard error of the mean of measurements from 4 hearts. *Data not presented.

Fig. 4. Mean CK release, heart rate and perfusion before, during and after infusion of 1 mg ISO, (▲); 50 mg ISO, (△); 100 mg ISO, (□), into isolated perfused rat hears, compared with control, (●). Each point is the mean ± S.E.M. of measurements from 4 hearts.

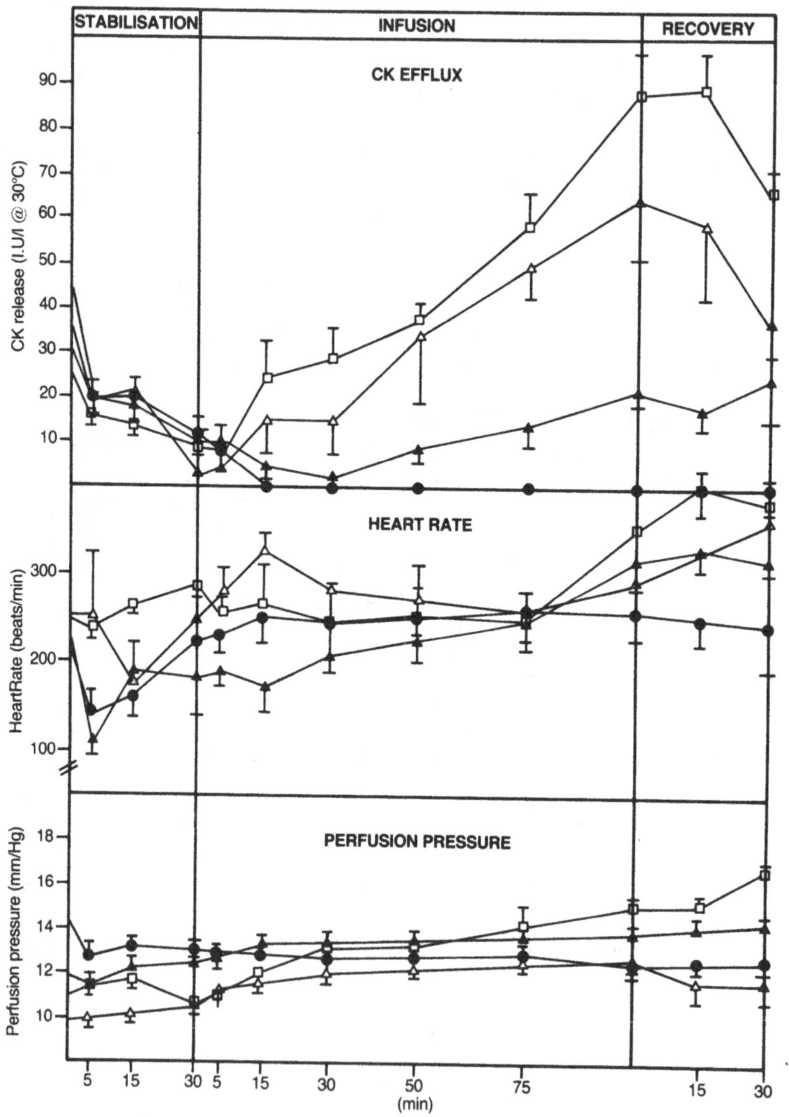

CK release. An increase in CK release occurred at each infusion level and with the exception of the lowest dose level began within 5 and 15 minutes of the start of the infusion and became maximal at the end of the period. At 50 and 100 mg enzyme release decreased subsequently during the recovery phase. With a 1 mg dose of ISO, enzyme efflux did not begin for 30 minutes following the start of the infusion and did not reduce during the recovery period.

Heart rate. Effects on heart rate were variable and not dose related. Close inspection of the data from individual experiments where heart rate was monitored continuously at intervals during the first 5 minutes of infusion, showed that a transient period of tachycardia occurred within half a minute of the commencement of the ISO infusion. This lasted for no more than 4 minutes and is in agreement with the findings of Brus and Drzewiecki (1973). At the highest infusion level, an initial mean decrease in heart rate occurred with subsequently stabilised close to control levels.

Perfusion pressure. An increase of 2 to 4 mm/Hg in perfusion pressure took place over the 100 minute ISO infusion period.

Electrocardiograms. Within the first 30 seconds of infusion, ISO induced an approximately dose related elevation in the ST segment of each ECG complex, in conjunction with increases in T-wave amplitude. These changes were associated with a transient but marked increase in heart rate. As this tachycardia diminished, a notable reduction in the ST segment elevation occurred over the following 30 minutes, despite a renewed though gradual increase in heart rate. Subsequently, the ST segment again became progressively more elevated with time. It is probable that the increases in R wave amplitude reflect the direct positive inotropic effects of ISO. However, at dose levels of 50 mg and above marked arrhythmia occurred within 15 minutes of the commencement of infusion. The changes, clearly demonstrated in Figure 5 show that fine ventricular fibrillation, observed 15 minutes after the commencement of infusion, progressed to ventricular fibrillation, after 50 minutes. This serious arrhythmia led to ventricular flutter during the recovery period.

Fig. 5. Bipolar ECG traces and heart rate (HR) recorded from the isolated perfused rat heart perfused with 100 mg ISO over 100 minutes. (Recorded at 25 mm/sec on AVL)

TIME (min)	ECG PROFILE	HR	TIME (min)	ECG PROFILE	HR
Stabilis-ation	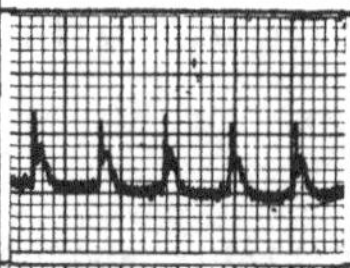	260	+50	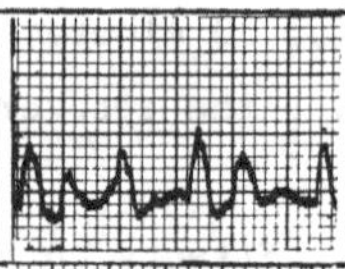	*
Infusion +5	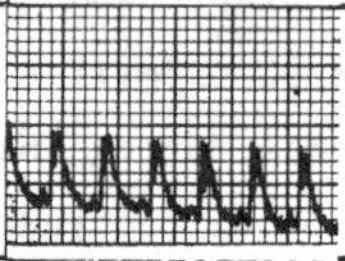	280	+75	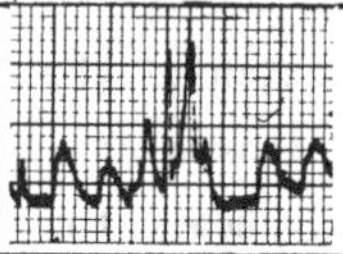	*
+15	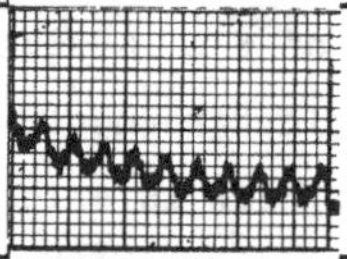	+	+100	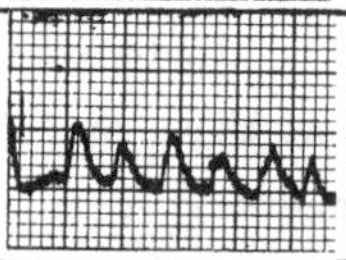	*
+30	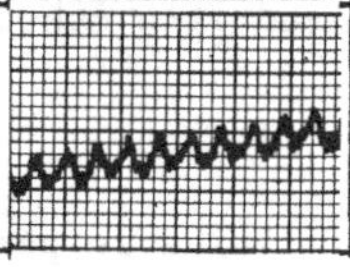	+	Recovery +30	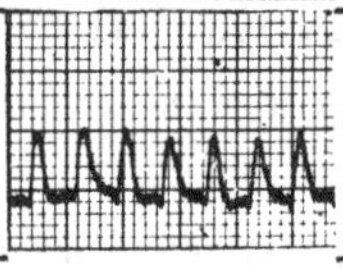	**

+ = FINE VENTRICULAR FIBRILLATION
* = VENTRICULAR FIBRILLATION
** = VENTRICULAR FLUTTER

Occurrence of cardiac swelling. Despite considerable inter-heart variation in the degree of 'oedema' formation for a given dosage, the group mean values for increases in heart wet weight at the end of the experiments were relatively consistent: Control 20.7%, 1 mg ISO 25.4%, 50 mg ISO 22.2% and 100 mg ISO 21.8%.

3.2 Response to ischaemia induced by gaseous emboli

Ischaemia has been defined as that reduction in flow which provides an oxygen supply insufficient to meet oxygen demand (Jennings et al, 1975). In the heart, such a situation commonly results in the formation of an infarct zone following coronary occlusion by a thrombus. Because of the good collateral circulation, an infarct is generally restricted to an area of myocardium adjacent to the occluded coronary vessel, and the resulting ischaemia is, therefore, described as regional.

In the isolated heart, homogenous or whole heart ischaemia can be induced by reducing flow rate to the point at which an imbalance exists between oxygen supply and demand; moreover - this can be graded and reproduced under controlled conditions. Alternatively, large areas of the heart can be rendered ischaemic by carefully ligaturing the left or right coronary vessels. Neither technique, however, mimics the regional ischaemia resulting from myocardial infarction in intact animals or man. Furthermore, both procedures have inherent disadvantages. Thus to create whole heart ischaemia in the isolated heart model, it would be necessary to reduce or stop perfusion. With the alternative manipulation of coronary ligation, myocardial damage and hence enzyme leakage would occur.

In consequence, to simulate the regional ischaemia resulting from coronary thrombosis a small bubble of air is introduced into the aortic cannula which in turn enters the coronary vasculature and leads to embolisation (figure 6).

<u>Perfusion pressure</u>. Perfusion pressure increased immediately air entered the heart via the aortic cannula. This rise in pressure signified an increase in coronary resistance and was taken as evidence of coronary occlusion by gaseous emboli.

Fig. 6. Typical examples of the response of the isolated perfused rat heart to air emboli in terms of increased perfusion pressure (▲) and CK (●) release.

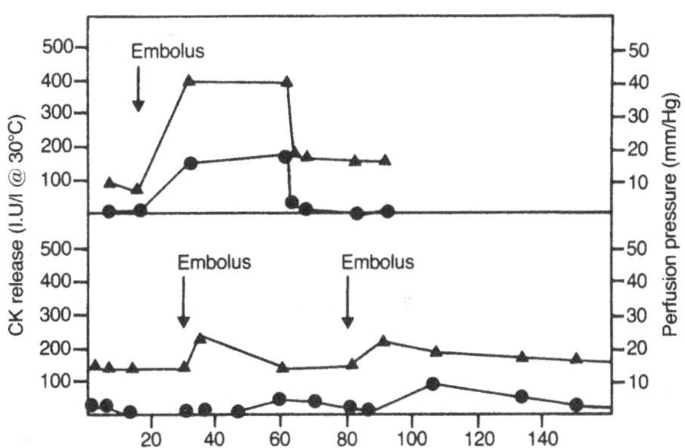

Enzyme release. Increased myocardial CK release occurred within 5 to 15 minutes of embolisation and was considered to be due to ischaemic damage.

Subsequently, the degree and profile of enzyme release was broadly related to the extent of coronary occlusion as demonstrated by changes in perfusion pressure. A reduction in perfusion pressure was followed by a decrease in enzyme release within 10 minutes. No significant increase in CK release occurred at perfusion pressures of 20 mm/Hg or less.

Heart rate. There was no clearcut pattern of heart rate response to increases in perfusion pressure. In three experiments, the rate decreased as perfusion pressure increased while in two experiments heart rate increased.

Electrocardiograms. In three of the five experiments, marked conduction disturbance arrhythmias occurred. The changes included paired beating and ventricular fibrillation, the latter occurring within 6 minutes of the onset of ischaemia. No ECG waveform changes were seen in the remaining two hearts.

Occurrence of 'oedema'. A mean increase of 11% in heart wet weight was obtained albeit with considerable intragroup variation. The fact that this increase was at the bottom of the range for control hearts indicated a possible difference, i.e. less oedema occurred than 'normal'. This may well have been accounted for by the poorer perfusion of ischaemic tissue due to occluding coronary emboli and hence lower overall fluid retention.

3.3 Response to Physical Damage

Immediately after the 30 minute recovery period, each heart was lanced once through the ventricular apex with a 21 gauge needle. The perfusate was then collected for up to 5 minutes and subsequently assayed for CK activity. The objectives were two-fold. Firstly to determine whether CK, as a biochemical marker, increased in the perfusate following severe physical injury, as might be expected, and secondly, if this was the case, to use this response to validate grossly the analytical aspect of each experiment. In this context it is relevant that a characteristic enzymatic response is seen clinically following cardiac catheterisation (Lucena et al, 1974) and endomyocardial biopsy (Harmjanz, 1975).

Time Course of Enzyme Release (Figure 7). During the first minute, the enzyme activity was 20 to 30-fold greater than control values. Within 5 minutes the values fell to 5 to 10 times control. In studies where 2 adjacent areas of the ventricular apex were lanced, approximately twice the amount of enzyme leakage occurred in the first minute following injury compared with that following single insult.

Fig. 7. Mean CK release after lancing the ventricular apex once with a 21 gauge needle. Each bar represents the mean ± S.E.M. of measurements from 5 hearts.

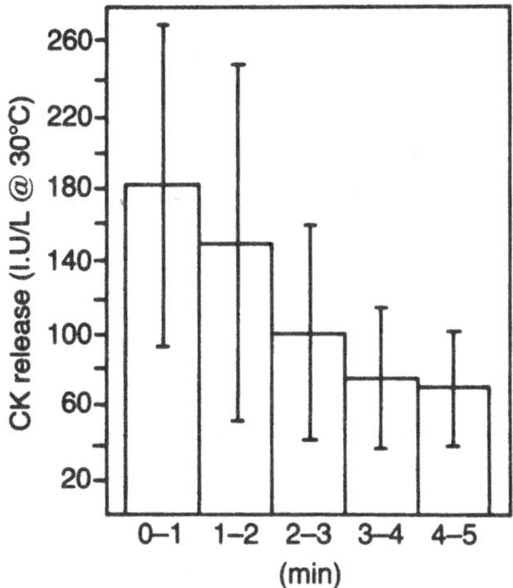

CK assay validation. In view of the clearcut increase in enzyme activity after lancing the heart, all assays were arbitrarily considered valid where CK activity after a single insult by lancing was a minimum of five-fold (40 I.U./l) the corresponding control pre-lancing value. On the occasions when CK values in excess of 40 I.U./l were obtained during the infusion and recovery period, and lower values on lancing were then obtained, the former results would be admitted as evidence of assay integrity. In this way each experiment contained the necessary in-built control to provide reassurance of the presence of intracellular CK, its ability to leak into coronary perfusate, its relative stability in the perfusion medium and of the analytical procedure employed for its measurement.

4 DISCUSSION AND CONCLUSIONS

Iatrogenic cardiopathies are by no means confined to the use of drugs for the treatment of heart disease. Drugs for many other indications also produce equally varied and potentially life-threatening cardiac side effects (Aviado, 1975; Deglin et al, 1977). This problem is compounded by the lack of reliable predictive *in vivo* techniques which is partially due to difficulties in singling out effects on the heart *per se*.

Against this background, a major advantage of the isolated heart is the fact that cardiac response can be seen and measured directly. This applies not only to acutely acting compounds such as ISO, but also to subacute cardiotoxins like the anthracyclines (Breed et al, 1979). While a major concern regarding all *in vitro* procedures is the uncertain extrapolation of findings, it is noteworthy that the isolated heart model described in this Chapter has been validated by responding to diverse insults in a similar way to the intact animal. With ISO, inotropic and chronotropic responses were observed at low infusion levels giving way to marked arrhythmia and fibrillation at high infusion concentrations. Structural damage was indicated by CK release and functional impairment by ECG changes. Using gaseous emboli to induce coronary occlusion as a model for human myocardial infarction, increases in CK in the perfusate from the isolated heart indicated its sensitivity to ischaemic damage. Similarly, a large but short lived increase in enzyme efflux resulted from mechanical damage to the isolated heart, thus directly correlating tissue injury with enzyme release.

In modifying the Langendorff perfusion technique, care was taken to select the minimum numbers of parameters consistent with obtaining an early insight into the nature of any drug induced cardioactivity. Thus perfusion pressure, heart rate and ECG (Sahyoun and Hicks, 1978) were measured to detect alterations in function, while CK release was measured as an index of structural damage (Hearse et al, 1973; Lott and Stang, 1980). Dreyfus et al, (1960) were the first workers to recognise the potential diagnostic advantages of CK. Studies by Wexler and Kittinger (1963 a and b) and Wexler and Judd (1970), showed that ISO induced myocardial necrosis in the rat is accompanied by marked increases in plasma CK and moreover that the degree of change in activity was commensurate with the extent of the myocardium infarcted. Hearse and Humphrey (1975) have additionally shown that the anoxic isolated rat heart leaks CK at a faster rate and in larger quantities than aspartate aminotransferase (AST), αhydroxybutyrate dehydrogenase (αHBDH ≡ LDH1), glyceraldehyde-3-phosphate dehydrogenase (GADPH) and myokinase (MK): this may be due to its cytoplasmic location. Moreover, Osborne and Dent (1973) concluded that CK was by far the most reliable and sensitive index of damage to cardiac tissue in the Beagle dog. In addition to these advantages, the specificity of CK determinations conducted on perfusate leaving the isolated heart contrasts favourably with *in vivo* plasma sampling where isoenzyme studies are necessary to confirm with certainty a cardiac source.

A significant disadvantage of many of the existing *in vivo* cardiotoxicity models is that the techniques employ known cardiotoxins in addition to the drug under test, either to increase the susceptibility of the heart by pre-treatment, or to challenge the treated heart. In routine toxicology studies acute myocardial damage can be missed due to the subacute timing of routine investigations. Subsequently, the heart may develop resistance to further damage. With subacute cardiotoxins such as the anthracyclines a period of several weeks dosing may be necessary to induce diagnosable indications of cardiac damage. These factors have led other workers, who have found the predictive value of existing screening techniques to be unreliable, to the isolated heart. Hale and Poklis (1984) studied the ECG and heart rate response of a racemic mixture of thioridazine-5-sulfoxide, while Mosinger and co-workers (1977) showed that irreversible morphological changes following catecholamine treatment were preceded by increased lactate dehydrogenase release into the effluent. The changes became apparent usually after 4 hours of perfusion and appeared as small foci or streaks on the ventricles which coalesced into opaque patches. Similar lesions were also found in transverse sections of the heart. Light and electron microscopy showed disruption of the myocytes analogous to myocardial infarction but lacking the infiltration. Taylor and Bulkley (1982) have successfully used light and electron microscopic techniques to visualise the very early changes seen in isolated hearts with adriamycin. In 1973, Mir et al were perhaps first to employ the isolated heart for screening purposes, quantitating flow rate, heart rate and force of contraction to establish a rank order for compounds having cardiodepressant activity. At the same time as the model described in this Chapter was developed (Cockburn, 1977), other workers (Aronson and Serlick, 1977) confirmed the utility of the isolated rat heart for the assessment of cardiotoxicity. However, data published in 1976 by Aronson and Serlick indicates several apparent deficiencies in their experimental procedure. In particular, the ischaemia seen histochemically by these workers was probably a consequence of the reduced heart rate and coronary flow rate which occurred with time due to the absence of any filtration of the perfusion fluid compounded by the fact that the freshly isolated hearts were not arrested in ice cold buffer as an 'oxygen sparing' procedure before perfusion. It should also be noted that the use of a heart clip penetrating the muscle of the ventricles will lead to tissue damage and is incompatible with the use of histopathology and the measurement of intermediary metabolites for assessing any but the most profound cardiac effect.

It is of relevance to consider briefly another application of the isolated rat heart which is of clinical significance. This involves its use for evaluating the efficacy of various interventions designed to regulate myocardial infarct size (Hearse and Humphrey, 1975; Garlick et al, 1975; Hearse et al, 1975). The rationale for these interventions is the concept that in addition to the potentially necrotic tissue of the central infarct zone, there is a surrounding area of jeopardized, but still viable, ischaemic myocardial tissue supported by the collateral circulation. This border zone is postulated to be a region whose survival hangs in the balance for several hours before irreversible damage occurs. There is now a general appreciation backed up by some experimental evidence, that appropriate and rapid mechanical, pharmacological, or biochemical interventions, or a combination of these, might save this border zone (Maroka and Braunwald, 1976; Lucchesi et al, 1976). In some respects the anoxic isolated heart model employed by these workers uses the opposite diagnostic principle to that described in the foregoing Chapter for cardiotoxins. Thus "protective agents" are detected by their ability to attenuate or delay the initially high enzyme release of the anoxic system, while cardiotoxins are detected by their ability to exacerbate the initially low levels of enzyme release in the normal system.

As an alternative to the isolated perfused organ, the cultured foetal mouse heart has been studied by Armstrong and Longmore (1973) and Hacker et al (1983) and shown to be sensitive and selective for the screening of cardiotoxic agents. Cultured myocytes from rats and other animals including man have been used extensively to investigate the comparative toxicities of a wide variety of cardiotoxic drugs. Surprisingly, incubation with ISO at concentrations known to be toxic to the intact animal or the isolated heart, did not induce changes in cell morphology or viability (Steen et al, 1982). This finding suggested that myocardial cells might not be the main target for ISO induced necrosis and that some alternative, possibly an indirect mechanism, may be involved. More recently Ramos et al (1983), have shown discrete evidence of early cell injury with ISO but only by utilising more sensitive parameters of cytotoxicity e.g., mitochondrial membrange fragility. Arrhythmias have been seen with tricyclic antidepressants (Acosta and Ramos, 1984) and alterations in beating rates and metabolism (Wenzel and Cosma, 1984) have been noted with the anthracyclines. Thus, with the potential of _in vitro_ techniques now being more fully exploited, the necessary data with which to make _in vitro_ to _in vivo_ correlations will increase accordingly. With this information the toxicologist will have at his disposal a range of sophisticated models with which to investigate different mechanistic aspects of cardiotoxicity.

In conclusion, the isolated heart provides an extremely flexible model for the evaluation of cardiotoxic potential, possible therapeutic interventions and the investigation of basic mechanisms. The system is inexpensive, simple to develop and use, and provides a rapid and sensitive method for the detection of structural and/or functional effects following cardiac insult. It is proposed that with the benefit of accumulated evidence from *in vitro/in vivo* correlations, the isolated heart system should provide a useful adjunct to routine toxicity studies for the early identification and study of drugs with side effects on the heart.

ACKNOWLEDGEMENTS

I am grateful to Beecham Pharmaceuticals for support and to those colleagues who have provided technical help or their valuable critical comments.

REFERENCES

Acosta, D. and Ramos, K. (1984). Cardiotoxicity of tricyclic antidepressants in primary cultures of rat myocardial cells. J. Tox. Env. Health., 14, 137-143.

Armstrong, S.R. and Longmore, D.B. (1973). The effects of cardioactive drugs on the performance of cultured foetal hearts. Nature, 243, 350-352.

Aronson, C.E. and Serlick, E.R. (1976). The effects of prolonged perfusion time on the isolated perfused rat heart. Tox. Appl. Pharmacol., 38, 479-488.

Aronson, C.E. and Serlick, E.R. (1977). Effects of chlorpromazine on the isolated perfused rat heart. Tox. Appl. Pharmacol., 39, 157-176.

Aviado, D.M. (1975). Drug Actions, reaction and interaction. II Iatrogenic cardiopathies. J. Clin. Pharmacol., 15, 641-655.

Bach, P.H. and Cockburn, A. In Press. In Subcellular Pathology of Systemic Disease. Ed. Peters, T.J. Chapter 1., Chemical Toxins in Experimental Pathology. Publ. Chapman and Hall, London.

Baker, J.B.E. (1951). An improved apparatus for mammalian heart perfusion. J. Physiol., 115, 30-32.

Balazs, T., Ohtake, S., Cummings, R.R. and Noble, J.F. (1969). Ventricular extrasystoles induced by epinephrine, nicotine, ethanol, and vasopressin in dogs with myocardial lesions. Tox. Appl. Pharmacol., 15, 189-205.

Breed, J.G.S. (1979). A Technique for evaluating the cardiac toxicity of anthracycline analogs. Cancer Treatment Reports., 63, no. 5, 869-873.

Brus, R. and Drzeswiecki, J. (1973). Effect of d.l. alprenolol on the isolated rat heart. Pol. J. Pharmacol. Pharm., 25, 429-434.

Chapple, D.J., Hughes, R. and Johnson, B.F. (1976). The relationship between cardiotoxicity and plasma digoxin concentration in conscious dogs. Br. J. Pharmac., 57, 23-27.

Cockburn, A. (1977). Cardiotoxicity screening in the isolated perfused rat heart. Ph.D. Thesis. Brunel University.

Deglin, S.M., Deglin, J.M. and Chung, E.K. (1977). Drug-induced cardiovascular diseases. Drugs, 14, 29-40.

De Leiris, J., Breton, D., Feuvray, D. and Coraboeuf, E. (1969). Lacticodehydrogenase release from perfused rat heart under the effect of abnormal media. Arch. Int. Physiol. Biochem., 77, 749-762.

Garlick, P.B., Hearse, D.J., and Shillingford, J.P. (1975). The effects of drugs on myocardial enzyme release. Proceeding of the Medical Research Society, Abstract 47.

Hacker, M.P., Newman, R.A., and Fagan, M.A. (1983). The fetal mouse heart: a potential model for anthracycline-induced cardiotoxicity. Drugs. Exptl. Clin. Res., IX (6), 393-401.

Hale, P.W. and Poklis, A. (1984). Thioridazine-5-sulfoxide cardiotoxicity in the isolated, perfused rat heart. Toxicology Letters, 21, 1-8.

Harmjanz, D. (1975). Problems of myocardial biopsy. Post. Grad. Med. J., 51, 291-292.

Hearse, D.J., Humphrey, S.M. and Chain, E.B. (1973). Abrupt reoxygenation of the anoxic potassium arrested perfused rat heart: A study of myocardial enzyme release. J. Mol. Cell. Cardiol., 5, 395-407.

Hearse, D.J. and Humphrey, S.M. (1975). Enzyme release during myocardial anoxia: A study of metabolic protection. J. Mol. Cell. Cardiol., 7, 463-483.

Hearse, D.J., Humphrey, S.M., Naylor, W.G., Slade, A., and Border, D. (1975). Ultrastructural damage associated with reoxygenation of the anoxic myocardium. J. Mol. Cell. Cardiol., 7, 315-324.

Herman, E.H., Balazs, T., Young, R., Earl, F.L., Krop, S., and Ferans, V.J. (1979). Acute cardiomyopathy induced by the vasodilating antihypertensive agent minoxidil. Tox. Appl. Pharmacol., 47, 493-503.

Jennings, R.B., Ganote, C.E. and Reimer, K.A. (1975). Ischaemic tissue injury. Am. J. Pathol., 81, 179-180.

Joseph, X., Bloom, S., Pledger, G. and Balazs, T. (1983). Determinants of resistance to the cardiotoxicity of isoproterenol in rats. Tox. Appl. Pharmacol., 69, 199-205.

Krebs, H.A. and Hensleit, K. (1932). Untersuchungen uber die Harnstoffbildung im Tierkorper. Hoppe-Seyler's Z. Physiol. Chem., 210, 33-66.

Lahtinen, R., Uusitupa, M., Kuikka, J., Lansimies, E. (1982). Non-invasive evaluation of anthracycline-induced cardiotoxicity in man. Acta Med. Scand., 212, 201-266.

Langendorff, O. (1895). Untersuchungen am uberlebenden Saugetierherzen. Pflug. Arch. ges. Physiol., 61, 291-332.

Lehr, D. (1972). In Myocardiology, recent advances on cardiac structure and metabolism. Ed. Bajusz, E. and Rona, G. Proceedings of the third annual meeting of the international study group for research in cardiac metabolism and of the conference on "Preventive Myocardiology" of the American College of Cardiology. University Park Press, Baltimore, 1, 526-550.

Lott, J.A. and Stang, J.M. (1980). Serum enzymes and isoenzymes in the diagnosis and differential diagnosis of myocardial ischaemia and necrosis. Clin. Chem., 26 no. 9, 1241-1250.

Lucchesi, B.R., Burmeister, W.E., Lamas, T.E. and Abrams, G.D. (1976). Ischaemic changes in the canine heart as affected by the dimethyl quaternary analog of propranolol. J. Pharmacol. Exptl. Ther., 199, 310-312.

Lucena, G.E., Scheften, M., Azar, M., Adicoff, A. and Gobel, F.L. (1974). Serum enzyme activity following cardiac catheterisation and endomyocardial biopsy. J. Lab. Clin. Med., 84, 6-19.

Maroka, P.R. and Braunwald, E. (1976). Effects of metabolic and pharmacologic interventions on myocardial infarct size following coronary occlusion. Acta Med. Scand., 199, 125-137.

Marshall, F.N. and Lewis, J.E. (1973). Sensitisation to epinephrine-induced ventricular fibrillation produced by probucol in dogs. Tox. Appl. Pharmacol., 24, 594-602.

Marshall, F.N. and Lewis, J.E. (1973). Sensitisation to epinephrine-induced ventricular fibrillation produced by probucol in dogs. Tox. Appl. Pharmacol., 24, 594-602.

Mir, G.N., Lawrence, W.H. and Autian, J. (1973). Toxicological and pharmacological actions of methyl-acrylate monomers I: effects on the isolated perfused rat heart. J. Pharm. Sci., 62, 778-782.

Mosinger, B. Stejskal, J. and Mosinger B. (1977). Heart infarction-like effect induced by natural catecholamines in vitro. Exp. Path., Bd., 14, 157-161.

Osborne, B.E. and Dent, N.J. (1973). Electrocardiography and blood chemistry in the detection of myocardial lesions in dogs. Fd. Cosmet. Toxicol., 11, 265-276.

Ramos, K., Combs, A.B. and Acosta, D. (1983). Cytotoxicity of isoproterenol to cultured heart cells: Effects of antioxidants on modifying membrane damage. Tox. Appl. Pharmacol., 70, 317-323.

Rona, G. (1967). In Animal and clinical pharmacological techniques in drug evaluation. Ed. Siegler, P.E. and Moyer, J.H. Year Book Medical Publishers Inc. Vol II, Chap. 41, 464-470.

Ross, B.D. (1972). In Perfusion Techniques in Biochemistry. Clarendon Press Oxford.

Sahyoun, H.A., and Hicks, R. (1978). Electrocardiographic recording of normal and infarct bearing rat hearts in a perfused isolated preparation. J. Pharm. Met., 1, 351-360.

Singal, P.K., Yates, J.C., Beamish, R.E., Dhalla, N.S. (1981). Influence of reducing agents on adrenochrome-induced changes in the heart. Arch. Pathol. Lab. Med., 105, 664-669.

Steen, E.M., Noronha-Dutra, A.A. and Woolf, N. (1982). The response of isolated rat heart cells to cardiotoxic concentrations of isoprenaline. J. Pathology., 137, 167-176.

Taylor, A.L. and Bulkley, B.H. (1982). Acute adriamycin cardiotoxicity - morphologic alterations in isolated perfused rabbit heart. Laboratory Investigation, 47 no. 5, 459-464.

Tharp, G.D. and Folk, G.E. (1965). Rhythmic changes in rate of the mammalian heart and heart cells during prolonged isolation. Comp. Biochem. Physiol., 14, 255-273.

Umbreit, W., Burris, R.H., and Stauffer, J.F. (1964). In Manometric Techniques. Mineapolis: Burgess Publishing Co., p.132.

Wenzel, D.G. and Cosma, G.N. (1984). A model system for measuring comparative toxicities of cardiotoxic drugs for cultured rat heart myocytes, endothelial cells and fibroblasts. II. Doxorubicin, 5-fluorouracil and cyclophosphamide. Toxicology, 33, 117-128.

Yates, J.C., Taam, G.M.L., Singal, P.K., Beamish, R.E. and Dhalla, N.S. (1980). Protection against adrenochrome-induced myocardial damage by various pharmacological interventions. Br. J. Exp. Path., 61, 242-255.

BRAIN REAGGREGATE CULTURES IN NEUROTOXICOLOGICAL INVESTIGATIONS

C.K. Atterwill, B.Pharm. PhD. M.P.S. (Dept. Toxicology, Smith Kline & French Research Ltd., The Frythe, Welwyn, Herts., U.K.)

(A) General Introduction

Rotation-mediated aggregating cultures constructed from single cell suspensions of foetal brain have so far proved extremely useful and informative in multi-disciplinary neurobiological and neuropharmacological studies. However they have not yet been as extensively used for neurotoxicological investigations as have monolayer and explant cultures. Brain reaggregates appear to restrict cellular division whilst enhancing biochemical and morphological differentiation (see Seeds et al, 1980) and more closely reflect the *in vivo* developmental process than primary monolayer cultures. In fact, in several instances they have been found to express systems found *in vivo* and not in surface culture such as some of the myelin-related enzymes.

In common with other tissue culture models there are several advantages over *in vivo* studies (see also section D), added advantages being firstly the high tissue yield for neurochemical analysis, and secondly their long survival in chemically-defined, serum-free media (Honegger & Lenoir, 1980; Atterwill et al, 1985) enabling detailed studies of hormone action to be carried out. Of interest is a report that the longevity of cells in brain aggregate cultures can be further enhanced by the addition of vitamin E.

The cells within these organotypic cultures change from a population of completely undifferentiated neuroepithelial cells to an integrated population of neurones, astroglia and oligodendroglia. The brain cells are generally mechanically dissociated (this is preferable to trypsinization, giving more viable cells) from 15-16 day rat foetuses and the cultures remain viable for around one to two months. Up until 11 days _in vitro_ (DIV) the aggregates remain relatively immature and between 11-17 DIV there is a rapid neuronal development with dendritic and axonal growth, and synaptogenesis which peaks at 21-30 DIV, whilst the myelination of axons continues (Trapp et al, 1979). Brain cell reaggregate cultures can be easily and successfully grown from telencephalon, mesencephalon-diencephalon and rhombencephalon and with more care from brain regions such as cerebellum, cerebral cortex, hypothalamus and the visual system. Certain areas such as cerebral cortex form larger aggregates compared with, for example, the cerebellum. Aggregation is age and species-dependent and tends to be greatest at an age when the 'starting' tissue shows active proliferation and cell migration. Mouse brain aggregates from all brain regions are consistently larger than those cultivated from chick brain.

Since the pioneering work of Moscona (1961 onwards:- see Garber and Moscona, 1972 I & II) in establishing the usefulness of this method much work has been done in characterizing various neurochemical, neuropharmacological and neurotoxicological aspects of the CNS using these cultures and some of these will be covered in a later section. From the developmental biology angle certain aspects of cell recognition, migration and morphogenesis have been elucidated which would not have been possible with developing embryos _in vivo_.

These parameters were first studied in embryonic avian and mammalian non-neuronal cells (Moscona, 1962) and then extended to neural retina and brain cells (see Garber & Moscona, 1972 I & II), and led to the isolation of specific "cell-aggregating" factors (such as the retinal cell-aggregating glycoprotein) which have been hypothesized to mediate cell-recognition and histotypic cell associations (see Seeds et al, 1980). Cell interaction in reaggregate development is also supported by studies showing synergistic effects on cholinergic development in aggregates prepared from chick optic tectum and retina (Ramirez et al, 1980). These studies suggest that early cell contacts may be important for normal CNS development and are thus potential 'targets' for neurotoxic xenobiotics.

More recently brain reaggregates have been successfully employed to study the synthesis, storage, release and binding of various putative neurotransmitter compounds (see Wolfe et al, 1981; Honegger & Richelson, 1979) in both normal and genetically deficient CNS material. Synaptogenesis, transition to adult isozyme expression, myelin formation, bioelectrical activity (Stafstrom et al, 1980) and the effects of hormones on these parameters (Atterwill et al, 1983, 1984, 1985) have also been studied in considerable detail.

In the following sections the practical aspects of growing rat brain reaggregate cultures will be covered first including methods for obtaining aggregates enriched in either neurones or glial cells. Readers are advised to refer to the author's individual publications for detailed information on neurochemical, morphological and immunocytochemical measurements. Secondly, examples of the neuropharmacological and neuroendocrinological work performed with reaggregates is discussed referring specifically to our own work on the effects of thyroid hormone (T_3) on neural function. In addition, the effects of the neurotoxic agents ascorbate and kainate will be considered (see Trapp & Richelson, 1980) as well as some recent work from our own laboratory on the novel cholinergic neurotoxin, elthylcholine mustard aziridinium ion (ECMA). Finally, the advantages and disadvantages of this culture type will be discussed along with descriptions of other available models for in vitro neurotoxicological investigations.

(B) Practical aspects

Method for growing rat whole-brain reaggregates

a) Cell Culture & Harvesting

Foetal brain reaggregating cultures are grown essentially by the method of Honegger and Lenoir (1980) and as described by Atterwill et al (1981, 1985 - see Fig. 1). Whole brains from 80-100 P16 rat foetuses (from approximately 12 female pregnant rats and yielding around 20 individual culture flasks) are dissected aseptically in a sterile solution of ice-cold, isotonic Hanks D2 solution (see below) containing gentamycin and then washed extensively in a nylon gauze bag (Nybolt - pore size 205μm). The tissue is then dissociated by extrusion through the gauze by gently stroking with a glass rod in 30ml Hanks D1 solution (+ gentamycin;

FIGURE 1 Method for preparing foetal rat brain reaggregate cultures.

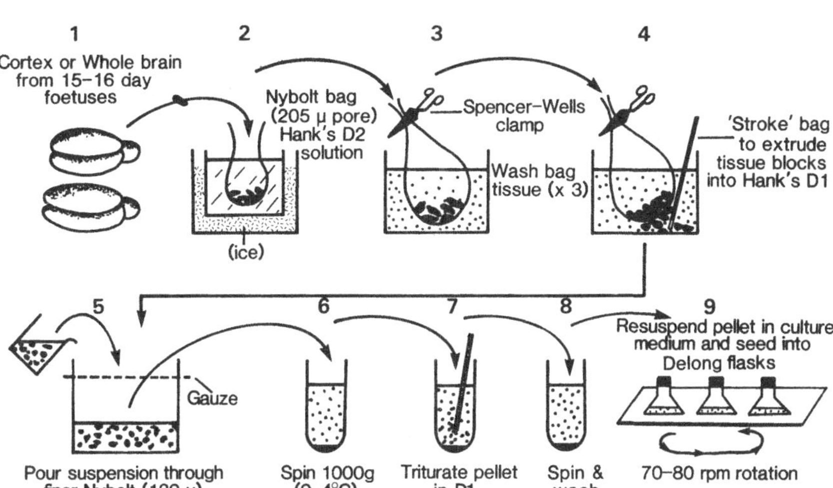

Ca^{2+},Mg^{2+}-free - see below). The suspension is then refiltered through Nybolt (130um pore size) and centrifuged at 100g x 6 min (0-5°C). Following gentle mechanical trituration of the tissue (10 passes through 5ml pipette) in 10ml D1 solution, the cells are centrifuged as above. This procedure is repeated twice. The final cell pellet is resuspended in culture medium (S+ = DMEM + 10% foetal calf serum + extra glutamine supplement (see Table 1 for preparation and details); or S- = medium based on the N2 medium of Bottenstein and Sato

(1979), which is a 3:1 mixture of DMEM and Hams F12 containing Insulin (5μg/ml), Transferrin (100μg/ml), Putrescine (10μm), Selenium (30nM) and Progesterone (20nM). Gentamycin (25ug/ml) and extra glutamine (final conc. = 300μg/ml) are also added to both the S+ and S- culture media.

Next 3.5ml of the cell suspension (10^4 cells/ml) is innoculated into 25ml Delong conical culture flasks and cultured for up to 28-30 days in a 9% CO_2/humidified air mixture (37°C) at a constant rotation of 70 rpm on a Luckham rotaset orbital shaker (orbit diameter = 1.0 in). The speed is gradually increased to 80 rpm. After 3 DIV the 'mini' aggregates are transferred to 50ml Delong vessels and 5ml fresh culture medium added. This is repeated on alternate days. If thyroid hormone (T_3; 30nM) is to be added, this was done at 2 DIV, and on alternate days thereafter. For ECMA addition this is performed usually at 9 DIV once only. Aggregates are harvested for neurochemical measurements by allowing them to sediment under gravity and washing x 3 with Dulbecco's phosphate buffer saline (PBS) at 25°C. The final cells are generally frozen in liquid N_2 and stored at -70°C prior to analysis. To perform morphological or immunocytochemical analyses readers should refer to Atterwill et al (1985) or Woodhams et al (1986).

b) <u>Preparation of neuronal or glial reaggregates</u>

Recently techniques have been developed for the preparation of reaggregates of either exclusively rat CNS glial cells (astrocytes) or neurones (Guntert-Lauber et al, 1984). In the case of glial reaggregates this firstly involves the preparation of astrocytic monolayers in S+ medium (containing 10% FCS) as described by Atterwill et al, (1985). This is effected using either 8 day postnatal rat cerebellum or 2 day postnatal cerebral hemispheres. Following 12 DIV in monolayer culture the cells are detached from the plastic dishes with 0.5mM EDTA in S- culture medium and cells forced to aggregate as described above using Delong flasks. For neuronal aggregates whole brain aggregates are prepared from 15 day foetal rat as described above in S- medium with the exception that 0.4μm cytosine arabinoside (an antimitotic agent to prevent glial proliferation/survival) is added at 0 DIV. Aggregation is then carried out normally as described for the mixed-cell cultures.

c) Dissection and Dissociation Media

Dissection (Hank's D2)

(Parentheses = final quantity or concentration in working solution-500ml final volume). NaCl (138mM), KCl (5.4mM), Na_2HPO_4 (0.17mM), KH_2PO_4 (0.22mM), $CaCl_2.2H_2O$ (1.8mM), $MgCl_2.6H_2O$ (0.8mM), phenol red (14μM), glucose (0.495g), sucrose (7.065g) and Gentamycin (10μg/ml). Adjust to pH 7.4 with sterile 0.05N NaOH.

Dissociation (Hank's D1)

As for D2 but omitting Ca^{++} and Mg^{++}. Then add 7.954g sucrose, 0.495g glucose per 500ml and 10ug/ml gentamycin.

Table 1

Culture Medium Type		Substance	Quantity	Dissolved in	Volume used	Added to	Final concentration
A) S- Aggregate	1.	Progesterone (L)	20µl	2ml F-12	64µl	-	20nM
	2.	Selenium (L)	i) 20µl ii) 40µl	2ml F-12 4ml F-12	3.2ml of ii)	-	30nM
	3.	Putrescine (S)	16mg	10ml F-12	3.2ml	-	10µM
	4.	Transferrin (S)	32mg	F-12	All	-	100ug/ml
	5.	Insulin (S)	10mg	1ml F-12 by addition 25µl 1M NaOH	0.16ml	-	5µg/ml
	6.	Hams F-12 + (1-5) (L)	-	-	80ml	240ml DMEM	-
	7.	L-Glutamine (S)	150mg	5ml H_2O	3.2ml	Medium	300µg/ml
	8.	50mg/ml Solution of of Gentamycin	-	-	0.16ml	Medium	25µg/ml
B) S+ Aggregate	1.	Foetal Calf Serum (complement inactivated)	50ml	450ml DMEM Medium	-	-	10% FCS in DMEM
	2.	Gentamycin (50mg/ml)	-	-	0.25ml	Medium	25µg/ml
	3.	L-Glutamine	150mg	5ml H_2O		Medium	300µg/ml

(L) Liquid (S) Solid

d) Morphological appearance of the whole-brain (mixed-cell) cultures

Plate 1 shows the light-microscopic appearance in toluidine blue stained 'semi-thin' sections of whole brain reaggregates (10 DIV) cultured in either S(+) or S(-) medium. There is a fairly well-ordered arrangement of cells within the aggregates with very little pyknosis at this developmental stage (slightly more pyknosis occurs in the S- medium). Larger cells are generally in the central zone of the aggregate with smaller ones nearer the edge. There is a relatively cell-free zone around the circumference where fibre-bundles are abundant as shown by immunoreactivity to neurofilament proteins. This immunoreactivity is generally denser in S- cultured cells. Another important difference between serum-supplemented (S+) and serum-deprived (S-) aggregates is the

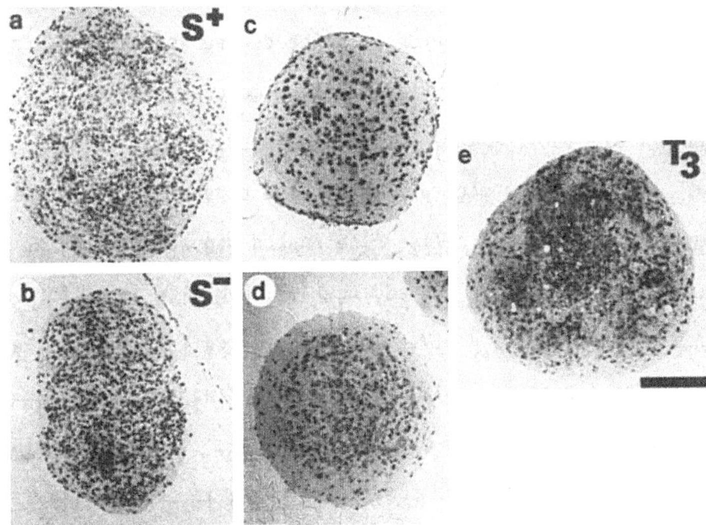

Plate 1

presence of a single-layer of cells present exclusively around the circumference of S+ aggregates which are immunoreactive for glial fibrillary acid protein (GFAP): a 'glia-limitans'. The neurotoxicological significance of this cell layer must be considered when assessing penetration of compounds into the reaggregates. By 28 days (21 DIV for S-) in culture aggregates start to display considerable central pyknosis and are not used for neurotoxicological or neurobiological experiments.

(C) Experimental examples

i) Neurobiological and Neurochemical Studies

More recent investigations of cell-sorting, migration and recognition in the CNS have shown that natural histogenetic mechanisms persist after dissociation where cerebellar cells will sort into aggregates with granule neurones in the centre and large neurones (e.g. Purkinje cells) near the surface (outer 'molecular' layer) thus generally reflecting the whole mature tissue (see Seeds et al, 1980; Orkand et al, 1984). Mutant Reeler mice with inherited cerebellar defects show malpositioning of these cells. The inward migration rates of the granule neurones can be monitored by adding [^{3}H] thymidine to preformed aggregates at around 3-4 DIV. This type of cell movement is aided by secretion of a protease, plasminogen activating substances which can also be detected using a fibrin overlay technique. Using mouse midbrain aggregates it has also been shown that there is a selective association of catecholamine-containing neurones measured by the Falck-Hillarp histofluorescence method. An unselective cell distribution is seen initially, followed by small clusters of fluorescent neurones at 48h. By 96h in culture a thick elongated band of reactive neurones is present along the margin followed by neurite extension.

It has also been shown that cells dissociated from foetal rostral mesencephalic tegmentum (RMT) and then reaggregated only contain dopaminergic neurones that elaborate processes and exhibit functional characteristics (e.g. stimulated dopamine release) when the RMT cells are cocultured with appropriate target cells from corpus striatum or frontal cortex (see Shalaby et al, 1984).

With respect to myelination in reaggregate cultures, this occurs between 18-19 DIV as assessed biochemically. Myelin basic protein (MBP) and myelin-associated glycoprotein (MAG) increase subsequently although their levels are less than the corresponding age *in vivo* (see Trapp et al, 1982). As oligodendrocytes develop a more differentiated fine structure, MBP and MAG antisera stain oligo-processes and myelin sheaths.

A developmental sequence of bioelectrical changes has been demonstrated in reaggregates (Staffstrom et al, 1980) which parallel those found biochemically and morphologically. There is a spontaneous bioelectrical activity which is occasionally rhythmic and shows a maximum amplitude just below the aggregate surface. The average amplitude of spontaneous discharge is decreased by Mg^{++} and increased by tetrodotoxin. Spontaneous activity is increased by the convulsants bicuculline, strychnine and pentylenetetrazol. There also appears to be a differential development of Na^+,K^+-ATPase isozymes during reaggregate development. Whilst steady state ratios of intracellular ion concentrations (Na^+ and K^+) seem to remain unaltered during development, the rates of ion fluxes increase markedly (see Marks & Seeds, 1982). In aggregates cultured in a serum-free medium (S-), Na^+, K^+-ATPase development has been shown to be retarded even though intracellular ion concentrations are maintained, indicating the ability of the neural cells to maintain an ionic homeostasis (Atterwill et al, 1985). Furthermore, the developmental retardation in Na^+,K^+-ATPase activity _in vitro_ is reflected more in one particular isoenzyme thought to reside predominantly in astroglial cells (Atterwill & Collins, 1986).

ii) _Neuropharmacological and Neuroendocrinological Studies_

We have already discussed some of the work carried out on dopaminergic neurones in reaggregates (see above section). In addition, several pharmacological investigations have been performed on monoamine neuronal function. Studies using the radioligand [^{125}I]Iodohydroxy-benzylpindolol have demonstrated a rapid increase in ß-adrenoceptor density between 6-22 DIV when a maximum receptor density is attained. When cultures are grown in presence of the ß-adrenoceptor agonist, isoprenaline ('chronic' exposure), receptor development is markedly inhibited. Isoprenaline has also been shown to stimulate cAMP production in aggregates following acute exposure and this response is blocked by the antagonist propranolol (see Wehner et al, 1982; Wolfe et al, 1981).

Majocha et al (1981) have demonstrated that accumulated [^{3}H] noradrenaline (NA) is released by exposure to depolarizing agents such as high K^+ and veratridine and that [^{3}H]NA uptake can be blocked by tricyclic antidepressants (e.g. desmethylimipramine, DMI) or the neurotoxin 6-hydroxydopamine (6-OHDA) _in vitro_. Autoradiographic techniques showed dense clusters of NA neurones in these cultures which may have corresponded to the locus coeruleus, an area from which forebrain NA processes project.

A little work has been done on amino acid transmitters in reaggregates especially in relation to the actions of the 'excitotoxin' kainic acid. This will be discussed in the next section (iii).

In contrast, a considerable amount of work has been carried out on the cholinergic system and the effects of thyroid hormone on the development of cholinergic neurones in culture. The development of the acetycholine (ACh) metabolising enzymes, choline acetyltransferase (ChAT-ACh synthesis) and acetylcholinesterase (AChE-ACh breakdown) has been examined in aggregates derived from different macro-areas of the foetal brain. Such cultures develop a pattern of enzyme activities that reflect the presumptive starting tissue *in vivo*. Thus, cultures relatively enriched in the cholinergic 'system' are obtained by growing telencephalon whilst growth of mesencephalon-diencephalon yields cultures relatively enriched in the catecholamine-metabolising enzymes (see Honegger & Richelson, 1977).

Honegger & Lenoir (1980, 1982) and Atterwill et al (1984) have shown that the development of the cholinergic system in aggregates is depressed when they are grown in a serum-free medium. Thyroid hormone (T_3) and Nerve Growth Factor (NGF) treatment will greatly enhance the developmental increase in ChAT activity (see Fig. 2) under these conditions. In the case of T_3, the more undifferentiated cells are more responsive to treatment. Muscarinic receptors predominantly located on neighbouring cells are also affected in the same way as ChAT activity (see Fig. 2).

FIGURE 2 Effect of T_3 treatment on enzyme and receptor activities in cultured brain reaggregates.

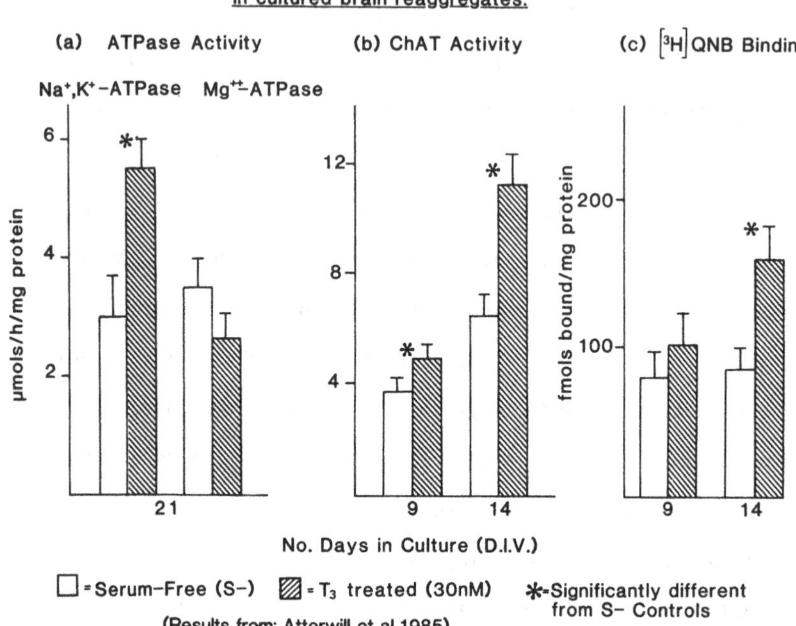

(Results from: Atterwill et al, 1985)

Brain reaggregates grown in presence of muscarinic receptor agonists such as oxotremorine show 'down-regulated' muscarinic receptors a phenomenon similar to that seen in vivo. Retinal aggregates show an independence of their nicotinic and muscarinic receptor regulation under such conditions (see Siman & Klein, 1983).

Honegger & Richelson (1979) have shown that brain aggregates can be 'prompted' to synthesize [^{3}H]ACh from [^{3}H]choline when a cholinesterase inhibitor is present, a 4h incubation with precursor is carried out and choline-depleted cells are used. Preincubation of the cultures with an inhibitor of ChAT (N-hydroxyethl-4(1-napthlvinyl)-

pyridinium bromide) results in a marked decrease in the amount of ACh recoverable from the cells. Under more 'normal' incubation conditions in our hands accummulated choline seems to be transported predominantly by a low-affinity transporter, is converted mainly to phosphorylcholine, not ACh, and may be localised in glial cells (see Atterwill et al, 1984). Further discussion of cholinergic function in reaggregates is carried out in section C (iv) where the actions of the cholinergic neurotoxin, ethylcholine mustard aziridinium ion (ECMA), are also considered.

Lastly, as for the cholinergic neurones in culture, we have been able to show that thyroid hormone (T_3) is probably an important serum component for the differentiation of neural plasma membrane function in brain. As mentioned earlier the activity of the plasma-membrane enzyme Na^+,K^+-ATPase is depressed under serum-free culture conditions (see Fig. 2). When S- cultures are treated with T_3 (30nM final concentration), it can be shown that the enzyme activity is restored to a level near that found in S+ cultures and _in vivo_ (Fig. 2; and see Atterwill et al, 1985).

iii) Neurotoxicological Studies

The effect of the vitamin, ascorbic acid on neurotransmitter-metabolizing enzyme activities has been tested in aggregating cultures of whole embryonic rat brain. Ascorbic acid (0.2mM) supplementation to the culture medium causes slight increases in ChAT, AChE, glutamate decarboxylase (GABA synthesis), catechol-o-methyltransferase (COMT) and monoamine oxidase (MAO:- monoamine catabolism) after 30 days incubation (see Trapp & Richelson, 1980). However, profound reductions in the catecholamine synthesizing enzymes, tyrosine-3- hydroxylase and aromatic L-amino acid decarboxylase are seen. This has been attributed to a possible toxic effect of vitamin C on catecholaminergic neurones caused by the intracellular generation of hydrogen peroxide. Other work has shown that exposure of explant cultures of newborn rat sympathetic ganglia to 1mM ascorbate causes damage to nerve fibres and cell bodies.

Kainic acid is a potent CNS excitatory cyclic analogue of glutamate (a putative excitatory neurotransmitter in brain) which when injected into the striatum of rats causes a specific degeneration of cholinergic and GABAergic neurones, while dopaminergic neurones (which innervate the striatum from the substantia nigra) remain relatively unaffected. Studies using rat brain reaggregates have demonstrated that treatment from 2-14 DIV with 5µM kainate causes no effect on neurotransmitter-metabolizing enzyme activity (Trapp & Richelson, 1980; Honegger & Richelson, 1977). When exposure is more prolonged (2-29 DIV), there are marked reductions in ChAT, AChE and GAD activities. At higher kainate concentrations effects are more pronouced and less cell-specific. A more detailed investigation showed that using cholinergic neurone-enriched telencephalic aggregates, treatment with 5µM kainate causes a greater reduction in cholinergic and GABA-related enzyme activites when the cells are exposed from days 11-19 in comparison to those exposed from days 5-11. Catecholaminergic enzymes are little affected. Thus kainic acid exhibits a selective and greater neurotoxicity on cholinergic and GABAergic cells in more differentiated aggregate cultures. This demonstrates the 'flexibility' and usefulness of this _in vitro_ model for investigating neurotoxic potential in the developing CNS.

Recently further work on cholinergic neurotoxicity using reaggregate cultures has been performed for the organophosphorus compounds. Wehner et al (1986) have demonstrated that treatment of mouse brain reaggregates with diisopropylfluorophosphate (DFP) at 17-24 DIV causes a 95% reduction in AChE activity by irreversible inhibition. By 24 hours following treatment 32% of control enzyme activity is returned and 'recovery' is complete within 7 days. This 'recovery' requires protein synthesis since cycloheximide prevents new AChE synthesis. In contrast, a reversible AChE inhibitor such as physostigmine allows full recovery of enzyme activity within 24h.

iv) Studies on the cholinergic neurotoxin ECMA in rat brain reaggregate cultures

Recent work in our laboratory has centred on the choline mustard analogues since these may be useful tools for causing selective neurotoxicity to central and peripheral cholinergic neurones. They can be potentially accumulated by the high and low-affinity choline uptake mechanisms which subserve cholinergic neuronal ACh synthesis. One such analogue, ethylcholine mustard aziridinium ion (ECMA) appears to be selective both *in vivo* and *in vitro*. Marked and persistent decreases in brain ACh levels and high affinity choline uptake in corpus striatum, cerebral cortex and hippocampus have been demonstrated following direct central administration of the compound and cholinergic-mediated behavioural and cognitive changes have also been found (see Walsh et al, 1984). Such studies suggest that lesioned animals may provide useful models for the dementing disorder Alzheimers Disease (see Archer & Fowler, 1985). Further _in vitro_ studies using a cholinergic neuroblastoma x glioma cell line (NG-108-15) have shown that ECMA acts as an irreversible active-site directed inhibitor of ChAT and possibly other enzymes recognising the ACh precursor, choline, such as choline kinase and AChE (Sandberg et al, 1985). In cell line culture models the onset of action of ECMA is relatively rapid and precedes the cytotoxic effects of the drug by several hours. Acutely, therefore, it may be useful for simply impairing cholinergic neurotransmission aside from its potential value as a neurocytotoxin against cholinergic neurones and in models of Alzheimers Disease.

There is, however, some _in vivo_ evidence suggesting that ECMA may not be entirely specific for central cholinergic neurones. Thus, further studies using impaired _in vitro_ systems such as the mixed-cell reaggregate cultures may both clarify the cellular specificity and provide further evidence for the mechanism of the ECMA-induced lesion. In this respect, obvious advantages are the ability to control carefully ECMA concentrations _in vitro_, to assess the toxic effect at different developmental stages and to study several neurochemical and morphological parameters simultaneously. An aim of the work was to establish an _in vitro_ model with cholinergic 'lesions' similar to those found in Alzheimer-diseased brain tissue and to assess agents which may alleviate the sequelae to central cholinergic lesioning. Another important consideration is that the cultures may permit identification of neurotrophic 'injury' factors secreted into the culture medium in response to neurotoxin exposure. Brain tissue does synthesize and utilize such factors (e.g. NGF) and in this context we have already used rat brain reaggregates cultured in serum-free media (Atterwill & Bowen, 1986) to 'bioassay' cholinergic neurotrophic factors produced from human brain tissue. It was shown in this work that both normal and Alzheimer human brain tissue contain factors which are capable of elevating ChAT activity in S- aggregate cultures. The action of cell growth factors

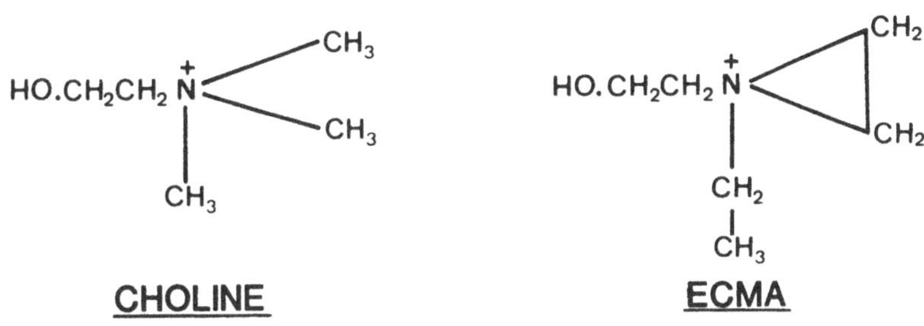

FIGURE 3 Effect of ECMA on cholinergic function (ChAT activity) in brain reaggregate cultures (S+).

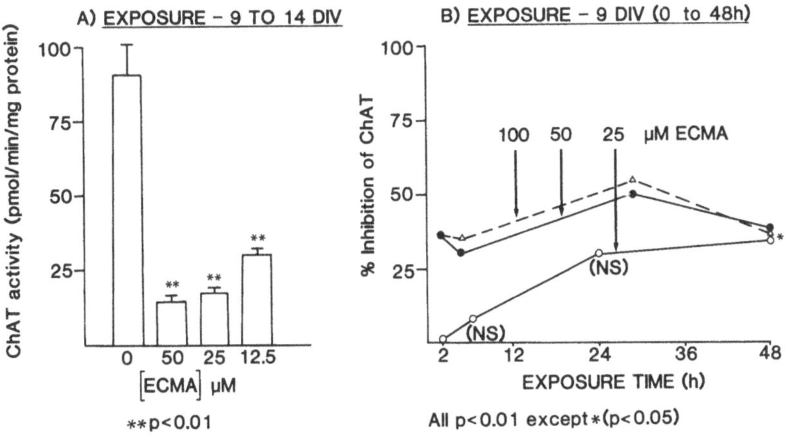

(Results from: Atterwill,Pillar & Prince: Brit.J.Pharmac.1986. In press)

such as insulin and insulin-like growth factors (IGF) has also been studied in reaggregates (Lenoir & Honegger, 1983) where their addition to serum-free reaggregates caused stimulation of DNA synthesis showing specific receptors for these peptides in the cultures.

Preliminary studies in our laboratory (see Fig. 3) have shown that ECMA added to the cultures at 9 DIV in concentrations ranging from 12.5-50μM causes 50-80% reductions in ChAT activity when examined at 14 DIV with no apparent dose-response relationship or morphological damage. When examined from 0-48 hours from ECMA addition the ChAT inhibition appears to be of rapid onset (within 2h) at 50μM ECMA and at 48h shows a 30-50% maximal reduction in activity. The reason for this difference in the degree of inhibition between short and long-term exposure is unknown but may suggest a progressive cellular toxicity response. The short-term neurotoxic effect on the cholinergic neurones _in vitro_ is also dependent on their accumulation of ECMA since pretreatment with hemicholinium prevented the reductions in ChAT activity. Some indication of specificity of this neurotoxin is provided by the finding that 12.5μM ECMA (9-14 DIV: which produces a maximal reduction in ChAT) does not reduce cholinergic muscarinic receptor binding and only produces small reductions in Na^+,K^+-ATPase activity. At higher concentrations both muscarinic receptors and Na^+,K^+-ATPase are affected. It appears, at this stage, therefore, that ECMA produces a cholinergic neuronal lesion _in vitro_ in this model which has time and dose-dependent characteristics. The exact degree of neural specificity of this effect now awaits investigation using additional neurochemical markers.

D) Discussion and Conclusions

Due to the functional and structural complexity of the central nervous system the detection of toxic effects probably poses more problems than with many other target organs and multidisciplinary *in vivo* (behavioural, neurochemical and neuropathological) and *in vitro* (*ex vivo* preparations such as brain slices and synaptosomes, and cell cultures) studies are essential for determining the nature and mechanisms of toxicity (see Dewar, 1981; Spencer & Schaumburg, 1980). Generally speaking, there are two main types of CNS toxicity, acute and chronic (Dewar, 1981), although exceptions to this rule exist. The former is usually reversible, occurs after a single dose, is due to functional changes and does not involve structural damage or degenerative changes. These acute effects are commonly due to pharmacological effects on, for example neural membranes or neurotransmitter metabolism. Most chronic neurotoxic effects, in contrast, involve structural and degenerative changes and are not readily reversible. Metabolic lesions of neural cells (neuronal cell bodies and their axons, astroglia and oligodendroglia) or interference with cerebral blood supply would be likely causes. Apart from the latter example most of the above factors can be investigated in cell culture systems following acute or chronic exposure.

It is still generally accepted that the primary use of cell-culture techniques in neurotoxicology is to perform detailed mechanistic studies once a neurotoxic potential has been identified from *in vivo* investigations. Cell culture models and in particular reaggregate (and other 'organotypic') cultures, can offer distinct advantages over *in vivo* studies (see below and Table 2) but the choice of culture and relevant measurements for solving a particular problem still requires careful consideration. In addition to their mechanistic and investigative potential in neurotoxicology CNS cultures may also have a place as pre-development screens for agents with interesting pharmacologic profiles plus neurotoxicity potential. In this respect, consideration of culture type again warrants careful consideration since certain models can be expensive and/or time consuming, although scaling-down procedures are possible. Cell-lines (derived from nervous system tumours) may still have an advantageous role and may suffice in this situation.

Some of the other important considerations for the design of toxicological studies with cultured cells (including reaggregates) are whether one should treat cells with neurotoxin during development and differentiation or at relative 'maturity', and whether the results obtained in one situation are applicable to the other. Developmental constraints are usually inherent to most CNS cell culture models and reaggregate cultures are no exception. The use of cell-lines also poses the problem of cellular de-differentiation and whether any result reflects that likely to be obtained from the brain *in situ*. The importance of metabolites must be considered and it is possible with cultures to determine whether the parent compound or one of its metabolites is responsible for the neurotoxic effect *in vivo*. For example, using organotypic CNS-PNS-muscle-tissue cultures, Spencer and Schaumburg (1975) have demonstrated that the primary neurotoxic agent in n-hexane and methyl-n-butylketone neuropathies is the metabolite 2,5-hexanedione. It is also of paramount importance to use realistic doses that span the clinically relevant age and from a technical standpoint to use the correct cell densities since some neurotoxicities in culture are cell-density dependent (see Schrier, 1982).

Nervous system culture types fall into six categories and all have been utilised for neurotoxicological investigations. It is far beyond the scope of this chapter to describe the compounds tested in these models and the reader is referred to reviews by Schrier (1982) and Yonezawa et al, (1980). The culture types include: a) dispersed cell cultures (including primary dispersed types, outgrowths from explants and secondary dispersed types) which offer good reproducibility for neurochemical studies and the ease of performing electrophysiological measurements on single cells; b) cell-lines (neuroblastomas, Schwanomas, hybrid lines, phaochromocytomas and gliomas) of which one can obtain large quantities of one cell-type for study; c) explant ('organotypic' cultures) which have been used extensively and successfully by Yonezawa et al (1980) and give good cytoarchitectural preservation for morphological studies; d) whole organ (eg peripheral autonomic ganglia - which offer the opportunity to culture from more 'mature' animals) (e) whole embryo cultures (a very specialized technique but giving an expected intact fetal metabolism and near-to-normal brain development); and f) reaggregation cultures.

Table 2

Advantages of reaggregates over other (a) in vitro systems and (b) in vivo models

a)
- Three-dimensional cytoarchitecture partially restored giving histogenetic asssociation between different cell types.
- Reproducibility of biochemical parameters better than e.g. explants and surface cultures. Plenty of tissue for analysis.
- Maturation more complete than dispersed cell cultures to allow neurotoxin testing during both development and maturation.
- Myelination occurs under carefully controlled conditions
- Glial multiplication limited (can be disadvantage in some systems).

---

b)
- Direct accessibility to compounds not penetrating blood-brain-barrier or metabolized to inactive metabolite peripherally. Thus, can treat acutely or chronically with well-controlled time courses and concentrations.
- Ability to test small quantities of potential neurotoxins in predevelopment screening and identify likely target structures.
- Can easily withdraw neurotoxin/drug from culture medium and monitor subsequent cell recovery.
- Can easily study effects on cell interactions, migration, sorting, and synaptogenesis.
- Can measure profile of released neuronotrophic factors in response to cellular injury or 'insult'.
- Toxic effects on other organs eliminated (e.g. vascular, immune). Therefore, study primary CNS effects.
- Can investigate hormonal effects more easily.

Table 3

Disadvantages of brain reaggregate cultures for investigative neurotoxicological studies

- Difficulty in predicting whole animal response or lesion, or compound's ability to reach an 'effective' concentration at certain brain regions/cells in vivo.
- Active peripherally-formed metabolites not accounted for.
- Must always take into account developmental changes when considering neurotoxin effect.
- Large number of 'timed' pregnant animals required (in contrast to surface cultures, and embryonic 'timing' more critical for good aggregation). Increased dissection time but good yield.
- Cannot be easily manipulated for small brain regions (smallest=hypothalamus) as can with monolayers (dispersed cultures). Degree of restoration of cytoarchitecture can vary between batches.
- Inability to perform routine electrophysiological examination since in suspension. However, can record spontaneous extracellular electrical activity.
- Secondary neurotoxic effects from other organs (e.g. endocrine) not accounted for.
- Complete 'mixture' of cell types under investigation. Sometimes need supplementary information from cell-type enriched surface cultures.

The latter class of culture which we have discussed extensively in this chapter has definite advantages over some of the culture models described above and over some in vivo techniques in general. This information is summarized in Table 2. However, there are inevitably some disadvantages of reaggregate cultures compared with certain culture models together with the inherent difficulties of all culture types over in vivo neurotoxicological studies. These are also considered in Table

3. It is, therefore, important to balance out all the factors in Tables 2 and 3 whether designing experiments for investigating neurotoxicity mechanisms at the cellular level, or choosing a model to act as a neurotoxicological pre-development screen for pharmacologically interesting drug candidates.

Acknowledgement

The author would like to thank all the collaborators involved in work described in this review, particularly Dr Alan Prince and Miss Alison Pillar with whom work on ECMA was carried out.

REFERENCES

Archer, T. & Fowler, C.J. (1985). In "Trends in Pharmacological Sciences (TIPS)" February 1985. p61 (Elsevier, Amsterdam).

Atterwill, C.K., Atkinson, D.J., Bermudez, I. & Balazs, R. (1985). Effect of thyroid hormone and serum on the development of Na^+,K^+-ATPage and associated ion-fluxes in cultures from rat brain. Neuroscience, 14, 361-373.

Atterwill, C.K. & Bowen, D. (1986). Neurotrophic factor(s) for central cholinergic neurones is present in both normal and Alzheimer brain tissue. Acta. Neuropathologica., 69, 341-342

Atterwill, C.K. & Collins, P. (1986). Development of Na^+, K^+-ATPase molecular forms in rat brain in vivo and in vitro. The Toxicologist, 6, (1) 772.

Atterwill, C.K., Kingsbury, A. and Balazs, R. (1983). Effect of thyroid hormone on neural development in vitro. In 'Drugs & Hormones in Brain Development'. Ed. Lichtensteiger, W. & Schlumpf, M.S., Karger, Basle.

Atterwill, C.K., Nicholls, J, Kingsbury, A. & Prince, A.K. (1984). Development of Markets for cholinergic neurones in reaggregate cultures of foetal rat whole brain in serum-containing and serum-free media: effects of triiodothyronine. Brit.J. Pharmacol., 83, 89-102.

Bottenstein, J.E. & Sato, G.H. (1979). Growth of rat neuroblastoma cell line in serum-free supplemented medium. Proc. Natl. Acad. Sci. (USA), 76, 514-517.

Cohen, S.R. & Murray, M.R. (1982). Myelin formation in rotation-mediated aggregating cell cultures : immunocytochemical, electron microscopic and biochemical observations. J. Neurosci., 2, 986-993.

Dewar, A.J. (1981). "Neurotoxicity testing - with particular reference to biochemical methods". In Testing for Toxicity. Ed. J.W. Gorrod, Taylor & Francis Ltd., London, pp 199-217.

Garber, B.B. & Moscona, A.A. (1972, II). Reconstruction of brain tissue from cell cuspensions. II. Specific enhancement of aggregation of embryonic cerebral cells by supernatant from homologous cell cultures. Devel. Biol, 27, 235-243.

Garber, B.B. & Moscona, A.A. (1972, I). Reconstruction of brain tissue from brain suspensions. Aggregation patterns of cells dissociated from different regions of the developing brain. Devel. Biol., 27, 217-234.

Guentert-Lauber, B. & Honegger, P. (1983). Epidermal growth factor (EGF) stimulation of cultured brain cells. II. Increased production of extracellular soluble proteins. Devel. Brain Res., 11, 253-260.

Honegger, P. & Lenoir, D., (1980). Triiodothyronine enhancement of neuronal differntiation in aggreating fetal rat brain cells cultured in a chemically defined medium. Brain Res. 199, 425-434.

Honegger, P. & Richardson, E. (1977). Kainic acid alters neurochemical development in fetal rat brain aggregating cell cultures. Brain Res. 138, 580-584.

Honegger, P. & Lenoir, D. (1982). Nerve growth factor (NGF). Stimulation of cholinergic telencephalic neurons in aggregating cell cultures. Devel. Brain Res., 3, 229-238.

Honegger, P. & Richelson, E. (1977). Biochemical differentiation of aggregating cell cultures of different fetal rat brain regions. Brain Res., 133, 329-339.

Lenoir, D. & Honegger, P. (1983). Insulin-like growth factor I (IGF-I) stimulates DNA synthesis in fetal rat brain cell cultures. Develop. Brain Res. 7, 205-213.

Majocha, R.E., Pearse, R.N., Baldessarini, R.J., Delong, G.R. & Walton, K.G. (1981). The noradrenergic system in cultured aggregates of fetal rat brain cells : Morphology of the aggregates and pharmacological indices of noradrenergic neurons. Brain Res., 230, 235-252.

Moscona, A.A. (1952). Cell suspensions from organ rudiments of chick embryos Exp. Cell. Res., 3, 535-539.

Orkand, P.M., Lindner, J. & Schachner, M. (1984). Specificity of histiotypic organization and synpaptogenesis in reaggregating cell cultures of mouse cerebellum. Devel. Brain Res., 16, 119-134.

Ramirez, G., Manrique, E., Barat, A. & Villa, S. (1980). From "Tissue Culture in Neurobiology". Ed. E. Giacobini et al., Raven Press, New York. p.129.

Sandberg, K., Schnaar, R.L., McKinney, M., Hanin, I., Fisher, A. & Coyle, J.T. (1985). AF64A: An active-stie directed irreversible inhibitor of choline acetyltransferase. J. Neurochem., 44, 439-445.

Schrier, B.K. (1982). "Nervous System Cultures as Toxicologic Test Systems". In Nervous System Toxicology. Ed. Sy. C.L. Mitchell, Raven Press, New York. pp 337-348.

Seeds, N.W., Haffke, S.C. & Krystosek, A. (1980). From "Tissue Culture in Neurobiology". ed. Sy. E. Giacobini et al., Raven Press, New York. p.145.

Shalaby, I.A., Hoffmann, P.C. & Heller, A. (1984). Release of dopamine from mesencephalic neurone in aggregate cultures: influence of target and non-target cells. Brain Res., 307, 347-350.

Simon, R.G. & Klein, W.L. (1983). Differential regulation of muscarinic and nicotinic receptors by cholinergic stimulation in cultured avian retina cells. Brain Res., 262, 99-108.

Spencer, P.S. & Schaumburg, H.H. (1980). Experimental and Clinical Neurotoxicology. Williams & Wilkins, Baltimore/London.

Staffstrom, G.E., Johnson, D., Wehner, J.M. & Sheppard, J.R. (1986). Spontaneous neural activity in fetal brain reaggregate cultures. Neuroscience, 5, 1681-1689.

Trapp, B.P., Honegger, P., Richelson, E. & Webster, H.F. (1979). Morphological differentiation of mechanically dissociated fetal rat brain in aggregating cell cultures. Brain Res., 160, 117-130.

Trapp, B.P. & Richelson, E. (1980). In "Experimental and Clinical Neurotoxicology". Ed. Spencer, P.S. & Schaumburg, H.H. (Williams & Wilkins, Baltimore/London) pp 803-819.

Walsh, T.J., Tilson, H.A., De Haven, D.L., Mailman, R.B., Fisher, A. & Hanin, I. (1984). AF64A: a cholinergic neurotoxin selectively depletes acetylcholine in hippocampus and cortex, and produces long-term passive avoidance and radial-arm maze deficits in the rat. Brain Res., 321, 91-102.

Wehner, J.M., Feinman, R.D. & Sheppard, J.K. (1982). Beta-adrenergic response in mouse CNS reaggregate cultures. Devel. Brain Res., 3, 207-217.

Wehner, J.M., Smolen, A., Ness-Smolen, T. & Murphy, C. (1985). Recovery of acetylcholinesterase activity after acute organophosphate treatment of CNS reaggregate cultures. Fund. Appl. Toxicology, 5, 1104-1109.

Wolfe, B.B., Augustyn, D.H., Majocha, R.E., Dibner, M.D., Molinoff, P.B., Baldessarini, R.J. & Walton, K.G. (1981). Effects of isoproterenol on the development of beta-adrenergic receptors in brain cell aggregates. Brain Res., 207, 174-177.

Woodhams, P.L., Atterwill, C.K. & Balazs, R. (1986) An immunocytochemical study of the effects of thyroid hormone in rat brain aggregating cultures. Neuropath. Applied Neurobiol. IN PRESS.

Yonezawa, T., Bornstein, M.B. & Peterson, E.R. (1986). "Organotypic Cultures of Nerve Tissue as a model system for neurotoxicity investigation and screening. In. Experimental and Clinical Neurotoxicology. Ed. Spencer., P.S. and Schaumburg, H.H., Williams & Wilkins, Baltimore/London. pp 788-802.

APPLICATION OF THRYOID CELL CULTURE TO THE STUDY OF THYROTOXICITY

C.G. Brown
Smith Kline & French Research Ltd., The Frythe, Welwyn, Herts., AL6 9AR, U.K.

INTRODUCTION

The technique of thyroid cell culture provides a novel approach to the study of potential adverse effects of compounds or drugs on the thyroid gland. An assessment of drug-induced thyrotoxicity *in vitro* can be achieved economically in terms of time, quantities of test compound and numbers of animals. Furthermore, good tissue culture models permit human thyroid cell culture studies to be performed.

Identification of thyrotoxicity *in vivo* is usually achieved by observations of histopathological changes in the thyroid glands. These changes may arise either by a direct action on the thyroid gland or indirectly by altering hypothalamic thyrotrophin releasing hormone (TRH) and pituitary thyroid stimulating hormone (TSH) secretion, or target tissue and hepatic thyroid hormone metabolism. An advantage of *in vitro* studies is that they allow the thyroid cells to be examined in isolation from the inevitably complex and undefined interactions with their environment *in vivo*.

Over the past fifteen years numerous thyroid *in vitro* systems have been developed including primary and continuous thyroid cell culture, tissue slices and cell suspension culture. This chapter will focus on the practical aspects of primary and continuous cell culture. For details of the other thyroid *in vitro* methods the reader is referred to the following papers: Nitsch, *et al*. (1984); Heldin, *et al*. (1985); Schuman, *et al*. (1976).

Integration of thyroid cells into a follicular epithelium is an essential prerequesite of normal thyroid function since, as a consequence of this integration, thyroid cells gain polarity, and directional transport of material takes place. A model system of thyroid cells in culture, able to reproduce the main functional characteristics of the thyroid gland, should therefore resemble in vivo thyroid follicles.

The major component of colloid, thyroglobulin, is synthesised in the rough endoplasmic reticulum and the Golgi apparatus, transported to the apical pole of the cell, iodinated, and packed in vesicles which, via exocytosis, discharge their contents into the follicular lumen. Storage and endocytosis of iodinated thyroglobulin cannot occur within isolated cells; the latter are only capable of partial thyroid function.

Conditions under which histiotypic organization into follicle-like structures can be obtained have been described for primary thyrocyte cultures initiated from a number of species including sheep (Mothershill, et al. 1984), pig (Fayet & Hovsepian, 1977), dog (Roger & Dumont, 1984) and human (Dickson, et al. 1981). These studies have concentrated on the application of this technique to elucidating pharmacological and biochemical responses of thyroid cells and establishing a bioassay for thyroid stimulating auto-antibodies.

Having considered the requirements for a thyroid culture model, the following sections will describe the biochemical parameters used to assess functional effects on thyroid cells and the optimum conditions for reconstructing porcine thyroid follicles in vitro. The continuous culture systems to be described are the rat FRTL and FRTL-5 cell lines. These cells are partially de-differentiated and do not form follicular structures in culture and consequently do not organify iodide. They do, however, retain responsiveness towards TSH, as determined by the accumulation of both intracellular cyclic AMP and inorganic iodide, and are of use in assessing effects of compounds on these intracellular processes. The application of these techniques to the identification and study of thyrotoxicity will be described.

PRACTICAL ASPECTS

a) Biochemical parameters of thyroid cell function.

The unique functional parameters of thyroid follicular cells are shown diagrammatically in figure 1. It is generally accepted that transport of iodide is linked to the activity of Na^+K^+ATPase and that there is a co-transport between Na^+ and I^- in the thyroid epithelial cell (Wolff & Halmi, 1963). The second messenger for TSH receptor stimulation is thought to be cyclic AMP and alterations in intracellular protein phosphorylation lead to stimulation of iodide uptake and organification by the thyroid peroxidase enzyme (see Tong, 1974). These biochemical responses can be used as indicators of thyroid cell function and interaction with these cellular processes could indicate potential thyrotoxicity.

Figure 1: Biochemical parameters of thyroid cell function

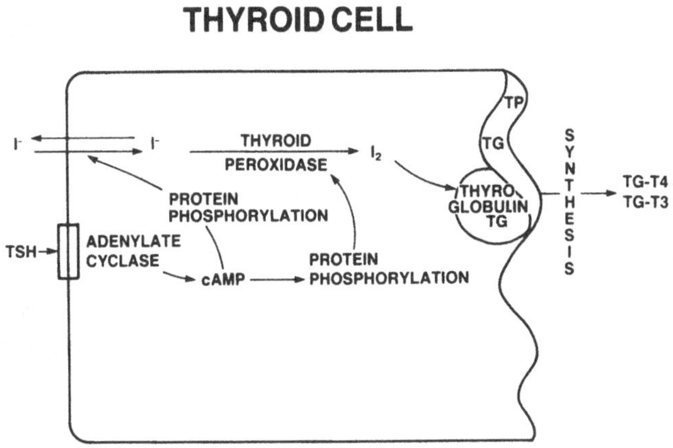

Thyrotoxicity could arise by alterations in cyclic AMP synthesis (Weiss, et al. 1984) or $Na^{+}K^{+}$ ATPase activity (ibid) which play an integral role in the capacity of the cells to concentrate iodide. Inhibitors of peroxidase also have profound effects on iodide metabolism in thyroid cells (Dickson et al. 1981). The site of action of the various compounds within the thyroid cells will determine at which point thyroid function is disturbed. Certain compounds such as anions (e.g. perchlorate and pertechnate), iodine containing compounds (e.g. iopanoic acid, amiodarone) or the $Na^{+}K^{+}$ATPase inhibitor ouabain will primarily affect iodide uptake, whereas peroxidase inhibitors affect iodide organification while having little effect on iodide uptake *in vitro*.

Reagents and Tissue Culture media

TSH has been reported to be an essential constituent of culture media, necessary to obtain the reorganization of cells into follicles (Winand & Kohn, 1975). In its absence, thyroid cells form a monolayer on the culture substratum and lose their capacity to concentrate and to bind iodide (Lissitzky, et al. 1971). Other hormone supplements necessary for optimum culture of thyroid cells have been characterised by Ambesi-Impiombato, et al. (1980). These include insulin, hydrocortisone, transferrin, glycyl-histidyl-lysine and somatostatin. Some reports have also indicated that a reduction of the serum concentration in, or its elimination from, the culture media has a permissive effect on the formation and the maintenance of thyroid follicles *in vitro* (Dickson et al. 1981; Ambesi-Impiombato et al. 1980).

The basic medium recommended for culture of FRTL and FRTL-5 cells and porcine thyrocyte culture is Ham's F12 (Flow Labs, Herts, U.K.) containing a hormone supplement: bovine TSH (10mu/ml, Sigma, Dorset U.K.), insulin (10µg/ml), cortisol (10^{-8} mol/l), transferrin (5µg/ml), glycyl-l-histidyl-l-lysine acetate (10µg/ml) and somatostatin (10µg/ml) (all from C P Laboratories, Herts, U.K.) and antibiotics penicillin (100u/ml) and streptomycin (100µg/ml). This medium is referred to as 6H or 5H when TSH is present or absent respectively. These hormones are made up as 60-100 fold concentrated stock solutions in Ca^{++} and Mg^{++}-free Hanks Balanced Salts Solution (HBSS, Flow Labs, U.K.) divided into aliquots and stored at -20°C until required. The complete medium is stored at 4°C for periods of no longer than 14 days.

Culture of porcine thyroid cells.

Porcine thyroid glands are obtained from a local abbatoir and transported to the laboratory within 1 hour of slaughter in ice-cold calcium and magnesium-free HBSS containing penicillin (200u/ml) and streptomycin (200µg/ml). Tissue is trimmed and chopped into $1mm^3$ pieces under sterile conditions and washed twice in HBSS and antibiotics. Cell dissociation is achieved by incubating in a trypsin (0.25%) collagenase (0.05%) and chicken serum (2%) mixture (CTC solution) for 1 hour at 37°C with constant stirring. The dispersed cells are filtered through sterile nylon gauze (150 mesh) and precipitated by centrifugation at 200 g for 5 minutes. Following 2 washes in 5H medium containing 5% newborn calf serum (Imperial Labs., Salisbury, Wilts., U.K.), the cells are resuspended in 5H medium containing either 50µU/ml TSH (or, when assessing the dose-response relationship to TSH, various concentrations from 5-500µU/ml TSH) and 0.5% newborn calf serum. Cell viability is typically >90% as determined by the exclusion of trypan blue dye (0.1% w/v). Cells are diluted in 5H medium to 2×10^6cells/ml and 500µl of cell suspension added to each well of poly-l-lysine (Sigma Chemical Co, Dorset, U.K.) pretreated (10µg/ml) 24-well culture plates (Linbro, Flow Labs, U.K.) and maintained under 5% CO_2 in air at 37°C in a water-saturated incubator. Following 3 days in culture, the cells are assessed for their ability to accumulate and organify iodide.

Culture of FRTL-5 cells

Rat FRTL-5 cells are obtained from Dr L Kohn, N.I.H., Bethesda, Maryland, U.S.A. as frozen cell suspensions. These are thawed and plated in Coon's modified Ham's F12 medium (6H medium) containing 5% newborn calf serum. Cells are maintained in 10cm polystyrene petri dishes (Falcon plastics) under 5% CO_2 in air at 37°C in a water-saturated incubator.

Sub-culture of FRTL-5 cells is achieved by dissociation in CTC solution. After centrifugation of the cell suspension at 200 x g for 5 minutes and washing in medium, cells are replated to a density of 2 x 10^5 cells/ml (0.5ml/well) in 24-well tissue culture dishes (Linbro, Flow Labs, U.K.) in 6H medium for 3 days. Culture is continued for a period of 7 days in TSH-free medium (5H-medium). On the 8th day of culture, cells are assessed for TSH responsiveness and the effect of test compounds. The medium in each well is replaced by medium containing various TSH concentrations (5-500μU/ml). After 24 hours in culture, the TSH-containing medium is removed and replaced with 5H medium for further 24 hours. Cells are then assessed for their ability to accumulate iodide (see below). Test compound is dissolved in medium or in dimethylsulphoxide (DMSO, BDH Chemicals Limited, Essex) in the case of poorly-water soluble compounds, and incubated with the cells either from the time of TSH stimulation to the iodide uptake experiment, or in the TSH-free 24 hour-period. DMSO is included in the medium (where necessary) at concentrations of up to 1% and the corresponding concentration is included in the control cultures.

The procedure for culture of FRTL cells is identical except for the serum concentration as mentioned above. These cells are commercially available from Flow Laboratories (ATCC No. CRL 1468).

<u>Appearance of rat and porcine thyrocytes in culture</u>

Following protease and collagenase digestion the porcine thyroid tissues are dissociated into mainly single cells with few clumps of approximately 10-20 cells. Generally no whole follicles are isolated. After 3 days in culture in TSH-containing medium, cells are fully reorganized into follicular-like structures (Figure 2). These structures are stable for about 7 days in culture. After this time or in TSH-free medium, cells begin to regress to a monolayer and 'domes' appear as a result of local detachment from the culture plate (Figure 3). The appearance of rat FRTL cells in culture is shown in Figure 4. These cells elaborate processes in response to TSH in the medium.

Figure 2: Reorganization of porcine thyroid cells into 'follices' is achieved within 3 days of initiation of culture. Follicle-like structures are indicated by arrows.

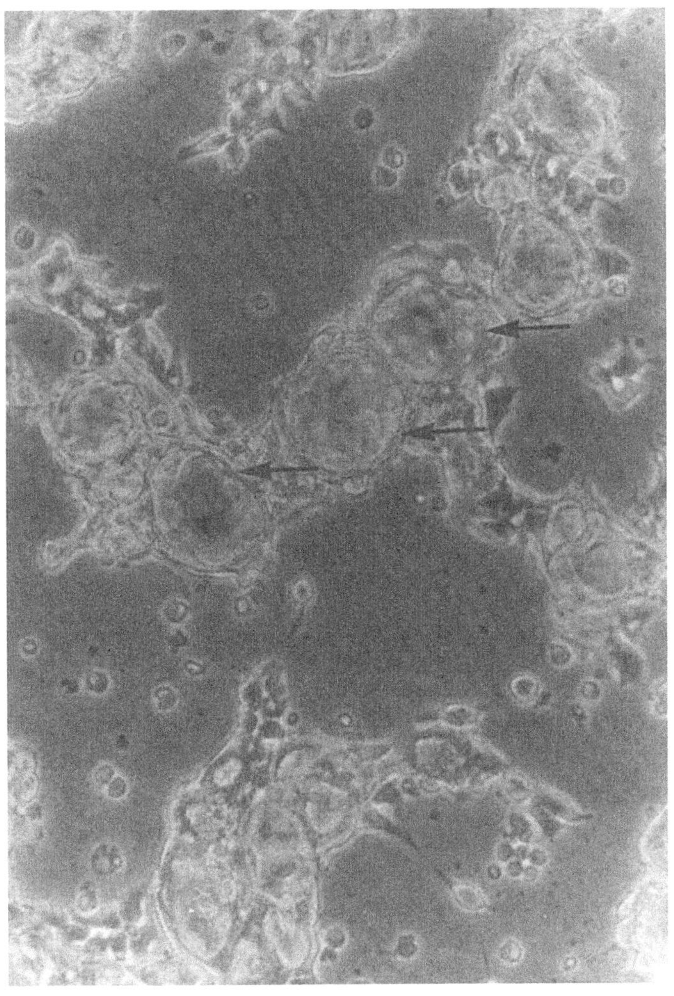

Figure 3: Regression of porcine thyroid cells into a monolayer occurs after approximately 7 days in culture.

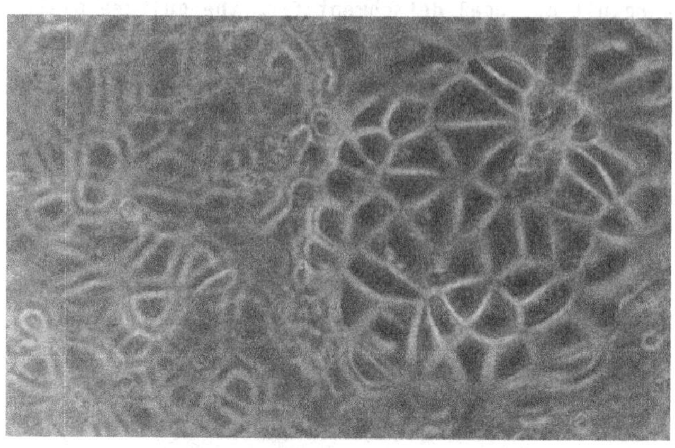

Figure 4: Appearance of rat FRTL cells in culture.

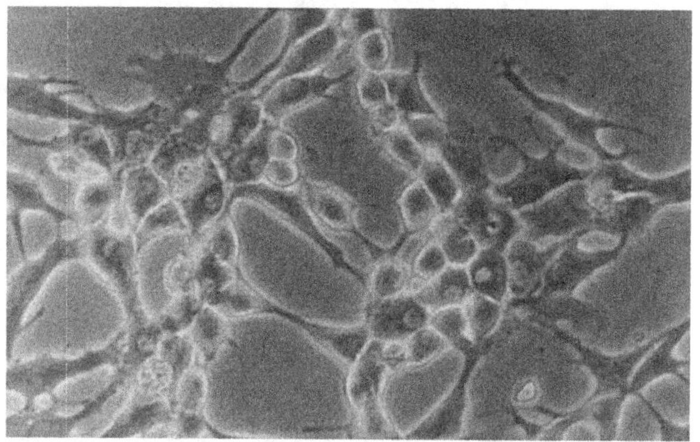

<u>Measurement of iodide uptake and/or organification</u>

Determination of iodide uptake is made by removing the medium from the cells and washing with 1ml of buffered HBSS. The assays are initiated by overlaying the cells with 500µl of buffered HBSS containing 0.1µCi carrier-free $Na^{125}I$ (Amersham International plc, Bucks, U.K.) and 10µM $Na^{127}I$. Incubations are carried out for 1 hour (rat cells) or 5 hours (porcine cells) after which the medium is aspirated and the cell layer washed once with ice-cold HBSS. For rat cells, cellular iodide is discharged by incubation with 1ml of 100µM $NaClO_4$ in HBSS for 1 hour at 37°C. γ-emission associated with 100µl aliquots of the perchlorate solution provides an estimate of ^{125}I-uptake. For porcine thyrocytes the cell layer is dissolved in 0.1M NaOH for approximately 20 hours. The γ-emission associated with this fraction provides an estimate of ^{125}I-uptake. The absolute amount of radioactivity taken up by the thyroid cells will vary according to cell plating density but normally, using this amount of radioactivity between 10-20 x 10^3 cpm will be taken up per well by cells stimulated by 100µl/ml TSH. Protein bound iodide (organified iodide) is precipitated with 10% trichloroacetic acid (TCA) solution and separated from free iodide by centrifugation at 1000 g for 5 minutes. The γ-emission in the TCA-precipitate represents iodide organification. Approximately 30-50% of iodide taken up should be organified. Test compounds were included in the medium during the ^{125}I-uptake experiment as appropriate.

Effects of test compounds on cell viability

It is important to differentiate between biochemical responses and cytotoxic effects of the compounds under investigation. Thyroid cells contain significant amounts of lactate dehydrogenase (LDH) (Wroblewski & Gregory, 1961) and leakage of LDH into the culture medium can be used as an indication of the integrity of the thyroid cell membranes. It should be noted however that a compound which affects iodide organification without effects on iodide uptake is unlikely to be affecting cell viability since the latter process is strictly dependent on the activity of membrane-bound ATPase and on complete integrity of the thyroid cell membranes.

Responses to TSH: iodide uptake and organification

Characterisation of the time-course and dose-response relationship of basal and TSH-stimulated ^{125}I-uptake by porcine thyrocytes is shown in Figures 5 and 6. ^{125}I-uptake is maximal at approximately 2 hours of incubation in the presence of $Na^{125}I$ (Figure 5). TSH stimulates ^{125}I-uptake in a dose-dependent manner (Figure 6). A significant increase in iodide uptake can be obtained with very low concentrations of TSH (5μU/ml). This concentration is equivalent to 0.125 ng/ml as this TSH has an approximate activity of 40IU/mg on bioassay. Since the physiological plasma levels of TSH in rats are between 1 and 5ng/ml the sensitivity of the thyroid cells to TSH is well within the physiological range.

Figure 5: Time course of ^{125}I-uptake by porcine thyrocytes. Mean ± s.e.m. of determinations in 6 culture dishes.

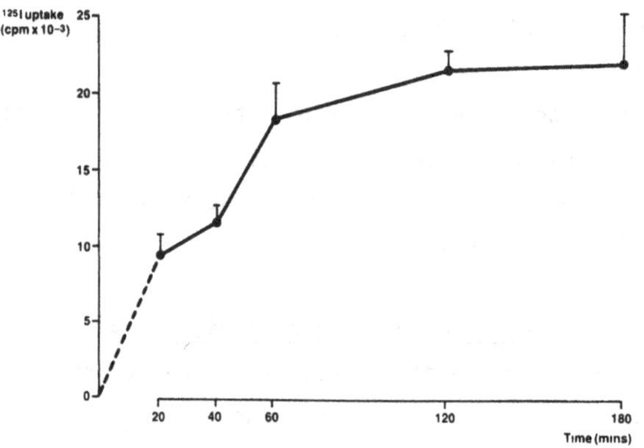

Figure 6: ^{125}I-uptake in response to TSH 0-500μU/ml alone or in the presence of sodium perchlorate (1mM).

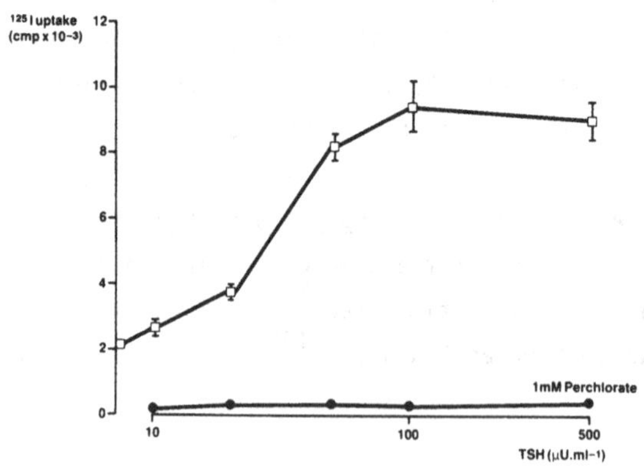

The experimental protocol for evaluating iodide uptake in FRTL-5 cells has been fully validated elsewhere (Bidey, et al. 1984). These cells show similar sensitivity to TSH to the porcine thyrocytes. Validation of this method can be further achieved by examining response to compounds such as perchlorate or methimazole (MTI) which are known to affect thyroid iodide metabolism directly. When evaluating effects of novel compounds it is useful to include compounds such as these in the experiments as 'positive controls' to confirm responsiveness of the thyroid cells.

EXPERIMENTAL EXAMPLES

Several compounds have been examined in this laboratory for their ability to perturb iodide metabolism in thyroid cells. One of these is an H_2-receptor antagonist SK&F 93479 (2-[2-(5-(-Dimethylamino-methyl)furan-2-ylmethylthio)-ethylamino]-5-(6-methylpyrid-3-ylmethyl) pyrimidin-4-one trihydrochloride). *In vivo* toxicity studies using this compound have indicated that oral administration of high doses of SK&F 93479 (400-1000 mg/kg) to rats for periods of 7 days or more is associated with thyroid histopathological changes (Harland, et al. 1985). These changes include hypertrophy and hyperplasia of thyroid epithelial cells, and depletion, and agglomeration of colloid in the follicular lumen, which are indicative of increased thyroid activity. Increased thyroid cell activity has been confirmed experimentally by observing increased ^{125}Iodide accumulation by rat thyroid glands *in vivo* (Harland et al. 1985). In order to determine if increased iodide uptake observed *in vivo* is a direct effect of the compound, the effects of SK&F 93479 on iodide metabolism on cultured thyroid cells have been studied.

Figure 7 shows that, in rat FRTL-5 cells, there was no effect of SK&F 93479 at concentrations of 1 or 10μM (concentrations estimated from the maximum plasma concentrations achieved at toxicological doses of SK&F 93479 in the rat), on either basal or TSH-stimulated ^{125}I-uptake. The positive control substance perchlorate (2mM) markedly attenuated iodide uptake.

Figure 7: Effect of SK&F 93479, 3-isobutyl-1-methylxanthine (IBMX) and sodium perchlorate on basal and TSH-stimulated ^{125}I-uptake by rat FRTL-5 cells. Values are mean ± s.e.m. of determinations in 4 culture dishes.

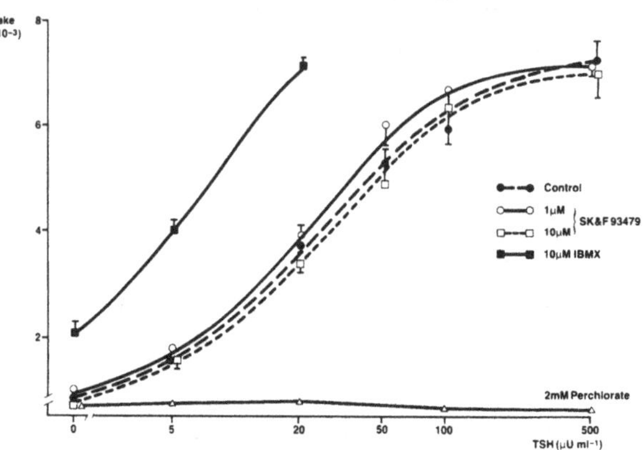

Figure 8: Effect of SK&F 93479, methimazole and propylthiouracil (PTU) on ^{125}I organification in porcine thyroid cells. Values are mean ± s.e.m. of n=4.

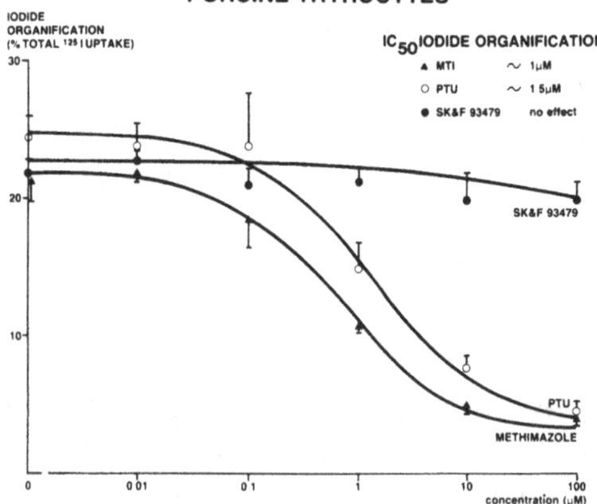

Iodide uptake by porcine thyrocytes was similarly unaffected by SK&F 93479 (data not shown). Iodide organification by these cells is shown in Figure 8. Whereas SK&F 93479 had no effect on iodide organification, MTI and propyl-thiouracil (PTU) produced a concentration-dependent inhibition of iodide organification at concentrations of between 0.01 and 100µM.

The lack of a direct effect of SK&F 93479 on the thyroid gland has been confirmed by studies indicating that the site of action of this compound in initiating a thyrotoxic effect is probably hepatic, by increasing thyroxine clearance. Subsequent increases in pituitary TSH release lead to the increased thyroid activity (Brown, et al. 1986).

An observation of additional interest was the effect of the phosphodiesterase inhibitor 3-isobutyl-1-methyl xanthine (IBMX, 10µM) which is also shown in Figure 7. By increasing the accumulation of intracellular cyclic AMP, this compound would be expected to augment basal and TSH-stimulated iodide uptake. These responses were seen in this experiment and may explain the goitrogenic effects of the methyl xanthines which have been reported in rats in vivo (Studer, et al. 1970).

Several neurotransmitters and putative neurotransmitters such as noradrenaline (NA) (Ahren, 1985), 5-hydroxytryptamine (5HT) (Melander & Sundler, 1972) and acetylcholine (Melander & Sundler, 1979) have been implicated in thyroid physiology. Consequently drugs interacting with these neurotransmitters or their receptors could also influence thyroid activity. The effects of NA, 5HT and effects of adrenergic blocking drugs on iodide metabolism in porcine thyrocytes have been examined in this laboratory.

Figure 9: Effect of propranolol (20μM, shaded histogram) on responses to 5-hydroxytryptamine, noradrenaline and salbutamol in porcine thyroid cells. Values are mean ± s.e.m. of determination in 3 culture dishes.

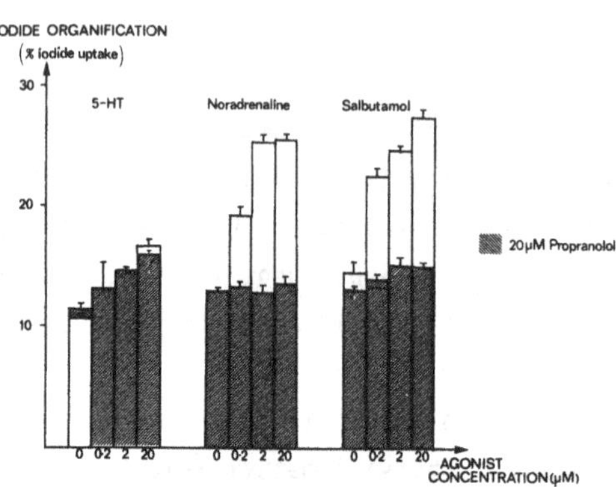

In these experiments agonist compounds were diluted in medium containing 10μM ascorbic acid (BDH Chemicals Ltd., Essex, U.K.) and this ascorbate concentration was also present in control cultures. NA and 5-HT both elicited concentration-dependent increases in iodide organification (Figure 9) whilst having little effect on iodide uptake (data not shown). Salbutamol had a similar effect to NA indicating that stimulation of iodide organification may arise by actions on the β_2-receptor subtype. In the presence of the β-antagonist propranolol (20μM, Sigma, U.K.) the responses to NA and salbutamol but not to 5-HT were abolished. Further support for the β-receptor mediated effect of NA comes from the observation that phentolamine (an α-adrenergic recepter antagonist) had no effect on the stimulation of iodide organification by NA.

Although there are no detailed reports regarding the thyrotoxicity of salbutamol or propranolol, these observations on the effects of these agents are of interest considering the beneficial effect of β-adrenergic receptor blocking drugs in hyperthyroid patients (Verhoeven, et al. 1977), and the contraindication of salbutamol in thyrotoxicosis (Martindale 1982).

Another example of the application of thyroid cell culture in elucidating mechanisms of thyrotoxicity relates to studies on the anticonvulsant aminoglutethimide (AG). This compound was withdrawn from clinical use following reports of goitrous hypothyroidism in treated patients (Hughes & Burley, 1970). Subsequent studies in rats have indicated that AG increases thyroidal ^{125}I uptake and decreases protein-bound iodide release (Studer et al. 1970). Figure 10 shows that AG had marked effects on iodide organification in porcine thyrocytes, being similar in potency to MTI (compare Figure 8). This was in contrast to the structural analogue glutethimide, a major tranquilizer which had no effect on iodide organification (and has no effect on thyroid activity *in vivo*).

Figure 10: Effect of aminoglutethimide on iodide organification in cultured porcine thyroid cells. Values are mean ± s.e.m. of determinations in 4 culture dishes.

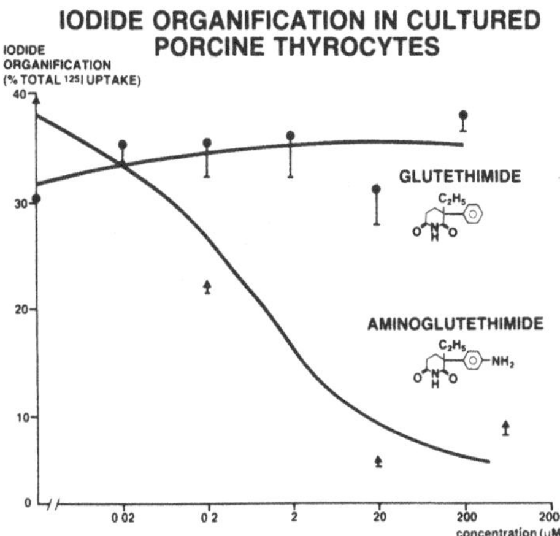

These results demonstrate both the specificity of drug effects on thyroid iodide metabolism *in vitro*, and the potential to examine structure activity relationships of a homologus series of novel compounds using this *in vitro* model.

DISCUSSION AND CONCLUSIONS

It is apparent from a consideration of the previous examples that many compounds can influence thyroid cells directly. The precise mechanism may be complex and may differ for each compound. However, the net result of the interaction is an alteration in iodide uptake and/or organification which is relatively simple to measure using the techniques described here. Other sites at which compounds could act which have not been addressed in this review include the coupling of mono- and di-iodotyrosines to form T_4 and T_3 and the release of thyroid hormones from thyroglobulin. It is unlikely that present day assay systems would have sufficient sensitivity to detect and quantify drug-induced alterations in thyroid hormone release into the culture medium. In this case, another *in vitro* technique such as thyroid slices (Shuman, *et al*. 1976) or thyroid superfusion (Mashita, *et al.* 1982) would be more appropriate.

Two different types of thyroid cell culture have been described: primary (porcine) cell culture and continuous (FRTL) cell culture. Whilst the maintenance of FRTL-cell lines is relatively straight-forward, they are only capable of partial thyroid cell function i.e. they do not organify iodide. To assess effects of compounds on iodide organification it is necessary to use primary cell culture. This procedure is technically more demanding than maintaining a cell line, in addition, these cells do not proliferate in culture and loose responsiveness to TSH within about 7 days. Clearly each culture type has advantages and disadvantages although the study of both cell types can provide useful information regarding potential thyrotoxicity.

A summary of the effects of the compounds discussed in this chapter, together with comparative data from *in vivo* studies is given in Table 1. The effects of the compounds tested *in vitro* on iodide metabolism in the thyroid cells relate closely with *in vivo* data and so far, no false positives or negatives have arisen using this method.

Several of the compounds mentioned have been used in man (MTI, PTU, perchlorate, AG, propranolol and salbutamol) where similar findings have been recorded (i.e. inhibition or stimulation of thyroid activity). Therefore, although species differences in thyroid susceptibility to drugs may exist, the studies reported here indicate that these animal models could provide a good predictive test for potential adverse thyroid effects in man.

The antithyroid activity (peroxidase inhibition) of certain compounds can often be predicted on the basis of chemical structure alone e.g. for the sulphur containing compounds of the thioamide class, methimazole and sulphonamides. However, this is not always the case. Structurally unrelated compounds may also affect thyroid peroxidase activity e.g. aminoglutethimide (Studer, *et al*. 1970) and aminotriazole (Sturm & Karnovsky, 1971). The comparative activities of aminoglutethimide and glutethimide given in this report illustrate that relatively small structural differences can lead to markedly differing antithyroid effects. In addition these results demonstrate the potential of this *in vitro* system for use in examining structure activity relationships. In this respect, where thyrotoxicity has been detected in conventional toxicity studies, this *in vitro* test may aid selection of a 'back-up' from a series of structurally related compounds. This conclusion must come with the caveat that it is only the parent compound or identified metabolites

Table 1: In Vitro/In Vivo correlations

COMPOUND	IODIDE UPTAKE IN VITRO	IODIDE ORGANIFICATION IN VITRO	IN VIVO	REFERENCE
TSH	+	+	Stimulates thyroid activity e.g. Graves disease.	Hall, Smith, Mukhtar (1975)
Perchlorate (K^+ClO_4)	-	No direct effect	Antithyroid compound	Martindale (1982)
Methimazole	No effect	-	Antithyroid compound	Martindale (1982)
Propyl-thiouracil	No effect	-	Antithyroid compound	Martindale (1982)
IBMX	+	+	Potentiates TSH effects→ goitrogenic in rats	Wolff and Varrone (1969)
SK&F 93479	No effect	No effect	No direct effect (rats)	Harland et al (1985)
Noradrenaline (NA)	No effect	+	Stimulatory innervation of thyroid gland (rats)	Melander, Sundler and Westgren (1975)
Salbutamol	No effect	+	Contraindicated in thyrotoxicosis	Martindale (1982)
Propranolol (on NA-stimulated thyrocytes)	No effect	-	1) Lowers thyroid hormone levels (man) 2) Inhibits B_2-receptor-stimulated colloid droplet formation (mouse)	Franklyn et al (1985) Melander et al (1975)
5-hydroxytryptamine	No effect	+	Stimulatory innervation of thyroid gland (rats)	Melander and Sundler (1972)
Aminoglutethimide	No effect	-	Antithyroid effects in man	Santen et al (1977)
Glutethimide	No effect	No effect	No reports of thyroid effects in vivo.	------

which can be studied using these *in vitro* methods, although it may be possible to culture thyroid cells in the presence of a cell preparation (liver S9-fraction) which is capable of metabolic activation (or inactivation) of compound.

Finally it must be noted that there are at present few studies relating to thyroid toxicity *in vitro* and it is the *potential* of this test to be predictive of *in vivo* thyrotoxicity which has been stressed here. A role for thyroid cell culture in toxicology studies must await further correlations of *in vivo* and *in vitro* thyrotoxicity.

REFERENCES

Ahren, B., (1985). Effects of α-adrenoceptor agonists and antagonists on thyroid hormone secretion. Acta. Endocrinol. 108, 184-191

Ambesi-Impiombato, F.S., Parks, L.A.M. & Coon, H.G. (1980). Culture of hormone-dependent functional epithelial cells from rat thyroids. Proc. Natl. Acad. Sci. USA, 77, 3455-3459.

Bidey, S.P., Chiovato, L., Day, A., Turmaine, M., Gould, R.D., Ekins, R.P. & Marshall, N.J. (1984). Evaluation of the rat thyroid cell strain FRTL-5 as an in vitro bioassay for thyrotrophin. J. Endocrinol, 101. 269-276.

Dickson, J.G., Hovsepian, S., Fayet, G & Lissitzky, S. (1981). Follicle formation and iodide metabolism in cultures of human thyroid cells. J. Endocrinol 90, 113-124.

Fayet, G & Hovsepian, S. (1977). Active transport of iodide in isolated porcine thyroid cells, application to an in vitro bioassay of thyrotrophin. Moll. Cell. Endocrinol. 7, 67-78.

Franklyn, J.A., Wilkins, M.R., Wilkinson, R., Ramsden, D.B. & Sheppard, M.C. (1985). The effects of propranolol on circulating thyroid hormone measurements in thyrotoxic and euthyroid subjects. Acta Endocrinol., 108, 351-355.

Hall, R., Smith, B.R. & Mukhtar, E.D. (1975). Thyroid stimulators in health and disease. Clinical Endocrinol., 4, 213-229.

Harland, R.F., Brown, C.G., Salmon, G.K. & Atterwill, C.K. (1985). Effect of an H_2-receptor antagonist on thyroid function. J. Endocrinol 104, Supplement p. 57.

Heldin, N-E., Karlsson, F.A. & Westermark, B. (1985). Inhibition of cyclic AMP formation by iodide in suspension cultures of porcine thyroid follicle cells. Molecular and Cellular Endocrinology 41, 61-67.

Hughes, S.W.M., & Burley, D.M. (1970). Aminoglutethimide: a 'side-effect' turned to therapeutic advantage. Postgraduate Medical Journal 46, 409-416.

Lissitzky, S., Fayet, G., Giraud, A., Verrier, B & Torresani, J. (1971). Thyrotropin-induced aggregation and reorganization into follicles of isolated porcine thyroid cells I. Mechanism of action of thyrotropin and metabolic properties. Eur. J. Biochem. 24, 88-99.

Martindale (1982). The Extra Pharmacopoeia. 28th Edition. Eds. J.E.F. Reynolds, A.B. Prasad, Pharmaceutical Press, London.

Mashita, K., Kawamura, S., Kishino, B., Kimura, H., Nonaka, K. & Tarui, S. (1982). Effects of iodide and propylthiouracil on the relase of 3,5,3,^{1}-triiodothyronine and of cyclic adenosine 3^{1},5^{1}-monophospate from perifused rat thyroids; Endocrinology 110, 1023 - 1029.

Melander, A., Ranklev, E., Sundler, F. & Westgren, U. (1975). β_2-adrenergic stimulation of thyroid hormone secretion. Endocrinology 97, 332-336.

Melander, A. & Sundler, F. (1972). Interactions between catecholamines, 5-hydroxtryptamine and TSH on the secretion of thyroid hormone. Endocrinology 90, 188 - 193.

Melander, A. & Sundler, F. (1979). Presence and influence of cholinergic nerves in the mouse thyroid. Endocrinology, 105, 7-9.

Melander, A., Sundler, F. & Westren, U. (1975). Sympathetic innervation of the thyroid : Variation with species and with age. Endocrinol., 96, 102-106.

Mothershill, C., Seymour, C. & Malone, J.F. (1984). Maintenance of differentiated sheep thyroid cells in primary culture for three months. Acta Endocrinolgica 107, 54-59.

Nitsch, Li, Taccheti, C., Tramonato, D., & Ambesi-Impiombato, F.S. (1984). Suspension culture reveals a morphogenic property of a thyroid epithelial cell line. Experimental Cell Research 152, 22-30.

Roger, P.P. & Dumont, J.E. (1984). Factors controlling proliferation and differentiation of canine thyroid cells cultured in reduced serum conditions: effects of thyrotrophin, cyclic AMP and growth factors. Molecular and Cellular Endocrinolgoy, 36, 79-93.

Santen, R.J., Wells, S.A., Cohn, N., Demers, L.M., Misbin, R.I. & Flotz, E.L. (1977). Compensatory increase in TSH secretion without effect on prolactin secretion in patients treated with aminogluthethimide. J. Clin. Endo. Metab., 45, 739-746.

Shuman, S.J., Zor, U., Chayoth, R & Field, J.B. (1976). Exposure of thyroid slices to thyroid-stimulating hormone induces refractoriness of the cyclic AMP system to subsequent hormone stimulation. Journal of Clinical Investigation, 57, 1132-1141.

Studer H., Kohler, H., Burgi, H., Dorner, E., Forster, R. & Rohner, R. (1970). Goiters with high radioiodine uptake and other characteristics of iodine deficiency in rats chronically treated with aminoglutethimide. Endocrinolgy. 87, 905-914.

Strum, J.M., & Karnovsky, M.J. (1971). Aminotriazole Goiter: Fine Structure and localization of thyroid peroxidase activity. Laboratory Invest. 24, 1-12.

Tong, W. (1974). Actions of thyroid-stimulating hormone in Handbook of Physiology Section 7, Vol. III. Eds. Greer, M.A., Solomon, D.H., Am. Physiological Society, Washington.

Verhoeven, R.P., Visser, T.J., Docter, R., Henneman, G., & Schalekamp, M. (1977). Plasma thyroxine, $3,3^{1}$, 5-triiodothyronine and $3,3^{1}5^{1}$-triiodothyronine during ß-adrenergic blockade in hyperthyroidism, J. Clin. Endo. Metab., 44, 1002-1005.

Weiss, S.J., Philp, N.J., Ambesi-Impiombato, F.S., & Grollman, E.F. (1984). Thyrotropin-stimulated iodide transport mediated by adenosine-3'5'-monophosphate and dependent on protein synthesis. Endocrinology 114, 1099 - 1107.

Winand, R.J. & Kohn, L.D. (1975). Thyrotropin effects on thyroid cells in culture. Effects of trypsin on the thyrotropin mediated cyclic 3'5' AMP changes. J. Biol. Chem., 250, 6534-6540.

Wolff, J. & Halmi, N.S. (1963). Thyroidal iodide transport. The role of $Na^{+}K^{+}$ activated, ouabain sensitive adenosinetriphosphatase activity. J. Biol. Chem., 238, 847-851.

Wolff, J., & Varrone, S. (1969). The methyl-xanthines a new class of goitrogens. Endocrinology 85, 410-414.

Wroblewski, F. & Gregory, K.F. (1961). Lactic dehydrogenase isozymes and their distribution in normal tissues and plasma and in disease states. Ann. N.Y. Acad. Sci., 94, 912-932

In Vitro Methods to Investigate Toxic Lung Disease

A Poole
Smith Kline & French Research Ltd. The Frythe, Welwyn, Herts

R C Brown
MRC Toxicology Unit, Carshalton. Surrey SMF 4EF

INTRODUCTION

The lungs are a major route of entry into the body and as such are constantly exposed either inadvertantly or (as in the case of tobacco smoke) deliberately to a wide range of toxic materials. Some toxicological changes result not from an agent being innately or specifically toxic to the lung but simply because lung cells are the first target encountered. Some materials may then become trapped and accumulate in the respiratory tract. Other substances, such as paraquat and 4-ipomeanol, apparently demonstrate a selective toxicity for specific target cells in the lung. This latter type of lung toxicity may occur even if the route of entry into the body is by a non-pulmonary route.

In addition to respiration the lung is involved in the synthesis, release and removal from the circulation of various mediators such as the prostaglandins and kinins. Insult to the lung is capable of perturbing any of these pulmonary functions. In clinical practice radiography and tests of respiratory function are the usual methods used to assess the structural and functional state of the lungs. For this reason alterations in lung function are rarely detected before the pulmonary architecture is damaged sufficiently to affect x-ray appearance or gas exchange. However, even these classical methods of detecting lung damage in humans are not widely available for use with experimental animals. Even on the rare occasion where some simplified version of them is available their use may not help the experimentor understand those biological processes which ultimately result in the observed pathological effect.

For this reason many workers have turned to the use of in vitro methods in order to investigate the mechanisms underlying the development of toxic endpoints in the lung. Theoretically such techniques allow the investigator to study the action of toxic materials on lung cells in a somewhat more defined environment than that occuring in the intact animal. The use of viable cells (or tissue) in culture also has many advantages over perfused lung preparations which last at most only a few hours and begin to deteriorate in minutes.

PRACTICAL ASPECTS

The lung consists of upwards of 40 different cell types (for examples see Figure 1 & 2), the proportion of which varies considerably in different anatomical regions, this heterogeneity complicates any attempts to isolate pure cell populations and maintain them in culture.

Despite the problems there are numerous references to the application of tissue culture to lung research. In general, the methods which have been used are similar to those used by other investigators studying less heterogeneous organs. Naturally in a short review such as this it is impractical to discuss and precis all the many approaches and techniques which have been published. However, many of the methods which have been used successfully for the isolation and study of lung cells from the various regions of the lung are described below.

We have included a description of studies on cells which although isolated from the lung are not organotypic. These have been regarded by some authors as especially useful in the study of pulmonary toxins simply because of their origin. While we consider this approach to be debatable (see discussion) a consideration of such studies is included for completeness. No attempt has been made

Figure 1

The bronchiolar epithelium, consisting of ciliated (C) and non-ciliated (N) cells, overlies fibroblasts (F) and smooth muscle cells (M) of the lamina propria. Erythrocytes (R), platelets (P) and a lymphocyte (L) are present in the adjacent alveolar septum. The alveoli are lined by Type I pneumocytes (I) and the capillaries are lined by endothelial cells (E).
bar = 10µm.

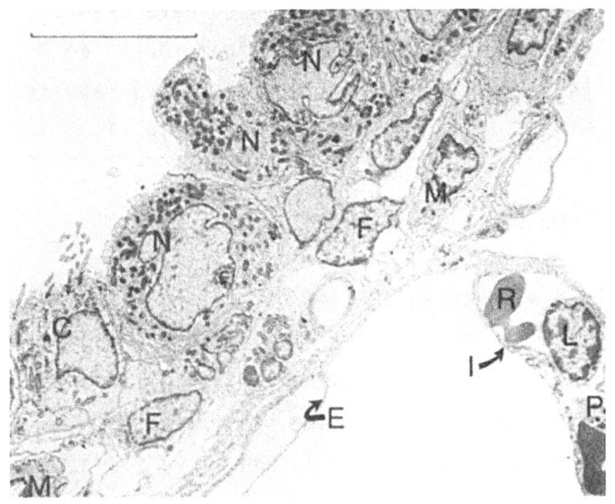

Figure 2

A Type II pneumocyte (II), fibroblasts (F) and associated collagen (C) at the junction of two alveolar septa. A macrophage (M) overlies the Type I pneumocytes (I) lining the alveoli (A) and an erythrocyte (R) is present within one of the capillaries lined with endothelial cells (E).
bar = 1µm.

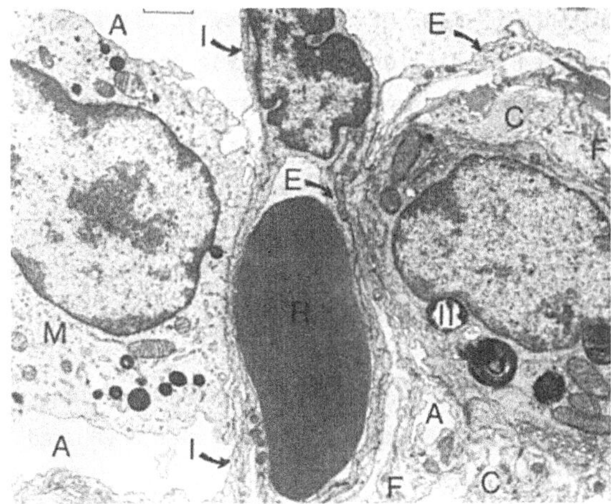

(Figures courtesy of Dr D Dinsdale)

to include the literature on the isolation, growth and use of malignant cells of pulmonary origin.

EXPERIMENTAL EXAMPLES

For this review the lungs have been divided into three regions: the airways, alveoli and pleura. The methods which have been used for the isolation and study of tissue and cells from these regions are described below. (A summary of methods for isolating lung cells and their use in toxicological studies is shown in Table 1).

Cells and tissues from the airways

The airways are lined with an epithelium consisting largely of ciliated and mucous cells with, at the level of the bronchioles, a significant number of non-ciliated (Clara) cells. Scattered in the epithelium are glands (whose location and number varies with species), several types of endocrine cell and nerve fibres. Under the epithelium is a layer of connective tissue with cartilaginous plates at the level of the trachea.

In vitro studies of toxic effects on the cells making up the airways have mainly used organ culture systems (as described by Trowell, 1959) or explant cultures. Many of the methods in use today resemble those developed by earlier workers (for review see Aydelotte, 1965). The modern experimenter can however exploit such methods more fully; the availability of commercial tissue culture equipment, media and medium supplements, and the use of powerful analytical tools (such as image analysis, radioactive and immunological assays) has enabled more data to be extracted from experiments that now require less effort than was formerly the case.

In order to study the activities of the airways epithelium explants have been placed in culture and then epithelial cells allowed to grow out of the tissue to form monolayers (Nevo *et al*, 1975). Such cultures, in common with explants from other tissues, also contain fibroblasts from the connective tissue and because of the slow

Table 1

Lung Cells in Tissue Culture and Their Use in Toxicology - A Summary

Cell Type	Major method of isolation	References	Uses and Limitations
Bronchial epithelium	Organ culture Explant culture Enzymic digestion and gradient centifugation	Aydelotte (1965) Stones *et al*, (1980) Goldman *et al*, (1980)	Useful cells for studies in airway secretion and neoplastic changes.
Clara cells	Enzyme digestion and elutration	Devereux *et al*, (1980) Jones *et al*, (1982) Minchin *et al*, (1985) Sonstergard *et al*, (1979)	Studies in the detoxification and activation of endogenous and exogenous substances.
Neuroendocrine cell	Explant Enzymic dissociation with gradient centrifugation	Curtz *et al*, (1985)	Due to shortage of data difficult to be precise about how useful such cells will prove - in theory could be of value for studying lung cancer and lung injury as well as basic biology of lung endocrine function.
Type I pneumocytes	Gravity separation on a 3-6% Ficoll gradient	Piccianno *et al*, (1978)	Primarily an air tissue barrier with little specialised function - of little interest to the experimental toxicologist.
Type II pneumocyte	Enzymic digestion and density gradient centrifugation	Witschi, (1976) Smith (1977) Li *et al*, (1983)	Large number of specialised functions including xenobiotic and pulmonary surfactant metabolism. The establishment of cell lines with there properties make such cultures very valuable in tox studies.

Table 1 (cont'd)

Lung Cells in Tissue Culture and Their Use in Toxicology – A Summary

Cell Type	Major method of isolation	References	Uses and Limitations
Fibroblasts	Explant cultures enzymic dispersion	Bradley *et al*, (1980)	Lung fibroblasts do not appear to have any specific functional properties or quantitative differences which make them any more useful than similar cells derived from other tissues or continuous cell lines.
Endothelial	Enzymic dispersion	Johnson (1980) Habliston *et al*, (1979)	There is no evidence of a specific function of pulmonary endothelial cells not seen in cells from other organs. Nevertheless endothelial cells, irrespective of their source of origin, are most useful in a variety of studies investigating metabolism aspects of endothelial function.
Macrophages	Bronchoalveolar lavage	Brain *et al* (1985)	It is difficult to obtain large numbers of alveoli macrophages for experimental purposes.
Mesothelial	Mechanical dispersion	Jaurand *et al* (1981)	Have little specialised function and of little use.

growth of the epithelial cells the fibroblasts gradually become dominant. Attempts have therefore been made to remove underlying tissue from the epithelium and then maintain the epithelial layer as explant cultures. Cells maintained as primary explants can reportedly retain some differentiated functions for up to 6 months (Stones 1980). Cells derived from such cultures reportedly have mucin vesicles and cilia and secrete both acidic and neutral glycoproteins into the culture medium (Mossman _et al_, 1980).

Chilton _et al_ (1981) produced a population enriched in basal and mucosal cells by using a pronase digestion of the epithelial surface followed by gravity sedimentation. These investigators did not, however, attempt to maintain these cells in culture but conducted their experiments on the freshly isolated cell suspensions.

The discovery that monooxygenase activity in the lung is concentrated mainly in the non-ciliated Clara cells (Boyd _et al_, 1977; Minchin and Boyd, 1983) provided a major impetus for attempts to isolate populations of this cell type. A number of researchers (Devereux and Fouts, 1980; Jones _et al_, 1982; Sivarajah _et al_, 1983) used pronase digestion, followed by mincing and filtration to produce cell suspensions from which Clara cells have been concentrated by centrifugal elutriation. For example Minchin _et al_ (1985) used collagenase digestion and elutriation to produce 7 different populations of lung cells including a Clara cell fraction.

The isolation and preparation of other cells from the epithelium has posed more difficulties. For example, there are a few reports of attempts to isolate and study neuroendocrine cells _in vitro_. Sonstegard _et al_ (1979) reported both morphological and metabolic studies on these cells using lung explants from foetal rabbits. More recently Curtz _et al_ (1985) isolated neuroendothelial cells from foetal rabbit lung using mechanical and enzymatic dissociation followed by separation and enrichment on a Percoll gradient. They reported that the neuroendocrine cells, which could be maintained in culture for up to seven days, were suitable for investigations into the role and function of the pulmonary neuroendothelial cell system. Difficulties in identifying neuroendocrine cells and their relative infrequency has, however, ensured that such studies remain a rarity.

The lung parenchyma

In some studies no attempt has been made to purify the cells after isolation, for example Tompa and Langenbach (1979) studied benzo (a) pyrene metabolism in cultures consisting of epithelial cells, endothelial cells and macrophages. They reported significant differences between metabolism in such cultures and ones derived from the liver. Organ cultures of lung, consisting mainly of parenchyma, has contributed a great deal to our knowledge of pulmonary biochemistry. Again this is particularly true of the metabolism of xenobiotics (Cohen et al, 1981)

The isolation of cells and their subsequent use is again complicated by the wide variety of cell types making up this region of the respiratory tract. Only six of these will be considered in the present review. A more detailed description of some other types and methods of isolation may be found in Smith (1985).

Pneumocytes The epithelial layer lining the alveoli consists of two main cell types usually known simply as type I and type II pneumocytes. The type I pneumocyte (squamous epithelial cell, membranous pneumocyte or small alveolar cell) has been regarded as primarily providing the air/tissue barrier and very few specialised functions have been ascribed to these cells. The type II cell (granular pneumocyte, large alveolar cell or great alveolar cell) is larger, contains numerous multivesicular and multilamellar bodies. This type of cell is responsible for the synthesis and secretion of pulmonary surfactant and is capable of metabolising numerous xenobiotics.

Many attempts have been made to isolate pure populations of alveolar cells usually using mild enzymic digestion and further centrifugal purification of the resulting cell suspension either on density gradients (reviewed by Witschi, 1976 and Finkelstein 1982) or including elutriation (Devereux and Fouts, 1981). Type I cells seem to be end cells incapable of division _in vivo_ and thus unsuitable for growth _in vitro_. There have, however, been a number of successful efforts to produce nearly pure, metabolically active suspensions of type II cells, though these nave involved different methods and have started with different species of laboratory animal.

A number of cell lines have been established which retain many of the features of type II pneumocytes even after prolonged periods in culture. Douglas and Kaign (1974) established the L2 line which retained differentiated morphological features for up to 6 passages. A continuously cultured line of human type II cells was established from an alveolar cell tumour by Lieber _et al_ (1976). This line (designated A549), used in the present authors' laboratories, resembles the parent type II cell even after several hundred passages _in vitro_. A549 cells have also retained the ability to metabolise some xenobiotics including polycyclic aromatic hydrocarbons. This cell line can form glucuronide conjugates from phenols (Table 2.) though we have been unable to detect sulphate conjugates at normal sulphate concentrations.

Li _et al_ (1983) established a line (LEC cells) from adult Fischer 344 rats that in many respects resembles the L2 line. This line has also remained morphologically differentiated and like the A549 cell line it has retained some xenobiotic metabolism.

The finding that differentiated characteristics are so resilient in three separate lines derived from the same cell type suggests that this might be a property of these cells. Lung damage commonly leads to type II cell hyperplasia suggesting that these cells possess a high reproductive capacity even _in vivo_. However, in the animal this differentiated state is not retained, the proliferation of type II cells leads to the production of undifferentiated cuboidal epithelium. In the case of acute injury these cuboidal cells may differentiate and regenerate a normal squamous epithelium consisting of type I cells.

Table 2.

Formation of Glucuronide Conjugates from 1-Naphthol in Cultures of Human Type II (A549) Cells Exposed to Crocidolite Asbestos.

	Nmoles of naphthol glucuronide formed per mg of protein. Time (hours) of exposure to naphthol		
	1h	3h	6h
Control Cultures	5.9	64.2	134.0
Cultures treated for 24h with 50µg/ml crocidolite asbestos.	4.5	27.0	74.5
Cultures treated for 72h with 50µg/ml crocidolite asbestos.	13.7	43.4	124.5

Cultures were grown to confluency in 75 square cm tissue culture grade plastic flasks. They were treated with crocidolite asbestos for either 24 or 72 hours and then exposed to 20µM ^{14}C 1-naphthol (1µCi/ml) for either 1, 3 or 6 hours.

The culture medium was then removed from the cells, the protein precipitated with ice-cold ethanol and the supernatant evaporated to dryness under vacuum. The residue was taken up in a small amount of 30% ethanol, neutralised with HCl and examined by HPLC (Brown et at 1983).

The figures in the table are expressed as nmoles of napthol glucuronide formed per milligram of protein in the times shown. Each figure represents the mean of duplicate cultures. The results demonstrate that the addition of crocidolite asbestos to cultured A549 cells produces a temporary inhibition of glucuronide formation.

Lung Fibroblasts Both outgrowth and enzymic digestion methods have been used to isolate fibroblasts from adult and foetal lung. In the former method the lungs are chopped into pieces of about 1-3mm^3, pieces of this mince can then be anchored to the base of Petri dishes by plasma clots or more simply on scratches made in the base with a sterile scalpel. Fibroblasts grow from the edges of the explants and these can be harvested by trypsinisation after removing the explants with forceps. For the enzymic isolation of lung fibroblasts the minced lungs need only be exposed to trypsin/EDTA, the released cells harvested by filtration and centrifugation, and then plated out in a suitable medium. Various detailed differences in the concentrations of trypsin, times of treatment etc have been used, a useful review may be found in Bradley *et al* (1980).

Human and animal lung fibroblasts have been used in numerous *in vitro* investigations. Most workers have considered these to be "model cells" and have used them in studies of aging, cytogenetics, virology, and general or genetic toxicology. Only rarely have they been considered specifically as lung cells. Indeed it has been generally assumed that fibroblasts in culture are functionally similar whatever their tissue of origin. It has been reported that although there are few, if any, features that can be used to distinguish between foetal fibroblasts obtained from different tissues there are clear differences between fibroblasts from different adult tissues (Bradley *et al*, 1980).

The comparison of lung and other fibroblasts reveals differences in growth characteristics, life span and DNA/RNA ratios. Lung derived cells may also differ in glycosaminoglycan production (Sjoberg and Fransson, 1977) and in their production of "minor" proteins that are possibly lung specific. They may also have different nutritional requirements (Ham, 1980). The relevance to any toxicological investigation of these biochemical differences between morphologically similar cells remains unknown.

Endothelial cells The lungs contain a particularly well developed vasculature and receive the entire output of the heart. Any damage to the integrity of the blood/gas interface can result in a number of pathological conditions. A common result of lung injury is the development of pulmonary oedema and this is commonly due to damage to the endothelial cells. As well as material entering from the airways these cells are exposed to circulating chemicals which may themselves be toxic or may be toxic metabolites of agents activated in other organs. A good example of this latter group is provided by the pyrrolizidine alkaloids (e.g. Huxtable _et al_, 1978). Pulmonary endothelial cells seem to have several specialised functions; substances such as serotonin and prostaglandins are removed from circulation and some peptides are hydrolysed (angiotensin I and bradykinin). These metabolic functions of pulmonary endothelial cells are reviewed by Junod (1982).

A number of workers have isolated endothelial cells from the lung. Johnson (1980) dissected pulmonary veins and arteries down to the level of the third or fourth branching points and after freeing the cells with collagenase this author found metabolic differences between the endothelial cells from veins and arteries. It, however, remains to be discovered if endothelial cells have properties specific to the tissue of origin and thus if damage by circulating toxins to the pulmonary vascular bed is due to metabolic peculiarities or simply because of anatomical position.

Alveolar Macrophages Macrophages are probably the cell that has been most used to study the effects of materials that are toxic or potentially toxic to the lungs. However, the cells used have not always been of pulmonary origin but have frequently been isolated from the peritoneal cavity. The differences between macrophages from these different sources are unclear. Alveolar cells are more aerobic and differ slightly in ultrastructure from other macrophages, but results obtained from studies using peritoneal and alveolar cells seem mostly similar.

The most common method for isolating alveolar macrophages is bronchoalveolar lavage. This technique has been practiced both on laboratory animals (alive or more commonly dead) or on humans (dead or more commonly alive). The various methods available for lavage are reviewed by Brain and Beck (1985). The maximum yield of macrophages is obtained using a calcium and magnesium free saline as lavage fluid and the yield may be increased by adding substances such as lignocaine.

The cells contained in the lavage fluid consist mainly of polymorphonuclear leukocytes, lymphocytes and macrophages with the numbers and proportions these cells providing valuable information on any inflammatory response in the lung. The isolated cells are usually harvested by centrifugation and then plated in various tissue culture media into Petri dishes. Vigorous washing of the cultures 1-2 hours later removes the non-adherent cells such as lymphocytes. The macrophages will survive in culture for several days while PMN will rapidly die.

Cultures of these cells have been used mainly for the study of particulates, in particular they are specially sensitive to silica and various silicates (see for example, Brown _et al_, 1980).

A number of cell lines have been established which have many of the properties of macrophages and these have been used in numerous studies in place of primary cells. The most widely used of these lines (P388D1) arose as a variant in cultures of the P388 murine lymphoma line. Although non of the cell lines originated from alveolar cells they have been successfully used to study the action of pulmonary toxins such as asbestos (Brown and Poole, 1984).

Mesothelial cells

There have been a number of reports on the _in vitro_ study of mesothelial cells. Some cells from human pleural effusions have been maintained in culture for short times (see for example Castor and Naylor, 1969). The identity of the actual cells surviving has been problematic, particularly in the case of malignant effusions, where tumour cells could be expected to survive better in culture and might overgrow any normal cells present in aspirated fluid.

Jaurand *et al* (1981) published a method for the isolation and maintenance of pleural mesothelial cells in long term culture. Monolayers of these cells could be subcultured and retained their morphological characteristics. These cells have been used to study the pathological effects of asbestos.

DISCUSSION AND CONCLUSION

From the preceding partial review it may be seen that it is possible to isolate, maintain and even subculture a wide variety of pulmonary cells *in vitro*. Many studies have used such cells to investigate the pulmonary toxicity of a wide range of chemical and physical agents. However, in many cases it is not necessary to use cells isolated from a particular target organ to study the mode of action of a toxicant simply because that agent is known to damage this organ after *in vivo* exposure.

While some cell types, such as the type II pneumocyte and Clara cell, are peculiar to the lungs many others (e.g. fibroblasts and endothelial cells) are also found in most other organs. Any specialised organotypic functions of these cells seem to be subtle and possibly derive from the environment in a particular anatomical location. Since these environmental factors will be removed on isolation and cultivation *in vitro* one might expect cells from different organs to become more uniform once in tissue culture.

After prolonged cultivation with repeated passaging any organ specific features will certainly be lost, some cells such as the V79-4 line were derived from the lung but now do not even resemble the cell type of origin. It is however not uncommon to see the effect of inhaled material studied in these cells as if they are particularly suited to this purpose. Arguments of this type are especially common on applications for financial support, where the supposed relevance of the model system will impress the grant-giving-body.

As mentioned in the introduction organ specific toxicity might arise for any of several reasons. For example the lungs may be the route of entry of a particular material. If the material is highly reactive then it may damage the first cells encountered, this is the situation occuring with corrosive or irritant gases. Similarly if the toxicant is not cleared from the lung then this is where the effects will be seen. Thus the effects of mineral dusts are usually seen in the lungs; however the accidental contamination of the peritoneal cavity by talc from surgeons' gloves will produce fibrosis, and this is presumably caused by the same mechanisms as those causing pulmonary talcosis after inhalation.

There is thus very little justification for requiring the use of pulmonary cells in studies of the effect of these materials. Morgan and Alison (1980) concluded that the biochemical responses of macrophages to mineral dusts were similar whether peritoneal or alveolar cells were used. Other investigators have found that macrophage like cell lines may be as useful as freshly isolated cells (Wade et al, 1976; Brown and Poole, 1984). Similarly the literature contains many papers on the use of pulmonary fibroblasts or indeed foetal lung fibroblasts to study fibrosis due to mineral dusts, bleomycin or other agents. We would suggest that these types of cell show a similar response to many insults whether they are derived from the lungs or from any other organ.

In addition to a toxic response due to the deposition of inhaled material it may be the anatomical location, density and interrelationship of cells within the lung that makes them particularly susceptable to some agents. The entire circulatory blood supply may pass through the lungs as much as 5 times a minute (Witschi, 1976). Toxic materials absorbed in the intestine may be activated in the liver and then exert a toxic effect on the first extensive capillary bed encountered - that of the lung.

Clearly none of the above arguments should preclude the study of lung derived cells if they can be obtained easily and in sufficient quantity. However, these considerations do mean that care must be taken not to dismiss studies of pulmonary toxins using cells from other organs. Of course some toxic processes do affect mainly those cell types that are unique to the lungs and for the meaningful study of these it is necessary to use well defined, metabolically active cells closely resembling those occuring *in vivo*.

Some of the best examples of this type of lung specific damage are provided by the sensitivity of Clara cells to agents such as 4-ipomeanol and methylfuran. The toxicity of some xenobiotics is due to them being activated at the site of subsequent damage and in the lung the Clara cell is probably the cell type most capable of this type of metabolism. It has been shown to be a major site of pulmonary cytochrome P450. Research, using both whole animals and isolated cells, has shown that the reason for these cells sensitivity to 4-ipomeanol is probably this metabolic competence (for reviews see Boyd, 1980 and Minchin and Boyd, 1983).

While type II pneumocytes are also capable of some drug metabolism these cells are specially adapted for the synthesis and secretion of dipalmitoyl lecithin. This material acts as a surfactant and facilitates the expansion of the alveolae. Excess secretion of this material has been reported in acute lung damage due to poison gas and both increases and decreases have been reported after exposure to a whole range of toxic materials. Several *in vitro* systems including organ culture (Douglas *et al*, 1980; Engle *et al*, 1980) and primary and continuous cell lines (Smith, 1977; Li et al, 1983) have been used as models for the study of surfactant synthesis, and its response to physiological changes as well as toxic insult. In some cases a source of the excess surfactant could be the hyperplastic response of the type II cells referred to above.

The lungs play a wide variety of physiological roles and consist of more cell types than do most other organs. They are exposed to airborne and circulating toxic materials and their position in the circulatory system means that they contain the first major capillary bed encountered by metabolites produced in the liver. This complexity makes the analysis of lung function and its response to damage difficult in the intact animal and only marginally easier in isolated organ systems.

All of these considerations make the use of isolated cell cultures attractive for the analysis of any pulmonary response to toxic materials. A great deal of progress has been made in the development of methods of isolating differentiated lung cells and then growing these in culture; however such methods may not be necessary in all studies of toxic lung damage.

Some of what appears to be organ-specific lung damage may be caused by effects on common cell types located at sites where exposure to, or accommodation of, the toxic material occurs. Such damage may be modelled _in vitro_ using cells isolated from tissues far more ameniable to experimental manipulation than is the lung. In the other cases toxic damage is to cells that are unique to the lung and the mechanisms responsible for this damage must be studied in cell or organ cultures containing these cells maintained in a differentiated state.

The only way to decide which of these situtions obtains in a particular case is by a critical examination of the data from animal experiments or human cases. In most cases the original evidence for a particular type of damage will come from histological examination of appropriate tissue.

Thus we see the role of _in vitro_ studies in pulmonary toxicology as being the provision of simplified systems for the analysis of mechanism. Eventually some screening role for these studies will be possible if only within groups of closely related compounds that could be expected to act by a common pathway.

References

Aydelotte, M.B. (1965). Respiratory tract. In Cells and Tissues in Culture, Methods, Biology and Physiology, ed. E.N. Willmer, pp 569-588. Academic Press Inc.

Boyd, M.R. (1977). Evidence for the Clara cell as a site of cytochrome P-450-dependent mixed-function oxidase activity in lung. Nature, 269 : 713-715.

Boyd, M.R. (1980). Biochemical mechanisms in chemical-induced lung injury: roles of metabolic activation. Critical Reviews in Toxicology, 7 : 103-176.

Bradley, K.H., Kawanami, O., Ferrans, V.J. and Crystal, R.G. (1980). The fibroblast of human alveolar structures: A differentiated cell with a major role in lung structure and function. In Methods in Cell Biology. Volume 21A. pp 37-64. Academic Press Inc.

Brain, J.D. and Beck, B.D. (1985). Bronchoalveolar lavage in Toxicology of Inhaled Materials eds. H.P. Witschi and Brain, J.D. pp 203-220 Springer-Verlag, Berlin, Heidelberg, New York, Tokyo.

Brown, R. C., Fleming, G. T. A. and Knight. A. I., (1983). Asbestos affects the in vitro uptake and detoxification of aromatic compounds. Environ Health Perspectives, 51: 315-318.

Brown R.C. and Poole, A. (1984). Arachidonic acid release and prostaglandin synthesis in a macrophage-like cell line exposed to asbestos. Agents and Actions, 15 : 336-340.

Brown, R.C., Chamberlain, M. Davies, R., Morgan, D.M.L., Pooley, F.D. and Richards, R.J. (1980). A comparison of 4 "In Vitro" systems applied to 21 dusts. In The In Vitro Effects of Mineral Dusts, eds. R.C. Brown, I.,P. Gormley, M. Chamberlain, R. Davies, pp 47-52. Academic Press Inc.

Castor, C.W. and Naylor, B. (1969). Characteristics of normal and malignant human mesothelial cells studied in vitro. Lab. Invest. 20 : 437-443.

Chilton, B.S., Kennedy, J.R. and Nicosia, S. (1981). Isolation of basal and mucous cell populations from rabbit trachea. Am. Rev. Respir. Dis 124 : 723-727.

Cohen, G. M. Gibby, E. M. and Mehta, R (1981). Routes of conjunction in normal and cancerous being. Nature. 291: 662-664.

Curtz, E., Yeges, H., Wong, V., Bienkowski, E. and Chan, W. (1985) In Vitro Characteristics of Pulmonary Neuroendocrine Cells Isolated from Rabbit Fetal Lung. 1. Effects of Culture Media and Nerve Growth Factor. Lab. Invest. 53:672-682.

Devereux, T. and Fouts, J.R. (1980). Isolation and identification of Clara cells from rabbit lung. In Vitro, 16 : 958-968.

Devereux, T.R. and Fouts, J.R. (1981). Xenobiotic metabolism by alveolar type II cells isolated from rabbit lung. Biochemical Pharmacology, 30 : 1231-1237.

Douglas, W.H.J. and Kaighm, M.E. (1974). Clonal isolation of differentiated rat lung cells. In Vitro. 10 : 230 - 237.

Douglas, W.H.J., Sanders, R.L. and Hitchcock, K.R. (1980). Maintenance of human and rat pulmonary type II cells in an organotypic culture system. In Methods in Cell Biology Volume 21A, pp 79-94. Academic Press Inc.

Engle, M.J., Sanders, R.L. and Douglas, W.H.J. (1980). Type II alveolar cells in organotypic culture: a model system for the study of surfactant synthesis. Biochimica. et Biophysica Acta, 617: 225-236.

Finkelstein, J.N. and Shapiro, D.L. (1982). Isolation of type II alveolar epithelial cells using low protease concentrations. Lung, 160 : 85-98.

Gail, D.B. and Lenfant, C.J.M. (1983). Cells of the lung : biology and clinical implications. Ames. Rev. Respir. Dis., 127: 366-387.

Habliston, D.L., Whitaker, C., Hart, M.A., Ryan, U.S. and Ryan, J.W. (1979). Isolation and culture of endothelial cells from the lungs of small animals. Am. Rev. Respir. Dis., 119 : 853-868.

Ham, R.G. (1980). Dermal fibroblasts In Methods in Cell Biology Volume 21A. pp 255-276. Academic Press Inc.

Hayflick, L. and Moorhead, P.S. (1961). The serial cultivation of human diploid cell strains. Exp. Cell Res., 25 : 285-621,

Huxtable, R., Ciaramitaro, D., and Eisenstein, D. (1978). The effects of a pyrrolizidine alkaloid, monocrotaline, and a pyrollidihydrometroneane on the biochemical functions of pulmonary endothelium. Mol Pharmacol, 14: 1189-1203. .

Jaurand, M.C., Bernaudin, J.F., Renier, A., Kaplan, H. and Bignon, J. (1981). Rat Pleural Mesothelical Cells in Culture. In Vitro, 17 : 98-106.

Johnson, A.R. (1980). Human pulmonary endothelial cells in culture. J. Clin. Invest. 65 : 841-850.

Jones, K.G., Holland, J.F. and Fouts, J.R. (1982). Benzo (α) pyrene hydroxylase activity in enriched populations of Clara cells and alveolar type II cells from control and ß-naphthoflavone pretreated rats. Cancer Research, 42 : 4658-4663.

Junod, A.F. (1982). Metabolic aspects of the pulmonary endothelium In Proceedings of the Fifth Course, of the International School of Thoracic Medicine. Cellular Biology of the Lung. eds. C. Cumming and G Bonsignore. pp 367-380. Plenum Press, New York and London.

Last, J.A., Kaizu, T. and Mossman, B.T. (1979). Glycoprotein synthesis by an established cell line from hamster tracheal epithelium. Exp. Lung. Res.

Li, A.P., Hahn, F.F., Zamora, P.O., Shimizu, R.W., Henderson, R.F., Brooks, A.L. and Richards, R. (1983). Characterisation of a lung epithelial cell strain with potential applications in toxicological studies. Toxicology, 27 : 257-272.

Lieber, M., Smith, B.T., Szakal, A., Nelson-Rees, W and Todaro, G. (1976). A continuous tumour cell line from a human lung carcinoma with properties of type II alveolar epithelial cells. Int. J. Cancer 17: 62-70.

Minchin, R.F. and Boyd, M.R. (1983). Localisation of metabolic activation and deactivation systems in the lung: Signifcance to the pulmonary toxicity of xenobiotics. Ann. Rev. Pharmacol. Toxicol., 23 : 217-238.

Minchin, R.F., McManus, E., Thorgeirsson, S.S., Schwartz, D. and Boyd, M.R. (1985). Metabolism of 2-acetyl-aminofluorene in isolated rabbit pulmonary cells. Drug Metabolism and Disposition, 13 : 406-411.

Morgan, D.M.L. and Allison, A.C. (1980). Effects of silica and asbestos on alveolar and peritoneal macrophages: A comparative study. In The In Vitro Effects of Mineral Dusts, eds. R.C. Brown, I.P. Gormley, M. Chamberlain, and R. Davies, pp 75-82. Academic Press Ltd.

Mossman, B.T., Adler, K.B. and Craighead (1980). Cytotoxicity and proliferative changes in tracheal organ and cell cultures after exposure to mineral dusts. In the In Vitro Effects of Mineral Dusts ed. R.C. Brown, I.P. Gormley, M. Chamberlain and R. Davies. pp 241 - 250 Adademic Press Inc.

Naum, Y. (1975). Growth of pulmonary alveolar macrophages in vitro : responses to media conditioned by lung cell lines. Cytobios. 14 : 211-216.

Nevo, A.C., Weisman, Z. and Sade, J. (1975). Cell proliferation and cell differentiation in tissue cultures of adult mico-ciliary epithelia. Differentiation, 3:79-80.

Naum, Y., Chang, C.M. and Houck, J.C. (1979). Pulmonary macrophage growth factor. Inflammation 3 : 253-260.

Picciano, P. and Rosenbaum, R.M. (1978). The type I alveolar lining cell of the mammalian lung. I Isolotation and enrichment from dissociated adult rabbit lung. Am. J. Pathol., 90 : 99-122.

Rosenbaum, R.M. and Picciano, P. (1978). The type I alveolar lining cells of the mammalian lung. 2 In Vitro identification via the cell surface and ultrastructure of isolated cells from adult rabbit lung A. M. J. Pathol, 90: 123-144.

Sivarajah, K., Jones, K. G., Fouts, J.R., Devereux, T., Shirley, J.E. and Eling, T.E. (1983). Prostraglandin synthetase and cytochrome P-450 dependent metabolism of benzo (α) pyrene 7, 8-dihydrodiol by enriched populations of rat Clara cells and alveolar type II cells. Cancer Research, 43, 2632-2636.

Sjoberg, I and Fransson, L. (1977). Synthesis of glycosaminoglycans by human embryonic lung fibroblasts. Biochem. J., 167 : 383-392.

Smith, B.T. (1977). Cell line A549. A model system for the study of alveolar type II cell function. Am. Rev. Respir. Dis. 115 : 285-293.

Smith, B.T. (1985). Pulmonary cell and tissue culture. In Toxicology of inhaled materials eds. H.P. Witschi and J.P. Brain pp. 181-202.

Sonstegard, K., Wong, V. and Cutz, E. (1979). Neuro-epithelial bodies in organ cultures of fetal rabbit lungs. Cell Tissue Res., 199 : 159-170.

Stoner, G.D., Katoh, Y., Foidart, J.M., Myers, G.A. and Harris, C.C. (1980). Identification and culture of human bronchial epithelial cells. In Methods in Cell Biology. Volume 21A pp 15-35. Academic Press Inc.

Tompa, A. and Langenbach, R. (1979). Culture of adult rat lung cells, benzo (alpha) pyrene metabolism and mutagenesis. In Vitro, 15: 569-578.

Trowell, O.A. (1959). The culture of mature organs in a synthetic medium. Exp. Cell Res., 16 : 118-136.

Wade, M.J., Lipkin, L.E. and Tuckes, R.W. (1976). Asbestos cytotoxicity in a long term macrophage-like cell line. Nature, 264: 444-446.

Witschi, H. (1976). Proliferation of type II alveolar cells : A review of common responses in toxic lung injury. Toxicology, 5: 267-277.

METABOLISM AND TOXICITY OF DRUGS IN MAMMALIAN HEPATOCYTE CULTURE

R.J. Chenery

Smith Kline & French Research Limited, The Frythe, Welwyn, Herts. England

INTRODUCTION

Drugs and xenobiotics exert toxic effects by a variety of mechanisms. The toxic response is often organ specific and may be caused by either parent drug or by metabolites of the drug. Information gained on the hepatic metabolism of drugs, therefore, is of general value in helping to understand toxicity caused by a drug because the liver is a major site of metabolic elimination of drugs and has a marked effect on determining the exposure of a specific organ to either parent drug or metabolite. Moreover, specific drugs may cause toxicity by directly acting on the hepatocyte or indirectly as a consequence of induction or inhibition of hepatic metabolic pathways.

For these and other considerations it is important to obtain information on the hepatic metabolism of new drugs as early as possible. In practice, metabolic and pharmacokinetic input in drug discovery is not usually substantial and the reasons for this are various, but generally centre on the resources and time required to develop and conduct appropriate metabolism studies.

One approach to this problem is to introduce *in vitro* methodology at an early stage of the analysis of drug metabolism and pharmacokinetics. Hepatocytes retain most of the metabolic capabilities of the intact liver (Abraham *et al*., 1983; Tsuru *et al*., 1982; Davis *et al*., 1983) and provide an opportunity to study both the pathways and extent of metabolism of novel drugs at a very early stage in the drug development process. One of the potential advantages of such an approach is the small amounts of unlabelled compound required to conduct a metabolism study. Generally parent drug can be separated from metabolites by analytical techniques such as h.p.l.c. (high performance liquid chromatography). It is also possible with this approach to address the question of species differences in drug metabolism, including the possibility of studying metabolism in human hepatocytes (Tee _et al_., 1985; Begue _et al_, 1983). In many respects, however, the hepatocyte system remains poorly characterised in two key areas: 1) The relationship between the rate of metabolism by hepatocytes _in vitro_ compared to that _in vivo_ and 2) The relationship of the metabolic profile of a drug produced by hepatocytes _in vitro_ compared to that _in vivo_.

Such information will provide valuable background data to help evaluate the utility of hepatocytes in cytotoxicity studies because the toxicity of many chemicals result from their metabolic conversion in the liver to reactive intermediates that cause cellular damage. Compounds such as paracetamol, cyclophosphamide, furosamide and aflatoxin B_1 are hepatotoxic _in vivo_ and can be shown to cause toxicity to hepatocytes _in vitro_ as a consequence of metabolic activation. Thus, the aim of this chapter is to present a limited number of examples which explore the relationships between metabolism and cytotoxicity _in vitro_ with that observed _in vivo_.

PRACTICAL ASPECTS

(i) Hepatocyte Preparation The production of isolated hepatocytes from a variety of species requires only a limited amount of equipment and cannot be considered to be unduly expensive. Hepatocytes are prepared in our laboratory by the technique of Strom _et al_. (1982) with a limited number of modifications. Simple perfusion equipment is required to enable a variety of different flow rates ranging from about 6 $ml.min^{-1}$ for the rat to about 100 $ml.min^{-1}$ for human tissue. Temperature must be maintained at 37°C either by a water bath or using a thermocirculator and heat exchange unit. Liver is removed and stored under ice-cold saline and lobes are removed with a scalpel and a major vessel of the lobe cannulated with a polyethylene catheter (16 gauge, Medicut). Perfusion is started immediately at a flow rate dependent on the species and results in a blanching of most of the lobe. The perfusate consisted of aqueous sodium chloride (NaCl, 142 mM), KCl (7 mM), HEPES (10 mM, pH 7.4) and EGTA (40 μM). After 3-5 minutes, the perfusate was changed to NaCl (142 mM), KCl (7 mM), HEPES (10 mM, pH 7.4), aqueous calcium chloride ($CaCl_2$, 1 mM) and 1 $mg.ml^{-1}$ collagenase and the perfusate recycled for 5-7 minutes.

The lobe was then removed from the perfusion apparatus and placed under cold buffer [NaCl (142 mM), KCl (7 mM), HEPES (10 mM, pH 7.4) containing 1% w/v BSA and 4 mg DNAase I per 100 ml]. The capsule was gently folded back and the hepatocytes released by gentle agitation of the lobe. The cell suspension was then filtered through a nylon mesh (64 μm) and centrifuged (approximately 100 g, 5 minutes, 4°C). Cells were resuspended in fresh buffer and the washing procedure repeated three times before resuspending the hepatocytes in buffer (final volume 10 ml). DNAase I was omitted from the final two washes. Hepatocytes were then counted in a haemocytometer in the presence of 0.04% trypan blue. Yields of 30-40 x 10^6 cells were commonly achieved from a lobe of rat liver with a viability in excess of 90%.

The hepatocytes can be studied in suspension in which case a simple shaking water bath would be adequate for metabolism studies. However, introduction of hepatocytes into monolayer culture (Figure 1) requires the availability of sterile laminar hoods, incubators and the application of sterile technique to the procedures. Alternative techniques would include the attachment of the hepatocytes to microcarrier systems again involving specialist techniques and procedures. In our studies hepatocytes were quickly diluted into culture medium consisting of Williams Medium E (WME) containing L-glutamine (4 mM), penicillin (100 $iu.ml^{-1}$) and newborn calf serum (10% v/v). The cell suspension was then seeded on to 35 mm wells (Falcon) which had been coated with soluble collagen. The hepatocytes were allowed to attach to the culture wells for 2 hours and then the culture medium was removed and replaced with WME containing dissolved drug. The WME used for the incubation stage was free from added protein and had phenol red excluded from the original formulation, thus preventing possible interactions of this pH indicator with glucuronidation reactions.

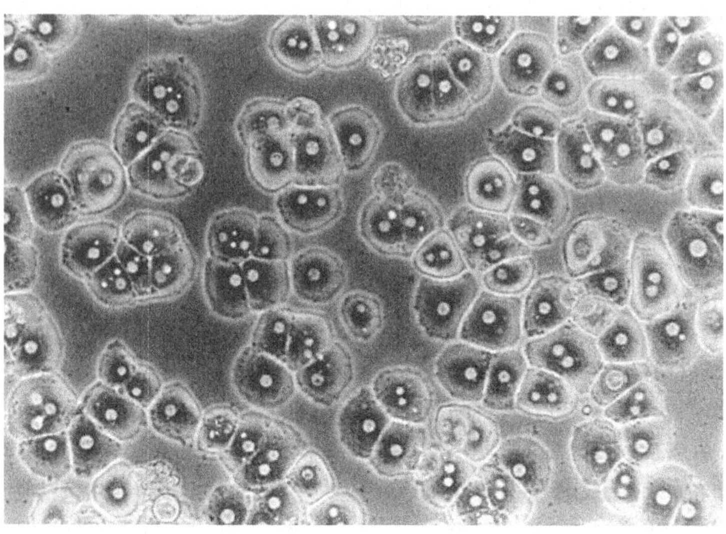

Figure 1. Rat Hepatocytes Cultured for 4 Hours as Described in Methods

(ii) Drug Metabolism Studies Drug and metabolite concentrations were analysed in the culture medium by h.p.l.c. Due to the kinetic approach that we have taken we have emphasised the development of automated, rapid separations which allow large numbers of samples to be analysed routinely. However, the detection and evaluation of novel metabolites produced by compounds in the early stages of development poses a number of problems which we have addressed in two ways. In many cases ultraviolet detection of peaks has been optimised by the use of diode-array detection systems such as the HP 1040A detector (Hewlett Packard) fitted with a data processing unit. The ability of this detector to provide U.V. spectra of metabolite peaks and to provide limited peak purity data greatly facilitates the establishment of rapid h.p.l.c. separation methods and reduces the number of injections required to evaluate a separation (Figure 2).

The recent introduction of the thermospray interface enables the application of l.c./m.s. (mass spectrometer coupled to h.p.l.c.) to be employed routinely on small size samples from hepatocyte incubations. A minimum of sample preparation is required for such samples but the range of mobile phases available with this technique is limited. The most acceptable appears to be ammonium acetate in combination with methanol or acetonitrile (pH >5.0). The assignment of structure with the thermospray interface is often fairly conclusive given the fact that the mass spectrum obtained contains little fragmentation data. Obviously, stereochemical information such as the exact location of sites of hydroxylation requires corroboration by other techniques such as n.m.r. (nuclear magnetic resonance).

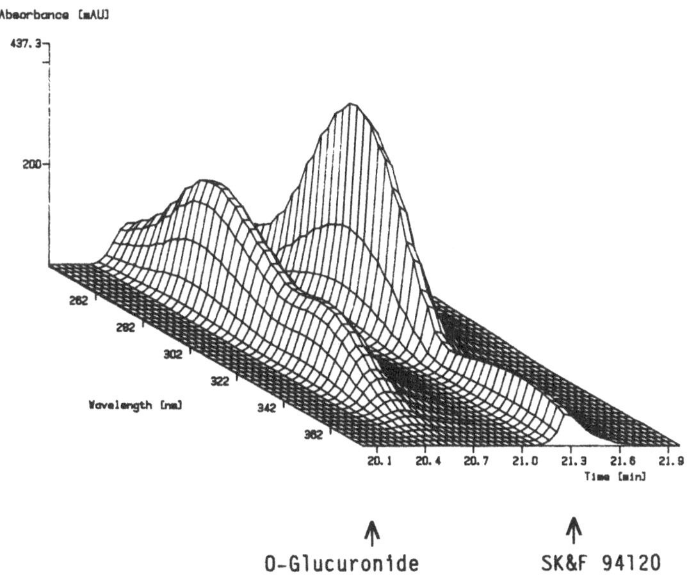

Figure 2 Separation of SK&F 94120 and an O-Glucuronide Metabolite.

(iii) Toxicity Studies Measurement of cellular viability is an integral part of performing drug metabolism studies but can also be the specific object of a study. In our laboratory we routinely employ measurements of membrane function such as trypan blue exclusion or determination of enzyme leakage. A wide variety of enzyme activities may be monitored. Lactic dehydrogenase activity (LDH) is a convenient marker because of the stability of the enzyme activity in the culture system. Enzyme activity in the culture medium is measured directly whereas the activity in the rat hepatocyte monolayer is measured after lysis with 0.2% triton X-100 added to the culture medium and waiting 5 minutes for complete cell lysis. In some cases other measurements of cellular function such as oxygen consumption and protein synthesis may be more discriminating.

Oxygen consumption in freshly isolated hepatocytes can be measured with an oxygen electrode (Rank Brothers, Cambridge) consisting of a perspex incubation chamber (2 ml) surrounded by a water jacket connected to a thermocirculator to maintain a constant temperature (37°C). The instrument was calibrated utilising phenylhydrazine in the presence of ferricyanide. Measurement of protein synthesis can be performed by the addition of ^{14}C-leucine (0.5 µCi) to a plate of rat hepatocytes (35 mm wells, final volume 2 ml; Villa et al.,1980). After 1 hour at 37°C medium was removed and the monolayer washed 6 times with ice-cold saline (2 ml) containing leucine (1 mg.ml^{-1}). Cells were then scraped from the plastic well and transferred into a plastic tube in the same medium and cell protein precipitated by addition of TCA. The precipitate was then centrifuged and washed twice with TCA (5%) before solubilisation in aqueous sodium hydroxide (1M). Radioactivity was determined by scintillation counting.

Changes in cell structure can provide considerable insight into the mechanism by which a drug or chemical causes toxicity. Such information can be provided by light or electron microscopy (Chenery *et al.*, 1981). Figure 3 shows scanning electron micrographs of rat hepatocytes maintained in culture for 24 h. In the control cultures the cells are flattened and covered with numerous microvilli whereas hepatocytes treated with toxic concentrations of paracetamol are rounded and exhibit numberous blebs and balloons.

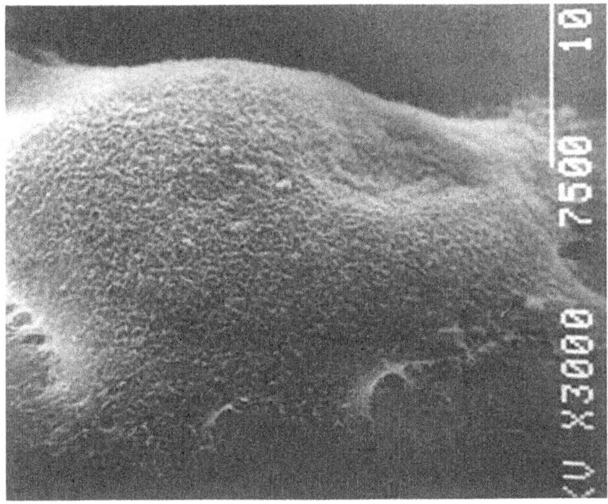

Figure 3a Scanning Electron Micrograph of Rat Hepatocytes Cultured for 24 h.

Figure 3b Scanning Electron Micrograph of Rat Hepatocytes Cultured for 24 h with 6 mM Paracetamol.

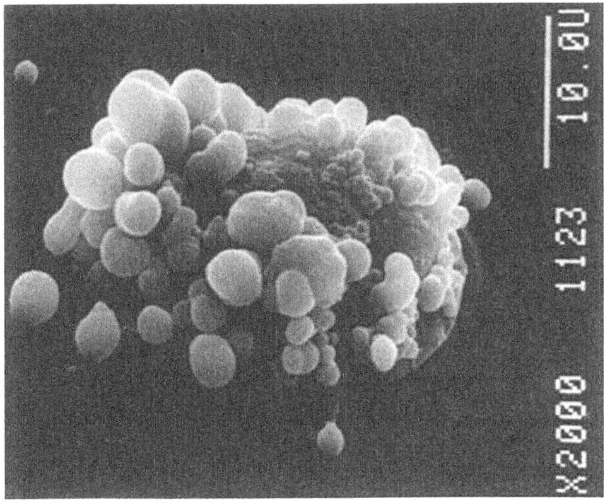

(iv) Maintenance of Differentiated Function One of the major limitations of the cultured hepatocyte system is the loss of differentiated function observed after extended culture. In particular, losses in cytochrome P_{450} levels are commonly observed within the first day of culture (Paine and Legg, 1978), although little information is available on the metabolism of drugs and xenobiotics by hepatocytes maintained in culture.

Table 1

Changes in Cytochrome P_{450} Levels in Cultured Hepatocytes

Source	Cytochrome P_{450} (Mean ± S.D.) (pmol.mg protein^{-1})	
	2 h	24 h
Rat	151 ± 18	67 ± 31
Rat (Phenobarbital treated)	576	351
Rat (ß-naphthoflavone treated)	228	87
Rabbit	305 ± 15	333 ± 106
Dog	138 ± 32	95 ± 7

The changes in total cytochrome P-450 content of cultured hepatocytes from rat, dog and rabbit are shown in Table 1. These data would suggest that the losses of cytochrome P-450 observed during the initial 24h of culture in rat hepatocytes were more marked in rat compared to rabbit and dog.

The impact of such losses of differentiated function can be investigated using probe drugs such as warfarin (Branchflower and Chenery, unpublished observations, Table 2) and paracetamol (Emery et al.,1985). Losses of total cytochrome P-450 were associated with a reduced ability to activate paracetamol as judged by covalent binding and glutathione conjugate formation and by a change in the metabolite profile of warfarin. In contrast, the changes seen in paracetamol conjugation reactions were a modest decline in sulphation and a stimulation of glucuronidation. This stimulation of glucuronidation of drugs has recently been reported to involve *de novo* protein synthesis (Grant and Hawksworth, 1985). Thus, it is clear that at present most hepatocyte culture systems can provide useful metabolic information for only a few days at most. Recent advances in this area will be discussed later.

TABLE 2

The Effect of Culture Period on the Hydroxylation of (R)-Warfarin in Rat Hepatocytes

Time in Culture (h)	Medium	Cytochrome P_{450} (pmol.mg $prot^{-1}$)	% Composition (Mean ± S.D.) 4'	6	7	8
1	A	250 ± 29	18±3	16±2	58±6	8±2
	B					
24	A	257 ± 26	19±2	14±3	59±7	8±2
	B	264 ± 52	24±1	17±3	50±5	9±2
120	A	29 ± 11	12±1	20±2	55±3	13±2
	B	94 ± 5	31±2	22±3	30±2	17±1

Medium A contains 25 mM nicotinamide
Medium B without cysteine/cystine

EXPERIMENTAL EXAMPLES

RATES AND ROUTES OF METABOLISM

(i) SK&F 94120 (Figure 4) has been shown to possess positive inotropic and vasodilator activity in animals and was being developed as a therapeutic agent in the treatment of congestive heart failure. This compound is rapidly and completely absorbed but is rapidly cleared (plasma clearance in the rat is 2.5 $l.kg^{-1}.h^{-1}$). Studies in the rat, mouse and dog indicate that a major route of hepatic elimination of the compound is by conjugation of the pyrazinone ring with glucuronic acid.

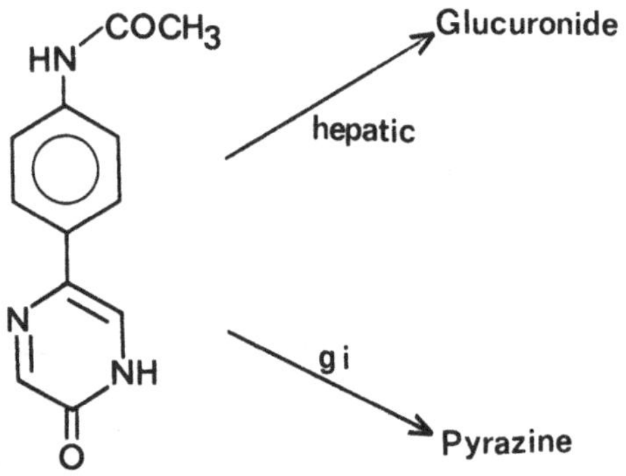

Figure 4. Structure of SK&F 94120

The glucuronide of SK&F 94120 was also the major metabolite produced by hepatocytes isolated from rat, rabbit and dog liver (Figure 2). In the case of the rat the glucuronide was the only metabolite produced by isolated hepatocytes. The kinetics of this transformation were characterised by initial rate and disappearance techniques in the rat system. Initial rate studies indicated that the Km for glucuronidation was 78.2 μM and the Vmax for glucuronidation was 20 $nmol.h^{-1}.mg\ protein^{-1}$. The disappearance of parent drug was rapid and appeared to be first-order throughout a 5 h incubation period. This disappearance was quantified in terms of clearance and was demonstrated to be equal to the ratio Vmax/Km for the glucuronidation reaction (Table 3). This clearance term is in fact the intrinsic clearance of free drug (Cl_{int}; Gillette, 1971).

Table 3

Summary of In Vitro Kinetic Constants for SK&F 94120

Parameter	Initial Rate	*Disappearance Data
Km (μM)	78.2	67.0
Vmax ($nmol.h^{-1}.mg^{-1}$)	20.0	25.0
Cl_{int} ($ml.h^{-1}.mg^{-1}$)	0.256	0.373

$$* \quad \frac{t}{Co-Ct} = \frac{1}{Vmax} + \frac{Km}{Vmax}\ \frac{(Ln\ (Co/Ct))}{Co-Ct}$$

Where Co is the initial concentration
Ct is the concentration at time t

(ii) Diazepam The concept of the intrinsic clearance of free drug has been applied in our laboratory to species differences in the rates and routes of metabolism of diazepam. Diazepam has been shown *in vivo* to be metabolised rapidly in experimental animals but only slowly in man (Guentert, 1984). Moreover, marked species differences in the types of circulating and urinary metabolites have been demonstrated. The extent to which the hepatocyte system reflects these differences depends not only on the rate of formation of the particular metabolite but also on the clearance of the metabolite from the system by subsequent metabolic steps. Thus, in the dog the major circulating metabolite is nordiazepam. In the rat, nordiazepam is present in the circulation at only very low concentrations. We have demonstrated that this difference can be attributed to a relative lack of reactions other than N-demethylation in dog hepatocytes. Nordiazepam is therefore produced rapidly by dog hepatocytes but is cleared only very slowly. In contrast, in rat hepatocytes, reactions such as hydroxylation in the 4'-position occur rapidly producing 4'-hydroxydiazepam rather than nordiazepam. In addition, nordiazepam is also cleared rapidly via metabolism in the rat hepatocyte system.

(iii) Paracetamol Species differences in the metabolism of paracetamol have been evaluated in the hepatocyte model (Moldeus, 1978). Paracetamol is metabolised by glucuronidation, sulphation and by cytochrome P_{450} mediated pathways in the rat and mouse. The *in vitro* system allows information to be obtained concerning the Km and Vmax of each of the pathways of metabolism and consequently provides a rational explanation regarding the relative susceptibility of rat and mouse to the toxic effects of paracetamol. Thus, a comparison of rat and mouse hepatocytes revealed that the mouse exhibits relatively low sulphate conjugation whereas the formation of the glutathione conjugate by cytochrome P_{450} mediated pathways was faster than the rat. These findings therefore provide an explanation for the observation that the mouse is more susceptible to the toxic effects of paracetamol than the rat, because more of dose is converted into the reactive metabolite in this species.

(iv) Tolbutamide The use of isolated hepatocytes as an *in vitro* model for *in vivo* comparative metabolism studies has been evaluated with tolbutamide (Gee et al, 1984). Hepatic metabolism of tolbutamide follows two major pathways, oxidation of the methyl group or dealkylation of the sulfonylurea group, leading to the formation of four primary metabolites. The major metabolite for the rat and squirrel monkey was hydroxymethyl-tolbutamide, whereas p-tolylsulfonylurea and p-tolylsulfonamide were the major metabolites found in the dog. Rabbit hepatocytes formed mostly carboxymethyl tolbutamide. Both the relative rates of metabolism and the metabolite profiles from hepatocytes from the rat, rabbit and dog correlated well with published *in vivo* data on tolbutamide half-lives and urinary metabolite profiles.

TOXICITY OF DRUGS IN CULTURED HEPATOCYTES

Isolated and cultured mammalian hepatocytes have been utilized in studies of hepatotoxicity on a considerable number of occasions (Acosta *et al*., 1985). In most cases drugs known to affect the liver in a dose related manner have been chosen and the emphasis has been to elucidate biochemical mechanisms associated with the lesion. Other authors have attempted to optimize the process of measuring drug toxicity in hepatocyte systems, and have concluded that no single parameter proved to be adequate for testing a range of different drugs. A combination of plasma membrane enzyme leakage and measurement of protein synthesis is probably preferred. Some chemicals may produce cellular injury without prior modification while others may be innocuous unless chemically activated by the cell (Gillette, 1981). Thus, toxicity has been evaluated with structures requiring metabolic activation (Chenery et al.,1981) and with agents acting directly (George *et al*.,1982).

(i) Oxmetidine Recently, we have investigated the toxicity of several histamine H_2-receptor antagonists in the cultured hepatocyte model (Oldham, *et al*., 1985; Figure 5). Oxmetidine is a potent histamine H_2-receptor antagonist and is efficacious in the treatment of peptic ulcers. During recent clinical trials in the United States a number of patients exhibited elevated serum transaminases which were reversible upon removal of the drug. These findings have resulted in the suspension of clinical trials and the eventual withdrawal of oxmetidine from further development. We have therefore investigated the use of cultured rat hepatocytes to study possible mechanisms by which oxmetidine may induce cell injury.

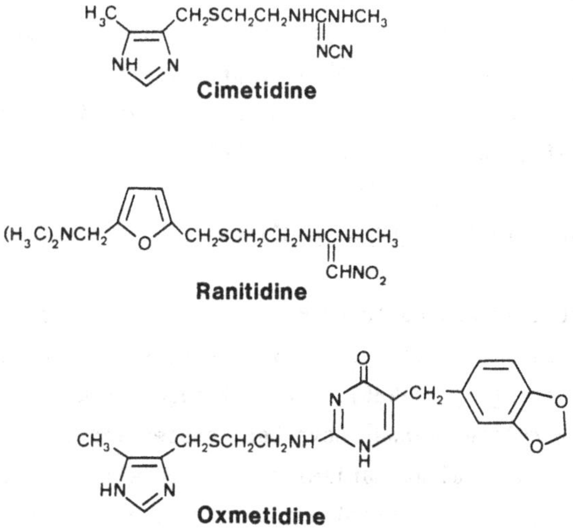

H_3C $CH_2SCH_2CH_2NHCNHCH_3$ NCN NH N

Cimetidine

$(H_3C)_2NCH_2$ O $CH_2SCH_2CH_2NHCNHCH_3$ $CHNO_2$

Ranitidine

O N CH_2 O O CH_3 $CH_2SCH_2CH_2NH$ N H HN N

Oxmetidine

Figure 5 Structure of Cimetidine, Ranitidine and Oxmetidine

Oxmetidine was found to be cytotoxic to primary cultures of adult rat hepatocytes. The criteria of cellular injury included leakage of cytoplasmic enzymes into the culture medium (Figure 6), inhibition of protein synthesis and measurement of oxygen consumption by freshly isolated hepatocytes. These parameters were correlated with morphological changes in the cells as judged by inverted phase-contrast microscopy. In contrast, two other histamine H_2-receptor antagonists used clinically, cimetidine and ranitidine, caused only minor changes in these parameters of cytotoxicity. The extent of injury observed with oxmetidine was both time and concentration dependent and was similar in hepatocytes maintained in culture for 2, 24 or 48 hours. Prior treatment of rats with phenobarbital or ß-naphthoflavone did not influence oxmetidine-induced cytotoxicity. Inhibitors of cytochrome P450-mediated monooxygenase activity had little effect on oxmetidine - induced injury with the exception of metyrapone, which was shown to inhibit the observed cytotoxicity by a mechanism other than inhibition of monooxygenase activity. In contrast, the injury could be potentiated by L-ethionine, an antimetabolite which reduces cellular ATP levels, suggesting that oxmetidine induces cytotoxic effects as a consequence of an interaction with intermediary energy metabolism. These studies have been extended by Rush _et al_. (1985) to indicate that the site of action of oxmetidine appears to reside in the inner mitochondrial membrane electron transport chain prior to ubiquinone oxidoreductase.

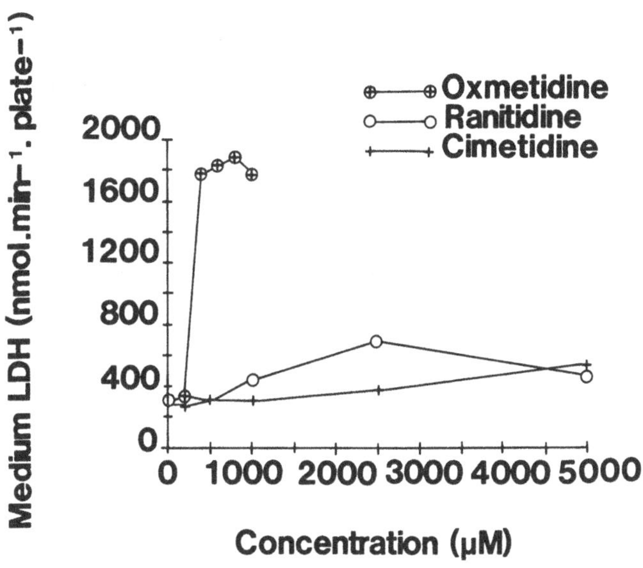

Figure 6 LDH Leakage from Rat Hepatocytes Treated with Oxmetidine Cimetidine and Rantidine.

(ii) Aflatoxin B_1 Aflatoxin B_1 is produced by the moulds Aspergillus flavus and Aspergillus parasiticus which grow on grains, nuts and other crops. Aflatoxin B_1 primarily affects the liver, where it is metabolised to a number of different products. Animal species differ markedly in their sensitivity to the toxic and carcinogenic effects of aflatoxin B_1; the rat being markedly more susceptible than the mouse despite the fact that liver microsomes from the mouse are more active than those from rat in metabolising aflatoxin B_1 to reactive metabolites. However, the mouse can detoxify these reactive metabolites more efficiently than the rat by conjugating the epoxide with glutathione. Hanigan and Laishes (1984) demonstrated that isolated hepatocytes accurately reflect this interplay between activation and detoxification, demonstrating a 1000-fold greater LD50 of aflatoxin B_1 for mouse hepatocytes than for rat hepatocytes.

(iii) Paracetamol The metabolism and cytotoxicity of paracetamol in hepatocyte preparations has been studied in several laboratories (Moldeus, 1978; Harman and Fischer, 1983). Green *et al*. (1984) studied the metabolism of paracetamol in hepatocytes from resistant and susceptible species. In agreement with whole animal studies, hepatocytes from hamsters were very susceptible to paracetamol-induced toxicity whereas hepatocytes from rat, rabbit and dog were resistant. Parameters of paracetamol metabolism generally correlated with *in vivo* species susceptibility to the drug. However, the substantial loss of glutathione (GSH) from dog liver cells in the absence of cytotoxicity suggests that further experimentation in this area would be of great value in understanding the detoxification of reactive metabolites in hepatocytes.

CONCLUSIONS

Although the potential for using isolated hepatocytes is often recognized there is little published data demonstrating their utility in drug metabolism and pharmacokinetics studies. Paine *et al*, (1985) have shown that in the case of pindolol and fluperlapine nearly all of the known metabolites of these compounds can be generated by rat hepatocyte cultures. We have extended previously reported observations in several significant directions. Our studies have shown that rat hepatocytes can distinguish between rapidly and slowly metabolised drugs. Rat hepatocytes metabolize diazepam at rates about 50-fold greater than antipyrine (Chenery et al., 1985). Disappearance of parent drug can be quantified in terms of clearance and we have demonstrated that this clearance term is in fact the intrinsic clearance (Cl_{int}) of free drug (Gillette, 1971) and in the case of SK&F 94120 was demonstrated to be equal to the ratio of Vmax/Km for the enzyme system responsible for the metabolic conversion.

In the case of drugs such as diazepam and tolbutamide (Gee et al, 1984) it has been possible to demonstrate that both the relative rates of metabolism and the metabolic profile of the drug in hepatocytes from the rat, rabbit and dog correlated well with published _in vivo_ data. In the case of a drug such as paracetamol _in vitro_ studies with hepatocytes provide a rational basis for the known differences in metabolism and toxicity in the rat, rabbit, hamster and mouse. Thus, the application of the hepatocyte system to the question of species differences in metabolism appears to be of considerable significance and relevance. However, a direct extrapolation of rates of metabolism from the hepatocyte system to duration of drug _in vivo_ will often not be possible because of the inability of the _in vitro_ system to predict the distribution of the drug _in vivo_. Clearly, the area of _in vivo_/_in vitro_ comparisons in metabolism and kinetics is an area requiring considerable systematic work.

Hepatocyte culture medium represents a very 'clean' system for the analysis of drugs and their metabolites. Moreover, the widespread use of rapid h.p.l.c. technology to separate drugs and metabolites, automatic injectors and sophisticated detection systems such as diode-array and LC-MS enables information on the metabolism of novel structures to be made available rapidly to drug discovery teams. This information should be of considerable value in discovering drugs with appropriate duration of action and in reducing the incidence of toxic metabolite formation. This _in vitro_ information should also be considered in the context of providing early _in vivo_ pharmacokinetic information about a drug using cold plasma assays. In this case the _in vitro_ data can be used to complement _in vivo_ data and to help select between candidate drugs for further study.

The hepatocyte system provides an excellent model to study the relationships between metabolism and toxicity and the factors responsible for activating molecules. In general, the degree of prediction for toxicity _in vivo_ will depend on a number of factors but in particular predictability will depend upon the mechanism of injury. True hepatotoxins (intrinsic, predictable) produce hepatocyte injury by acting directly on membranes or on cellular metabolic processes in both experimental animals and humans. Such compounds are by their nature more likely to elicit a response both _in vivo_ and _in vitro_. In contrast, idiosyncratic agents produce hepatic injury in susceptible individuals and the basis of the injury may be immunological or metabolic (Zimmerman, 1983). Thus, the greater variability of response _in vivo_ must make it more difficult in such cases to establish relationships with responses _in vitro_. The implication is that any screening procedure using hepatocytes to discover potential hepatotoxic problems with novel drugs or chemicals will require a large mechanistic element and to specifically include measurement of parent drug and metabolites in a variety of species including human hepatocytes if possible. Even if these aspects are considered then the pharmacokinetics of the drug _in vivo_ may prevent tissue concentrations of the drug ever achieving high enough levels to elicit a toxic response. However, if hepatocytes do not predict accurately the extent of an interaction it is clear that these systems have considerable value in evaluating a series of close structural analogues for trends in toxicity, for mechanism of toxicity and for species differences in metabolism and toxicity.

Losses in differentiated function are well documented in hepatocyte culture (Guguen - Guillouzo and Guillouzo, 1983) and are clearly a limitation to the ultimate usefulness of the hepatocyte system. In particular, losses in monooxygenase activity are often noted within the initial 24 hours of culture. These changes have been minimized in our studies by the use of short culture times of less than 8 hours, during which time losses in cytochrome P450 levels are not significant (Paine and Legg, 1978). The design of our experiments was such that clearance of parent drug was demonstrated to be constant throughout the period of incubation thereby indicating the stability of the drug-metabolising systems involved.

Improvements in culture techniques are constantly being made, however, including the development of co-culture systems which enable differentiated functions to be maintained in culture for considerable periods of time (Guillouzo et al.,1985). These and other improvements such as cryopreservation (Seddon, 1985) should considerably enhance the overall utility of hepatocyte systems.

REFERENCES

Abraham, R.T., Sauers, M.E., Zemaitis, M.A. and Alvin, J.D. (1983). Barbiturate N-demethylase Activity in Isolated Rat Hepatocytes. Anal. Biochem. 129, 235-244.

Acosta, D., Sorensen, E.B. Anuforo, D.C., Mitchell, D.B., Ramas, K., Santone, K.S. and Smith, A.M (1985). An In Vitro Approach to the Study of Target Organ Toxicity of Drugs and Chemicals. In Vitro Cell Devel. Biol. 21, 495-504.

Begue, J.M., Le Bigot, J.F., Guguen-Guillouzo, C., Kiechel, J.R. and Guillouzo, A. (1985). Cultured Human Adult Hepatocytes: A New Model for Drug Metabolism Studies. Biochem. Pharmacol. 32, 1643-1646.

Chenery, R., George, M. and Krishna, G. (1981) The Effect of Ionophore A23187 and calcium on Carbon Tetrachloride-Induced Toxicity in Cultured Rat Hepatocytes. Toxicol. Appl. Pharmacol. 60, 241-252.

Chenery, R.J.,Oldham, H.G.,Standring, P.,Norman, S.J. and Ayrton, A (1985) Drug Metabolism Kinetic Studies in an Hepatocyte Model. Int. Conf. Pract. IN VITRO Toxicol. p71

Davis, R.A., Highsmith, W.E., Mcneal, M.M., Schexnayder, J.A. and Kuan, J.C.W. (1983) Bile Acid Synthesis by Cultured Hepatocytes. J. Biol. Chemistry 258, 4079-4082.

Emery, S., Oldham, H.G., Norman, S.J. and Chenery, R.J. (1985) The Effect of Cimetidine and Ranitidine on Paracetamol Glucuronidation and Sulphation in Cultured Rat Hepatocytes. Biochem. Pharmacol. 34,1415-1421.

Gee, S.J. Green, C.E. and C.A Tyson (1984). Comparative Metabolism of Tolbutamide By Isolated Hepatocytes From Rat, Rabbit, Dog and Squirrel Monkey. (1984). Drug Metabolism and Disposition 12, 174-178.

George, M., Chenery, R.J. and Krishna, G. (1982) The Effect of Ionophore A23187 and 2,4-dinitrophenol on the Structure and Function of Cultured Liver Cells. Toxicol. Appl. Pharmacol. 66, pp 349-360.

Gillette, J.R. (1971). Factors Affecting Drug Metabolism . Anu. N.Y Acad. Sci. 179, 43-46.

Gillette, J.R. (1981). An Integrated Approach to the study of Chemically Reactive Metabolites of Acetaminophen. Arch. Intern. Medic 141, 375-379.

Grant, M.H. and Hawksworth, G.M.(1985). Conjugation Reactions in Primary Cultures of Rat Hepatocytes. Int. Conf. Pract. IN VITRO Toxicol. p70

Green, C.E., Dabbs, J.E. and Tyson, C.A. (1984). Metabolism and Cytotoxicity of Acetaminophen in Hepatocytes Isolated from Resistant and Susceptible Species. Toxicol. Appl. Pharmacol. 76, 139-149

Guentert, T.W. (1984). Pharmacokinetics of benzodiazepines and of their Metabolites. Progress in Drug Metabolism, Vol. 8, Chapter 5, 241-338

Guguen-Guillouzo, C. and Guillouzo, A. (1983). Modulation of Functional Activities in Cultured Rat Hepatocytes. Molecul. Cellul. Biochem. 53/54, 35-56.

Guillouzo, A., Beaune, P., Gascoin, M.N., Begue, J.M., Campion, J.P., Guengerich, P.F. and Guguen-Guillouzo, C.(1985). Maintenance of Cytochrome P-450 in Cultured Adult Human Hepatocytes. Biochem. Pharmacol. 34,2991-2995.

Hanigan, H.M. and Laishes, B.A. (1984). Toxicity of Aflatoxin B_1 in Rat and Mouse Hepatocytes In Vivo and In Vitro. Toxicology 30, 185-193

Harman, A.W. and Fischer, L.J. (1983). Hamster Hepatocytes in Culture as a Model for Acetaminophen Toxicity: Studies with Inhibitors of Drug Metabolism. Toxicol. Appl. Pharmacol. 71, 330-341

Moldeus, P. (1978). Paracetamol Metabolism and Toxicity in Isolated Hepatocytes from Rat and Mouse. Biochem. Pharmacol. 27, 2859-2863.

Oldham, H.G., Norman, S.J. and Chenery, R.J. (1985) Primary Cultures of Adult Rat Hepatocytes - A Model for the Toxicity of Histamine H_2-Receptor Antagonists. Toxicology 36, 215-229

Paine, A.J. and Legg, R.F. (1978). Apparent Lack of Correlation Between the Loss of Cytochrome P450 in Hepatic Parenchymal Cell Culture and The Stimulation of Haem Oxygenase Activity. Biochem. Biophys. Res. Comm., 81, 672-679.

Paine, A.J. and Hockin, L.J. (1982) The Maintenance of cytochrome P450 in Liver Cell Culture : Recent studies on P-450 Mediated Mechanisms of Toxicity. Toxicology 25, pp 41-45.

Paine, A.J., Maurer, G. and Van Wartburg, B.R. (1984). The Application of Hepatocyte Culture to the Identification of Pathways of Drug Metabolism. Studies with Pindolol and Fluperlapine. Biochem. Pharmacol., 33, 3111-3114

Rush, G.F., Ripple, M. and Chenery, R.(1985). The Mechanism of SK&F 92994 (Oxmetidine) Cytotoxicity in Isolated Rat Hepatocytes. J. Pharmacol. Exp. Ther. 233, 741-746.

Seddon, T., Bobbis, A.R. and Davies, D.S. (1985) Drug Metabolising Activity of Cryopreserved Rat and Human hepatocytes B.P.S. P41

Strom, S.C. Jirtle, R.A., Jones, R.S. Novicki, D.L., Rosenberg, M.R., Novotny, A., Irons, G., Mclain, J.R. and Michalopoulos, G. (1982). Isolation, Culture and Transplantation of Human Hepatocytes. J.N.C.I. 68, 771-778.

Tee, L.B.G., Seddon, T. Boobis, A.R. and Davis, D.S. (1985) Drug Metabolism Activity of Freshly Isolated Human Hepatocytes. Br. J. Clin Pharmac, 19, 279-294.

Tsuru, M., Erickson, R.R. and Holteman, J.R. (1982). The Metabolism of Phenytoin by Isolated Hepatocytes and Hepatic Microsomes from Male Rats. J. Pharmacol. Expt. Ther 22, 658-661.

Villa, P., Hockin, L.J. and Paine, A.J. (1980). The relationship between the ability of pyridine and substituted pyridines to maintain cytochrome P450 and inhibit protein synthesis in rat hepatocyte cultures. Biochem. Pharmacol. 29, 1773-1777.

Zimmerman, H.J. (1983). Hepatotoxic Evaluation Methodology. Diagnostic Procedures in the Evaluation of Hepatic Diseases, Chapter 13, 159-194.

IN VITRO EVALUATION OF HAEMIC SYSTEMS IN TOXICOLOGY

J S H Luke & G R Betton Dept. of Pathology,
Smith Kline & French Research Ltd., The Frythe,
Welwyn, Herts., U.K.)

GENERAL INTRODUCTION

The haemic system can be visualised as a dynamic three compartment model viz the bone marrow (generative) compartment, the vascular/lymphatic (distributive) compartment and the peripheral organ compartment. This is further sub-divided into cellular subsets comprising erythrocyte, platelet, polymorphonuclear, lymphocyte and monocyte. These cell lineages are defined on morphological, functional and clonogenic characteristics. The relationship of these cell lines to the three compartment model is shown in Figure 1. In addition, the micro-environment of the bone marrow compartment, necessary for normal haemopoiesis, and the haemostatic mechanisms of the peripheral blood compartment are considered parts of the haemic system. Toxic substances exert their effects on the haemic system in many ways. Some may affect only one cell line in one compartment, whilst others may affect all cell lines in all compartments or alternatively all cell lines in one compartment.

The principle compartments and cellular subsets in which haematotoxicity has been demonstrated by a range of compounds are described below. Since the breadth of scientific and technical information available far exceeds the scope of a single chapter, experimental methodology has been reviewed in detail for erythrocyte haemolysis and platelet aggregation tests only. The reader is referred to recent reviews cited in the bibliography for details of the many other various *in vitro* techniques available for the evaluation of the haemic system. The generation of T and B lymphocyte precursors in the bone marrow and the distribution (and recirculation) of lymphocytes and mononuclear phagocytes in the blood are important elements in immunotoxicology and are discussed elsewhere in this volume (Miller et. al.) and by Dean (1986).

Bone Marrow Compartment

Toxic substances exert their effect on bone marrow by destroying precursor cells, impairing cell growth, impairing cell differentiation or by preventing mature cells from leaving the bone marrow cavity. In the last decade there has been a massive increase in the number of *in vivo* and *in vitro* techniques reported for the identification and investigation of the toxic effects of chemicals on bone marrow. Long term marrow cultures using mouse and human cells have been used to study pluripotential stem cells and clonogenic assays using a wide variety of culture techniques have been used in the evaluation of colony forming cells from all lineages. Advances in flow cytometric analysis of blood and bone marrow cells offers the potential to evaluate the toxic effects of compounds on cell function, growth and differentiaton. Unfortunately it is outside the scope of this chapter to detail all of these techniques and the reader is referred to the recent reviews by McCulloch (1984), Golde and Takaku (1985) and Irons (1985).

Figure 1 : Compartmental Model of the Haemic System

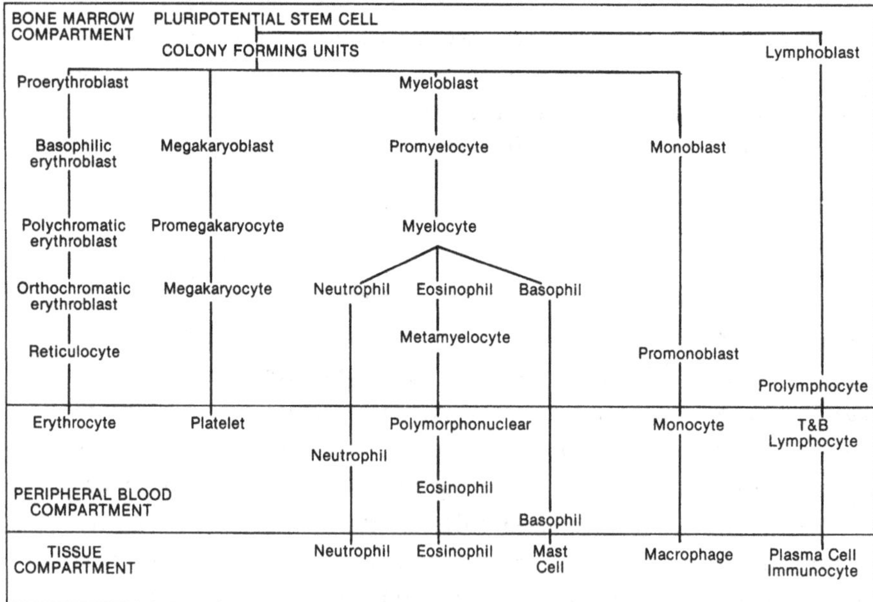

Peripheral Blood and Tissue Compartments

Haemostatic Mechanism The haemostatic mechanism is responsible for ensuring that cells such as erythrocytes, which function in the peripheral blood compartment, remain in that compartment until their functional lifespan is over. The haemostatic system depends on normal function and interaction between the vascular wall, platelets, the coagulation system and the fibrinolytic system. The effect of toxic substances on these factors results in a bleeding tendency, thrombosis or disseminated intravascular coagulation (Klocking 1985). Identification of toxic effects in these complex interactive pathways is at present confined to *ex vivo* techniques with animal subjects (Theus and Zbinden, 1984). The liver, as a source of a number of these factors, can secondarily impair coagulation following hepatotoxic episodes.

Cellular Constituents Toxic substances affect the cellular constituents of peripheral blood in two ways, by reducing the number of cells in the peripheral blood and/or by affecting the function of the cell. Premature destruction of cells in the peripheral blood compartment must be measured *ex vivo*, however the mechanism of cell destruction can be investigated using *in vitro* techniques, with the erythrocyte being the most studied.

Erythrocyte Toxicity - Toxicity towards the erythrocyte in the peripheral circulation is mediated by an effect either on the cell membrane, haemoglobin, red cell antioxidant protective mechanism or a combination of all three sites, resulting in loss of erythrocyte integrity or oxygen transport capability.

Any approach to analysing erythrocyte membrane damage should consider the membrane as an entire unit with cell membrane skeleton, lipid bilayer and cytoplasm interacting with each other (Sheetz, 1983). Parameters which are useful in detecting toxic damage to the erythrocyte membrane include erythrocyte haemolysis, potassium ion loss, autoxidation of membrane lipids, alteration in membrane fluidity, alteration in membrane deformability, membrane protein aggregates and measurement of changes in cell volume to surface area ratio.

Most drugs or toxic compounds exert their toxic effect on haemoglobin in the peripheral circulation by oxidising the haem iron of oxyhaemoglobin to form methaemoglobin, with or without denaturation of the molecule to haemichromes and ultimately "Heinz" bodies. Evidence of toxic damage to haemoglobin can be obtained by measuring the formation of methaemoglobin (Smith & Olsen 1973; Eyer et al 1975; Eckert & Eyer 1983, Linket al 1985), the formation of Heinz bodies (Winterbourn & Carrell 1973, Ward et al 1983), or the formation of haemichromes (Rachmilewitz 1974; Asakura et al 1977). The erythrocyte normally maintains several metabolic pathways to prevent the action of oxidising agents and to reduce methaemoglobin if it is formed. If these protective mechanisms are defective or the stress on the erythrocyte exceeds the reserve capacity of the protective enzymes, toxic damage will result. Reduced glutathione is important in maintaining a reduced intracellular environment and protecting the red cell from oxidant damage (Hill 1964; Awasthi et al 1983; Fujii et al 1984) therefore reduced glutathione is often measured as an indicator of toxic damage. Two of the most important enzymes involved in oxidant protection of erythrocytes are methaemoglobin reductase (Hegesh 1968; Beutler et al 1977; Choury et al 1983) and superoxide dismutase (Das & Nair 1980, Weiss 1980). Vitamin E has been measured as an indicator of oxidative damage (Bieri et al 1979; Gilbert et al 1984), but its role as an anti-oxidant protective agent is at present still not clear.

The direct toxic effect of drugs and chemicals on erythrocytes from the peripheral circulation can be measured, and the mechanism of the toxic effect investigated further using *in vitro* blood mixing studies, where defibrinated whole blood, anticoagulated whole blood or pure erythrocyte suspensions are mixed with drug or compound being tested under standard conditions of pH, temperature, mixing rate and tonicity.

Granulocyte Toxicity Drug-induced immune-mediated haematological toxicity has been extensively studied using *ex-vivo* techniques but, *in vitro* techniques have been of limited value. Tests of immune-mediated toxicity involve the detection of compounds or drug binding the erythrocyte surface (anti-globulin tests or isotopically-labelled drug binding studies) or alternatively treating an animal or in some cases a human volunteer with the drug or compound and then testing the serum *in vitro* for the presence of specific antibodies. *In vitro* tests to detect antibody-dependent cell mediated erythrotoxicity and antibody-dependant phagocytosis of erythrocyte opsonised complexes with penicillin by anti penicillin antibodies have been described (Yustet et al 1982).

In vitro studies to investigate drugs which affect cell function involve adding the drug or chemical in varying concentrations to isolated normal cells whose function is then measured. The important role of lysosomal enzymes and the superoxide generation system in bacterial killing following phagocytosis by neutrophil polymorphonuclear leukocytes can be disturbed with subsequent increased susceptibility to bacterial infection (Dean, 1986). Expression of granulocyte toxicity may therefore be as a neutropenia, for example following selective bone marrow toxicity by metiamide (Fitchen 1980) or as a functional impairment, e.g. chemotoxic, migration, phagocytoxis and microbiocidal activity. The toxic effects of drugs on the migration cascade and the killing cascade of the granulocyte have been extensively studied using *in vitro* techniques, for a review the reader is referred to the article by Marsh (1985).

Platelet Aggregation The adhesion of platelets to collagen fibres or to extravascular surfaces and subsequent aggregation is essential for normal haemostasis. The mechanism of platelet aggregration is complex and still incompletely understood. It involves membrane receptors, intracellular 3',5'-adenosine monophosphate (AMP), thromboxane synthesis, calcium ion availability, changes in membrane contractile proteins and release of substances stored in platelet organelles from the cell (Figure 2). In addition to platelet specific toxicity, tests of platelet function provide a sensitive means of detecting unpredicted pharmacological effects on several widespread pathways. Inhibitors of the cyclo-oxygenase pathway, for example, can be readily detected by platelet aggregation inhibition and may help to identify mechanisms of toxicity in other organs such as the gastric mucosa. *In vitro* tests to study the effects of novel drugs on platelet aggregation are of value in three circumstances, viz:

1. To detect the direct activation of platelets *in vitro* by novel drugs which can result in thrombocytopenia *in vivo*.
2. To detect inhibition of platelet aggregation by novel drugs which can lead to a bleeding diathesis *in vivo*
3. As an aid in the diagnosis and investigation of immune thrombocytopenia.

PRACTICAL ASPECTS

Apparatus

The instrumentation required to carry out the in vitro erythrocyte haemolysis test, a spectrophotometer and a bench top centrifuge, are usually available in research laboratories and the assay can be set up at minimal cost. The in vitro platelet aggregation test requires the use of a platelet aggregometer to measure the platelet aggregation activity. There are several manufacturers who supply a wide range of instrumentation in this field at varying degrees of cost from the basic single channel aggregometer to the dual channel lumi-aggregometer with ionised calcium measurement facility. (Chronolog, Payton, Biodata). Recent developments in the instrumentation available for studying platelet agregation responses include whole blood aggregometers (Chronolog) and the aquisition and analysis of information from the aggregometer by computer programs (Payton Instruments).

Figure 2 : Diagrammatic Representation of the Intracellular Pathways Involved in Platelet Aggregation

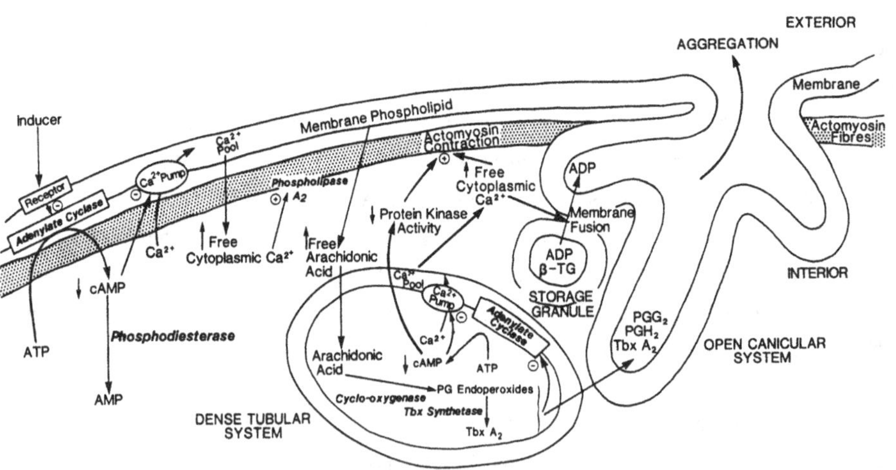

Choice of Species

Species differences exist when using red cells or platelets from animals for in vitro work. For example rat erythrocytes are less susceptible to haemolysis in vitro than dog erythrocytes which have a similar susceptibility to human erythrocytes. Platelets obtained from many species have been used in the study of platelet aggregation with the majority of research being done on rabbit platelets which respond to agonists in a similar manner to human platelets. Platelets from rats will respond to only a limited number of agonist under experimental conditions compared to human or rabbit platelets. In order to avoid these species differences, the use of human erythrocytes and platelets which are usually readily available from volunteer donors is strongly recommended.

Erythrocyte Haemolysis Test

Principle There are many modified protocols available in the literature for measuring erythrocyte haemolysis in vitro. The modifications are either to the erythrocyte preparation used in the test or the method used to measure the degree of haemolysis. Variation in erythrocyte preparation include the use of defibrinated whole blood, blood in heparin or citrate anticoagulant or washed erythrocyte preparations. The concentration of cells is standardised in one of a variety of buffer systems. Alternative methods for measuring the degree of haemolysis include radioactive labelling of the red cell preparation and measuring the residual radioactivity after haemolysis, converting the free haemoglobin lysed from the red cells into cyanmethaemoglobin and measuring the haemoglobin concentration against known standards or by directly measuring the haemoglobin in the haemolysate as its optical absorbance at 540nm.

The erythrocyte haemolysis test first proposed by Husa (Husa 1944) has been modified to minimise the effects of vehicle components on the absorbance or solubility of haemoglobin in the final solution (Reed and Yalkowsky 1985). The principle of the technique is that defibrinated red cells and solutions of test compound at varying concentration are mixed in a 1:1 ratio. The mixtures are incubated for a standard time and temperature before being made isotonic by the addition of a large excess of sodium chloride solution. After centrifugation, the supernatant is discarded and the haemoglobin remaining in the residual red cells released by lysis with distilled water. The concentration of haemoglobin is then measured as absorbance on a spectrophotometer.

Procedure - Blood (20mls) is taken by venepuncture from haematologically normal, healthy human volunteers, placed in sterile universal containers containing glass beads and defibrinated by gently rotating the container for 20 minutes. Defibrinated blood is then decanted into clean sterile universal container and gently inverted to aerate before use. 0.5mls of defibrinated blood is mixed with 0.5mls test compound and, a 100% standard (no haemolysis) is prepared by mixing 0.5mls of a 0.9% w/v sodium chloride solution with 0.5mls defibrinated blood. In the standard test each set of tubes is incubated at 37°C in a shaking water bath at 50 strokes/min for 2 mins. At the end of the incubation period 5mls sodium chloride solution is added to the tubes prior to centrifuging them at 150g for 10 minutes. The supernatant containing the haemoglobin lysed by the compound under test is discarded, and the residual haemoglobin in the cell pellet measured by lysing the remaining red cells with an excess of distilled water. The absorbance in the final solution is measured at 540nM on a spectrophotometer.

Results The % haemolysis induced by the compound under test can be calculated with reference to the 0.9 w/v sodium chloride tube and any positive reference agents incorporated.

In all in vitro techniques, the compound to be tested has to be in solution, and as many of the drugs are poorly soluble they require to be dissolved in cosolvents. A wide range of cosolvents have been tested for their haemolytic potential, dimethyl sulphoxide (DMSO), polyethylene glycol 400 (PEG 400), dimethyl isosorbide (DMI), ethanol (ETOH), dimethyl acetamide (DMA) and propylene glycol (PG) have been measured and the cosolvents placed in order of haemolytic potential (Reed and Yalkowsky 1985). Cosolvents such as DMI, DMA, PEG 400 and ETOH have a low potential to cause haemolysis, PG and DMSO have a high potential. The haemolytic effect of cosolvents in vitro was confirmed in vivo (Fort et al 1984) by testing cosolvent mixtures of PG ETOH: water; PG:ETOH: saline; and PEG 400: ETOH: water for their haemolytic effect in dogs and rats.

Platelet Aggregation Test

Principle Modifications to the platelet aggregation test are associated with the platelet preparation or the facet of aggregation to be measured. Alteration in the platelet cell preparation include washing the platelets in buffer systems, treating them with aggregation inhibitors such as aspirin, and labelling with fluorescence markers (Quin 2, Furan). A large number of parameters involved in platelet aggregation can be measured in vitro. An example of these parameters include release of ATP (luminescence), thromboxane ß2 synthesis (radio-immune assay) and movement of calcium ions (fluorescence markers). The agonist action of test compounds or known agonist on blood platelet aggregation can be measured by adding the compound under test to an aliquot of platelet rich plasma in a blood-platelet aggregometer and recording any increase in light transmission due to platelet aggregate formation by the method of Born (1962) (figure 3).

Figure 3 : Platelet Aggregation Responses to Collagen (5mg.ml), Adrenaline (10µm.l). Arachidonic Acid (O.mg.ml) and ADP (2 and 5 µm).

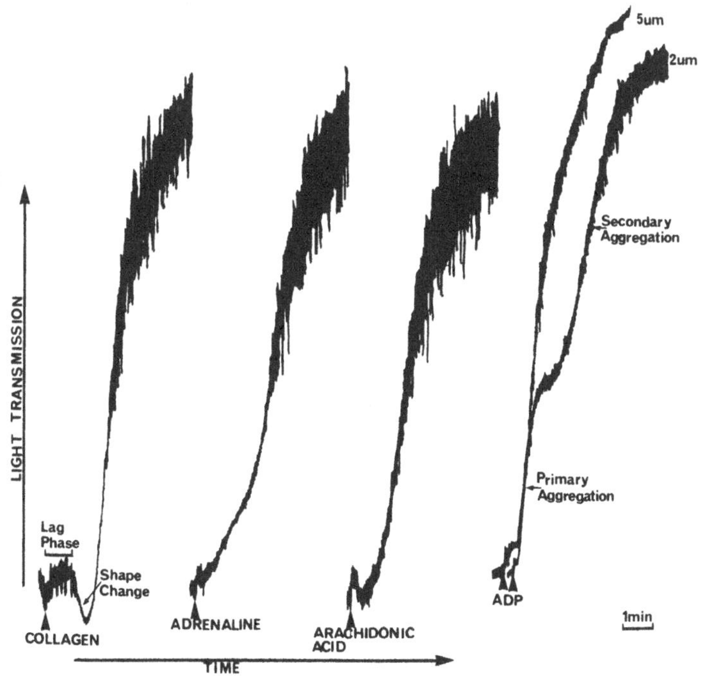

The antagonist action of test compounds on blood platelet aggregation can be measured by incubating the test compound with an aliquot of platelet rich plasma prior to adding an agonist with known aggregating activity to the mixture. The difference in aggregation response in the presence or absence of test compound is a measure of the inhibition or antagonism of platelet aggregation by the test compound.

Procedure

Platelet rich/platelet poor plasma - Blood from healthy donors who had not received medication for at least 14 days is mixed with 3.2% w/v trisodium citrate (9 parts blood : 1 part citrate). The samples are centrifuged at 150g for ten minutes and the supernatant, platelet rich plasma (PRP), removed. The sample is re-centrifuged at 500 g for 20 minutes and the supernatant, platelet poor plasma (PPP) separated into a clean plastic tube. Adjust platelet count in platelet rich plasma to 250 $\pm$ 50 x 10^9/l platelets by dilution with autologous platelet poor plasma.

Agonists Adenosine-5-diphosphate (ADP) - concentrations between 5 and 20 uM are prepared. Collagen - concentration 1.9 mg/ml Adrenaline - concentration 100 μM Arachidonic acid - concentration 5 mg/ml. ADP, and adrenaline are supplied by Sigma Ltd. The arachidonic acid is supplied by Biodata Corporation. Collagen suspension used in this method is lmg suspension equine collagen fibrils supplied by Hormon-Chemie. Munchen GMBH.

Activation Test 25μl aliquots of test compound, positive or negative control solutions are added to 225 μl aliquots of platelet rich plasma in an aggregometer at 37°C with a mixing speed of 900 rpm. The aggregation response is recorded until aggregation is complete or for a maximum of 5 minutes.

Inhibition Test 25μl aliquots of test compound, positive or negative control solutions are incubated with 225 μl aliquots of PRP in an aggregometer at 37°C for 3 minutes, mixing speed 900 rpm. After 3 minutes 25 μl of one of the agonists is added to each of the mixtures and the aggregation response recorded until complete or for a maximum of five minutes.

Results - The aggregation responses can be measured directly, as the % increase in light transmission at a predefined time after adding the agonist. Additional information about platelet aggregation mechanism can be obtained from these traces.

The effect of collagen on normal platelets is to cause the platelets to swell after an initial lag phase. The swelling is followed by the aggregation phase, these changes may or may not be observed with an other agonist, and may depend on the concentration of agonist used. At high concentration of ADP the aggregation appears to occur in one phase. However, at lower concentrations of ADP, aggregation is biphasic with the primary phase due to the exogenous ADP added to induce aggregation, and the secondary phase which is due to the release of ADP from granules within the platelet itself.

EXPERIMENTAL EXAMPLES

Erythrocyte Toxicity A large number of different types of compounds show haemolytic activity, these include anaesthetics, phenothiazide tranquillizers, antibiotics, saponins, animal venoms, anti-histamines and ß adrenoceptor blocking agents. Several large studies involving *in vitro* erythrocyte haemolysis tests have been carried out to measure the haemolytic potential of chemical compounds. In one series the haemolytic potential of 161 different compounds was measured, (Hammarlund and Pedersen-ßjergaard 1961), 90 compounds had no haemolytic effect in iso-osmotic solution and 71 showed varying degrees of haemolysis. In another study the haemolytic potential of 335 injectable drugs or solutions was tested (Oshida et al 1979). The study demonstrated that most injectables for intramuscular use showed severe haemolysis. The degree of haemolysis correlated with the severity of muscle lesions often seen with some i.v. injection. The haemolytic effect of phenothiazide tranquillizers has been extensively studied with *in vitro* erythrocyte haemolysis tests on human and animal red cells. Chlorpromazine is the most studied drug in this group and it has been shown *in vitro* that chlorpromazine can protect against hypotonic haemolysis at low concentration but cause haemolysis at higher concentration (Fievet et al 1971, Olaisen & Oye 1973, Ogiso et al 1981, Benga et al 1983).

ß adrenoceptor blocking drugs used in the control of hypertension (betaxolol, propranolol and practolol) have been shown to protect erythrocytes against hypotonic haemolysis at low concentration but to cause haemolysis at high concentrations (Olaisen and Oye 1973).

Using the in vitro erythrocyte haemolysis test previously described we have measured the haemolytic effect of SK&F 95018 (6-4-3-((3- (4-(2 - cyclopropyl (methoxyethyl) phenoxy -2-hydroxypropylamino) propionamido) phenyl - 4,5, -dihydro-5-methylpyridazin-3-(2H)-one) an antihypertensive compound with combined properties of ß adrenoceptor antagonism and vasodilation (Howson et al 1987). The haemolytic effect of SK&F 95018 was concentration dependent and from a graph of % haemolysis vs concentration (Figure 4), the concentrations of test drug required to cause 5%, 10% or 50% haemolysis (Hc 5, 10 or 50) were measured (table 1) as an indication of haemolytic potential. These measurements allowed us to compare the haemolytic potential of 17 structurally-related compounds before selecting the best candidate for further developmental studies (figure 5). The erythrocyte haemolysis test can be used to study the effects of varying concentration and time of exposure of erythrocytes to

Figure 4 : Haemolytic Effect of SK&F 95018 on Human Erythrocytes, Exposure Time 2 minutes at 37°C.

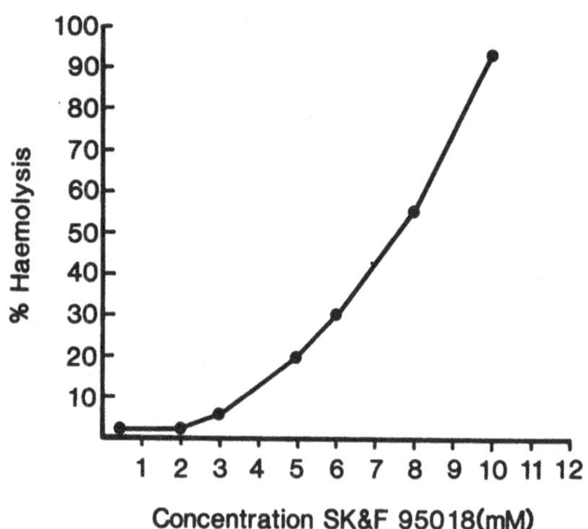

a drug causing erythrocyte haemolysis (Figure 6) and provide damaged erythrocyte for further investigative procedures such as electron microscopy and NMR studies.

In vitro experiments where compounds known to cause haemolysis are mixed with erythrocytes have been used to study the mechanism of haemolysis as opposed to the degree of haemolysis. The effects of compounds on membrane permeability have been studied, e.g. phenylhydrazine and polyethylene glycol (Nishio et al 1982) which cause erythrocytes to become osmotically fragile and non-selectively "leaky" to sodium and potassium. The formation of malondialdehyde, a secondary product of lipid peroxidation, can cross link membrane proteins with resulting loss of membrane fluidity and deformability causing cell

Table 1 : Haemolytic Potential of Compounds Structurally Related to SK&F 95018

Substituent Group				Haemolytic Concentration (mMol)		
R	R^1	R^2	x/n	H_C5	H_C10	H_C50
BENZIMIDAZOLES						
1-substituted						
H	4-CH_2CONH_2			>20	>20	>20
H	2-F,4-Cymoe			4	4	14.6
H	2_13_1-$(CH_3)_2$ –			5.2	6.8	14.0
CH_3	4 – Cymoe			10.0	11.0	18.0
2-substituted						
4-Cymoe	H		$(CH_2)_4$ NH –	1.65	2.5	8.0
4-Cymoe	H		CH_2 NH –	1.37	2.75	10.0
4-Cymoe	CH_3		CH_2 NH –	3.0	3.8	8.0
4-CH_2CONH_2	H		$(CH_2)_4$ NH –	>50	>50	>50
AMIDES						
	CH_3		2	2.0	2.75	4.4
	CH_3(R_1Sisomer)		2	1.5	1.9	4.2
	CH_3	N-C_3H_7	2	0.8	1.1	2.3
UREA						
2_13-$(CH_3)_2$				2.75	3.25	17.0
VASODILATORS						
H	CH_3	CH_3		30	100	100
CH_3	H	CH_3		>100	>100	>100
PRIZIDOLOL				27	100	>100
B ADRENOCEPTOR ANTAGONIST						
Betaxolol				25	25.5	40
Propranolol				6.5	13	>20

lysis in vitro (Evans & La Celle 1970, Morris & Williams 1979, Heath et al 1982 Mohandas et al 1983). Malondialdehyde formation has be shown by in vitro experiments to be part of the mechanism of erythrocyte toxicity due to diaminodiphenylsulfone, acetyl phenylhydrazine (Goldstein 1980) and hydrogen peroxide (Saubenan et al 1983, Aloisio et al 1982). Another mechanism of toxicity mediated by an effect on erythrocyte membrane is the insertion of drugs or compounds into the cell membrane with alteration in cell membrane surface area, volume, and structure. In an elaborate series of in vitro studies, Seeman et al (1969), measuring erythrocyte haemolysis and mean cell volume demonstrated that anaesthetics (1-pentanol, 1-nonanol, benzyl alcohol and chlorpromazine hydrochloride) could expand the erythrocyte membrane area, and above a "critical" concentration cause haemolysis. Below the critical concentration however they could protect the cell from osmotic lysis. Insertion of oxygenated sterol compounds (1ß-hydroxycholesterol, 22-ketocholesterol, and 20-hydroxycholesterol) into erythrocyte membranes cause a similar effect.

Figure 5 : General Structure of Compounds Related to SK&F 95018.

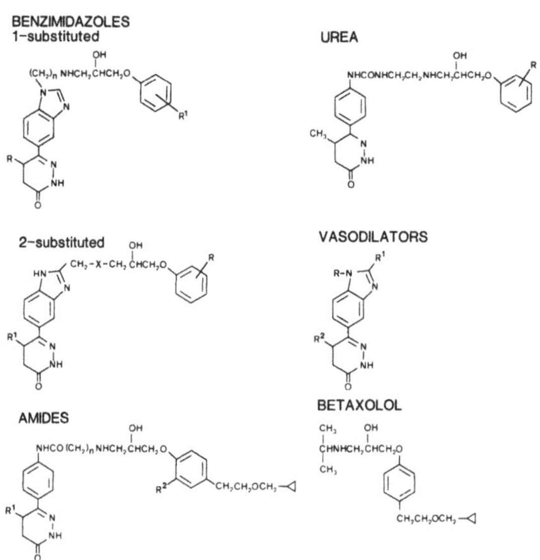

Haemoglobin Oxidation The conversion of oxyhaemoglobin to methaemoglobin by toxic compounds proceeds at a rapid rate and may be a transient phase leading to haemichrome formation and "Heinz" body formation. An *in vitro* technique has been developed for measuring the quantity and rate of methaemoglobin formation caused by 8-aminoquinolines (Link et al 1985). Other compounds which have been shown to induce methaemoglobin formation with or without haemolysis include dapsone, salazosulphapyridine, phenaphridine (Ward et al 1983), and phenacetin (Eckert and Eyer 1983) Cancer chemotherapeutic agents such as methotrexate, daunomycin, vincristine, BCNU, DTIC and L-asparaginase cause methaemoglobin formation *in vitro*.

Platelet Function

There are many compounds or drugs which have been shown to affect platelet function using *in vitro* techniques which reproduce the *in vivo* effects either in man or in animals. The agonist action of some of these compounds (ADP, arachidonic acid, collagen and adrenaline) is

Figure 6 : The Effect of Varying Exposure Time and Concentration of SK&F 95018 on Erythrocyte Haemolysis.

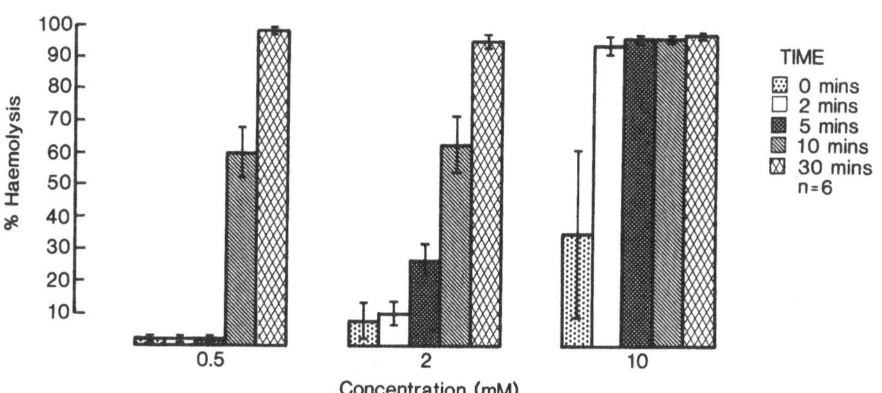

used to assess normal platelet function *in vitro* (Figure 3). Direct activation of platelet aggregation by ristocetin, an antibacterial agent derived from the fermentation broth of *Nocadia lurida* has been extensively studied (Gangarosa et al 1960). The mechanism of aggregation is believed to be by the direct action of ristocetin on factor VIII antigen and platelet membrane glycoproteins. Moreover platelets from subjects deficient in factor VIII antigen (Von Willebrands disease) or absence of platelet membrane glycoprotein complex lb (Bernard Soulier syndrome) do not aggregate with ristocetin (Hoyer 1976, Weiss 1980). Ristocetin has subsequently been withdrawn as an active drug and is used as a reagent in *in vitro* platelet aggregation tests to detect these disorders.

High molecular weight fractions of the anticoagulant heparin have been reported to cause platelet aggregation *in vitro* by a mechanism similar to ristocetin (Salzman et al 1980). Inflammatory mediators such as acetyl-glyceryl-ether-phosphorylcholine (AGEPC) or platelet activating factor (PAF) as it was called, are potent lipid mediators released from IgE sensitised mast cells (Hanahan et al 1980) which induce aggregation and release reaction in human platelets *in vitro* at micromolar concentrations (Marcus et al 1981). *In vivo*, AGEPC produces acute thrombocytopenia, granule release, intravascular platelet aggregation and platelet sequestration (McManus et al 1979).

As already stated many drugs inhibit platelet aggregation *in vitro* (antagonists) and it is possible to discuss only a few of the more important classes of compounds which do so. For review articles the reader is referred to the work of Holmsen (1976), Weiss (1972), and Rao and Welsh (1983).

Anti-inflammatory agents have been extensively studied since the discovery in the 1960's that aspirin inhibits second-phase platelet aggregation. This was subsequently found to be due to irreversible acetylation of cyclo-oxygenase in platelets. Aspirin is now widely used *in vitro* as a reagent which can block prostaglandin systhesis when investigating the platelet aggregation and release mechanism. Other non-steroidal anti-inflammatory agents such as indomethacin, phenylbutazone, ibuprofen, sulphyrazone, piroxican and naproxan have also been shown to inhibit prostaglandin metabolism, possibly by competitive inhibition of cyclo-oxygenase (Ali & McDonald 1978).

Adenylate cyclase activators inhibit platelet aggregation by increasing the levels of adenylate cyclase available to convert ATP to cAMP which inhibits aggregation. The reverse of this effect is inhibition of phosphodiesterase which normally converts cAMP to ATP. The most potent activators of adenylate cyclase are prostacyclin, PGE2, and PGD2 (Holmsen 1976). Adenosine, 2-chloroadenosine and isoprenaline elevate cAMP levels with inhibition of platelet aggregation, but to a lesser extent than PGE_1 (Huguette et al 1976).

Phosphodiesterase inhibitors include pyrimido-pyrimidine compounds (dipyridamole, RA 233, RA 433) used as vasodilators (Moncada and Korbutt 1978) and methylxanthines (caffeine, theophylline, aminophylline and papaverine) which inhibit platelet aggregation _in vitro_ (Burns & Dodge 1984) but at concentrations much higher than can be achieved _in vivo_. SK&F 94836 is a novel vasodilator, inotropic compound which inhibits phosphodiesterase type III. SK&F 94836 inhibits platelet aggregation stimulated by the agonists ADP, collagen and arachidonic acid (figure 7).

Antimicrobial drugs such as penicillin G, ampicillin, carbenicillin or cephalothin, when given in high doses _in vivo_ or mixed with platelets at high concentrations _in vitro_ can inhibit platelet aggregation possibly by coating the platelet surface and blocking membrane receptor sites in a non-specific manner (McClure et al 1970, Shatill et al 1980).

Many membrane-acting drugs, including local anaesthetics, tranquillizers, anti-depressants and antihistamines inhibit second wave platelet aggregation and release when present in high concentration. Cocaine, procaine and xylocaine have been shown to inhibit ADP and collagen-induced aggregation. Chlorpromazine, a phenothiazide with membrane stabilising properties, inhibits second wave aggregation induced by ADP or adrenaline, as do the dibenzazepine derivatives imipramine and desmethylimipramine (Mills & Roberts 1967).

Imidazole selectively inhibits thromboxane synthesis in platelets (Moncada et al 1977, Needleman et al 1977). Histamine and surprisingly histamine H_2-receptor antagonists have also been shown to inhibit second wave platelet aggregation _in vitro_. Imidazole derivatives, which act as histamine H_2-receptor antagonists, such as burimamide, metiamide, cimetidine and oxmetidine at high concentrations

Figure 7 : Inhibition of Platelet Aggregation by Aspirin (3mg), Oxmetidine (1mM), SK&F 94836 (1mM) and Imidazole (1mM), with Collagen (5μg.ml), Arachidonic Acid (0.5mg.ml) and ADP (2μM) as Standard Agonists.

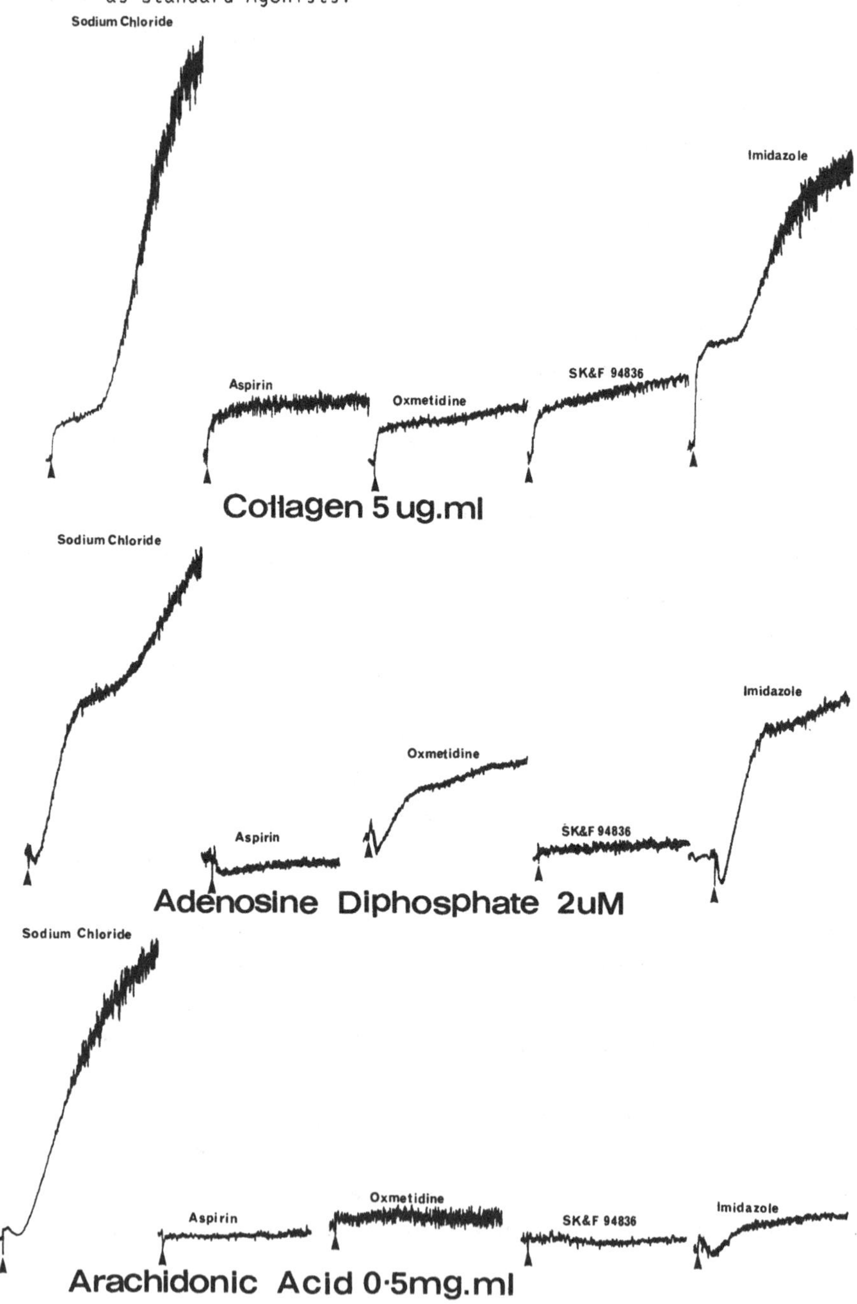

inhibit second wave aggregation induced by ADP, adrenaline, collagen or arachidonic acid (Allan & Eakin 1978, Gachalyi et al 1984, Horton et al 1983). We have confirmed the inhibition of second wave platelet aggregation by high concentrations of oxmetidine (Fig 7) in our laboratory using the in vitro aggregation test. Dazoxiben, an imidazole-derived selective inhibitor of thromboxane A_2 sunthesis, has also been shown to inhibit platelet aggregation in vitro (Bertele et al 1984).

A ß adrenoceptor blocking agent (propranolol) used extensively in the treatment of hypertension inhibits platelet aggregation, adhesion, serotonin uptake and release in vitro, probably by binding to membrane phospholipids at high drug concentration or inhibiting prostaglandin metabolism (Siess 1983).

In vitro tests of platelet aggregation are useful in detecting the presence of drug-dependant antibodies in subjects suspected of having drug-induced immune thrombocytopenia (Hackett, et al 1982). Although essentially an ex-vivo technique, it is important in the diagnosis of drug-induced thrombocytopenia as to warrant a mention. Essentially patient/subject serum (containing anti-drug antibody), drug and target platelets are mixed in vitro, and the mixture tested for clot retraction inhibition, platelet aggregation, platelet lysis or immunoglobulin binding. More recently developed techniques involve immunofluorescence, ^{51}Cr lysis, antiglobulin consumption or ^{125}I Coomb's test as indicators.

DISCUSSION AND CONCLUSIONS

In this short chapter we have attempted to introduce the reader to the concept of a dynamic haemic system, which by definition is difficult to reproduce completely in one simple in vitro test system. In order to investigate the system and devise alternative strategies for measuring the toxic effects of chemical compounds, it is necessary to divide the system into compartments with the consequence that some of the interaction between compartments may be lost in the in vitro test system. It has only been possible to discuss red cell haemolysis and platelet function fully. All aspects of the haemic system, are detailed in references to recent texts or reviews which will allow the interested reader to delve further into the fascinating study of the haemic system and the effects of drugs upon it. Tissue culture methods utilising both long and short term cultures with a variety of media have opened up the in vitro investigation of the bone marrow compartment. In particular, the functional or clonogenic identification of cell populations and their requisite growth factors which cannot be identified simply on morphological characteristics has been achieved. These assays are now being used to assess the effects of chemical compounds on the early progenitor cells with earlier prediction of bone marrow toxicity. Advances in cell identification and characterisation, including monoclonal antibodies and flow cytometric analysis, coupled with tissue culture techniques, have allowed the identification of toxic effects at the cellular and sub-cellular level to become a reality, although much work remains to be done to correlate the toxic findings at the cellular level with the clinical and pathological findings in the living animal.

Experiments where normal cells are mixed with chemical compound or drug under standard condition have been used extensively to study the peripheral blood compartment. These assays attempt to mimic the in vivo conditions under which drugs and blood cells interact by using protocols which control physical factors such as pH, temperature, blood mixing rate, concentration of drug in whole blood, cell suspension or plasma, and the time of exposure. The influence of time of exposure and drug concentration is well demonstrated in figure 4, where the haemolytic effect of SK&F 95018 at any concentration increased with time of exposure until all the remaining red cells were lysed. The difficulty arises in the interpretation of these data as applied to the in vivo situation and requires prediction of the exposure time of red cells to drug in a rapidly equilibrating blood flow situation to give some predictive indication of toxicity. The alternative to extrapolation from only in vitro indices is to carry out in vivo toxicology studies in small groups of animals to validate the data. This point raises the question of species specificity; care should be taken in the selection of species from which blood or bone marrow for in vitro analysis is taken. In our experience, wherever possible blood from normal human volunteers should be used if the effect of chemical compounds destined for human use of exposure is being studied. This approach avoids problems of interspecies extrapolation. Human sources of bone marrow are however limited. When the effect of chemical compounds on "abnormal" cells is being tested, it is often not possible to obtain human cells with the abnormal cell defect and an alternative animal model must be used.

With certain toxic substances, even although all the physical aspects of an *in vitro* test system mimic the *in vivo* situation, cell toxicity can only be demonstrated *ex vivo*. For example aniline, nitrobenzene or p-aminopropiophenone cause methaemoglobin formation *in vivo* but not in a direct *in vitro* test, whilst phenylhydroxylamine, nitrosobenzene and aminophenols can generate methaemoglobin formation both *in vivo* and *in vitro*. Metabolism of the first series of compounds probably accounts for their toxic effects. By coupling the direct *in vitro* test with a metabolising system such as short term hepatocyte cultures, it should be possible to increase the detection of cell toxicity in the peripheral blood compartment due to metabolites rather than the parent compound.

The availability of pharmacokinetic, plasma protein binding and metabolism data on the drug or compound being studied is essential to allow the concentration range over which the drug should be tested in any *in vitro* toxicity test to be selected. These data may also give an indication of whether the parent drug is easily metabolised, as a supply of metabolites for testing on cells from the haemic system may be required. Frequently toxic effects are observed at higher concentration of compounds under test than necessary to produce a pharmacological effect. The importance of these findings in relation to any toxic effect that such a compound will exert *in vivo* can only be assessed if the *in vitro* system has been properly validated with compounds of known toxicity *in vivo*, usually in animals models and/or human clinical experience.

The advantages of *in vitro* tests for the detection and investigation of toxic effects on the haemic system are many. Related compounds in drug development programs can be tested quickly and structure activity relationships established with the minimum use of live animals, and requiring only small quantities of test compounds. However, until *in vitro* systems can be devised which measure toxic effects of compounds on the integrated functions of all compartments of the haemic system there will always be a requirement for *in vivo* tests on animal models prior to clinical evaluation of novel compounds in man.

REFERENCES

Allan, G. and Eakins, K.E. (1978). Burimamide is a Selective Inhibitor of Thromboxane-A Biosynthesis in Human Platelet Microsomes. Prostaglandins, 15, No.4, 659-661.

Ali, M. and McDonald, J.W.D. (1978). Reversible and Irreversible Inhibition of Platelet Cyclo-oxygenase and Serotonin Release by Non-Steroidal Anti-Inflammatory Drugs. Thrombosis Research, 13, 1057-1063.

Alloisio, N. Michelon, D. Banner, E. Revol, A. Benzard Y. and Dalauney, J. (1982). Alterations of Red Cell Membrane Protein and Haemoglobin under Natural and Experimental Oxidant Stress. Biochimica et Biophysica Acta, 691, 300-308.

Asakura, T. (1977). Denatured Haemoglobin in Sickle Erythrocytes. Journal of Clinical Investigation, 59, 633-640.

Awasthi, Y.C. Misra, G. Rassin, D.K. and Srivastava, S.K. (1983) Detoxification of Xenobiotics by Glutathione-s-transferase in Erythrocytes : the Transport of the Conjugate of Glutathione and 1-chloro-2, 4-dinitro benzene. British Journal Haematology, 55, 419-425.

Benga, G. Ionescu, M. Popescu, O. and Pop, V (1983). Effects of Chlorpromazine on Proteins in Human Erythrocyte Membranes as Inferred from Spin Labelling and Biochemical Analysis. Molecular Pharmacology 23, 771-778.

Bertele, V. Falanga, A. Tomasiak, M. Chiabrando, C. Cerletti C., de Gaetano, G. (1984). Pharmacologic Inhibition of Thromobxane Synthetase and Platelet Aggregation : Modulatory Role of Cyclo-oxygenase Products. Blood, 63, No.6, 1460-1466.

Beutler, E. (1977). International Committee for Standardisation in Haematology : Recommended Methods for Red-cell Enzyme Analysis. British Journal of Haematology, 35, 331-340.

Born, G.V.R. (1962). Aggregation of Blood Platelets by Adenosine diphosphate and its Reversal. Nature, 194, 927-929.

Burns, G.B. Dodge, J.A. (1984). Theophylline Inhibits Platelet Aggregation, Prostaglandin and Thromboxane Production by a Mechanism which is Independent of Cyclic AMP. Agents and Actions, 14, No.1, 102-108.

Bieri, J.H. (1979). Determination of tocopherol and Retinol in Plasma and Red Cells by High Pressure Liquid Chromatography. American Journal of Clinical Nutrition, 32, 2143-2150.

Choury, D. Reghis, A. Pichard, A.L. and Kaplan, J.C. (1983). Endogenous Proteolysis of Membrane-Bound Red Cell Cytochrome b5. Reductase in Adults and Newborns: Its Possible Relevance to the Generation of the Soluble "Methaemoglobin Reductase" Blood, 61, No.5, 894-898.

Das, S.K. and Nair, R.C. (1980). Superoxide Dismutase, Glutathione Peroxidase, Catalase and Lipid Peroxidation of Normal and Sickled Erythrocytes. British Journal of Haematology, 44, 87-92.

Dean, J.H. Luster, M.L. Munson, A.E. and Amos, H. (eds) (1985). Immunotoxicology and Immunopharmacology. Raven Press.

Evans, E.A. and La Celle, P. (1975). Intrinsic Material Properties of the Erythrocyte Membrane Indicated by Mechanical Analysis of Deformation. Blood, 45, 29-35.

Eyer, P. Hertle, H. Kiese, M. and Klein, G. (1975). Kinetics of Ferrih emoglobin Formation by some Reducing Agents, and the Role of Hydrogen Peroxide. Molecular Pharmacology, 11, 326-334.
Fievet, C.J. Gigandet, M.P and Ansel, H.C. (1971). Haemolysis of Erythrocytes by Primary Pharmacological Agents. American Journal of Hospital Pharmacy, 28, 961-966.
Fitchen, J.H. and Koeffler, F.A. (1980). Cimetidine and Granulopoiesis: Bone Marrow Culture Studies in Normal Man and Patients with Cimetidine-associated Neutropenia. British Journal of Haematology, 46, 361-366.
Fort, F.L. Heyman, I.A. and Kesterson, J.W. (1984). Hemolysis Study of Aqueous Polyethylene Glycol 400, Propylene Glycol and Ethanol Combination In Vivo and In Vitro. Journal of Parenteral Science and Technology, 38, No. 2, 82-87.
Fujii, S. Dale, G.L. and Butler, E. (1984). Glutathione-Dependent Protection Against Oxidative Damage of the Human Red Cell Membrane. Blood, 63, No. 5, 1096-1101.
Gangarosa, E.J. Johnson, T.R. and Ramos, H.S. (1960). Ristocetin. Induced Thrombocytopenia : Site and Mechanism of Action. American Medical Association Archives of Internal Medicine, 105, 83-89.
Gilbert, H.S. Roth, E.F. and Ginsberg, H. (1984). Increased Erythrocyte Susceptability to Lipid Peroxidation in Myeloproliferative Disorders. Journal of Laboratory Clinical Medicine, 103, No.1, 6-13.
Golde, D. W. and Takaky, F. (1985). Hematopoietic Stem Cells. New York and Basel. Marcel Dekker.
Goldstein, B.D. Rozen, M.G. and Kunis, R.L. (1980). Role of Red Cell Membrane Lipid Peroxidation in Haemolysis Due to Phenylhydrazine. Biochemical Pharmacology, 29, 1355-1359.
Gachalyi, B. Tihanyi, K. Vas, A and Kaldor, A. (1984). In Vitro. Effect of Cimetidine on ADP Induced Platelet Aggreation and Thromboxane A_2 Synthesis in Man. Thrombosis Research, 35, 105-109.
Hackett, T. Kelton, H. and Powers, J.(1982). Drug-Induced Platelet Destruction. Seminars in Thrombosis and Haemostosis, 8, No.2, 116-137.
Hammarlund, E.R. and Pedersen-Bjergaard, K. (1961). Hemolysis of Erythrocytes in Various Iso-osmotic Solutions. Journal of Pharmaceutical Science, 50, 24-30.
Hanahan, D.J. Denopoulous, C.A. Liehr, J. and Pinckard, R.N. (1980). Identification of Platelet Activating Factor Isolated from Rabbit Basophils as Acetylglyceryl ether phosphorylcholine. Journal of Biological Chemistry, 255, 5514-5516.
Health, B.P. (1982). Deformability of Isolated Red Blood Membranes. Biochemical et. Biophysica Acta, 691, 211-218.
Hegesh, E. Calmanouici, N. and Avron, M. (1968). New Method for Determining Ferrihemoglobin Reductase (NADH - Methaemoglobin Reductase) in Erythrocytes. Journal of Laboratory Clinical Medicine, 72, No.2, 339-344.
Hill, A.S. Haut, A. Cartwright, G.E. and Wintrobe, M.M. (1964). The Role of Nonhaemoglobin Proteins and Reduced Glutathionein the Protection of Haemoglobin from Oxidation In Vitro. Journal of Clinical Investigation, 43, 17-26.

Holmsen, H. (1976). Classification and Possible Mechanism of Action of Some Drugs that Inhibit Platelet Aggregation. Seminars in Haematology, 8, No.3, 50-80.

Horton, M.A. Amos, R.J. and Jones, R.J. (1983). The Effect of Histamine H2 Receptor Antagonists on Platelet Aggregation in Man. Scandinavian Journal of Haematology, 31, 15-19.

Howson, W.A. Owen, D.A.A. Slater, R.A. Swayne, G.T.G. Eden, R.J. and Taylor, E.M. (1987). SK&F 95018, a Vasodilator/ß adrenoceptor Antagonist. Archives of International Pharmacology and Therapeutics (In Press).

Huguette, M. Caen, J.P. Born, G.V.R. Miller R. D'Auriac, G.A. Meyer, P. (1976). Relation between the Inhibition of Aggregation and the Concentration of cAMP in Human and Rat Platelets. British Journal of Haematology 33, 27-38.

Husa, W.J. and Adams, J.R. (1944). Isotonic solutions 11. Permeability of Red Cells to Various Substances. Journal of American Pharmacology Association, 33, 329-334.

Hoyer, L.W. (1976). Von Willebrands Disease. In Progress in Haemostasis and Thrombosis. vol 3 (ed) Spaet, T.H. pp 231-287. New York, Grune and Stratton.

Irons, R.D. (1985). Toxicology of the Blood and Bone Marrow. New York. Raven Press.

Klocking, H.P. (1985). Toxicologically Relevant Disturbances of Haemostasis. Archives of Toxicology, Suppl. 8, 142-147

Link, C.M. Theoharides, A.D. Anders, J.C. Chung, H. and Canfield, C.J. (1985). Structure-Activity Relationship of Putative Primaquine Metabolites Causing Methaemoglobin Formation in Canine Hemolysates. Toxicology and Applied Pharmacology 81, 192-202.

Marcus, A.S. Safier, L.B. Ullman, H.L. (1981) Effects of Acetyl glycerol ether phosphorylcholine on Human Platelet Function In Vitro. Blood, 58, 1027-1031.

Marsh, J.C. (1985). Chemical Toxicity of the Granulocyte. In Toxicity of the Blood and Bone Marrow, ed. Irons, R.D. Raven Press, New York.

McClure, P. Caserly, J. Monsier, C.H. and Crozier D. (1970). Carbenicillin - induced Bleeding Disorder. Lancet ii, 1307.

McCulloch, E.A. (1984). Clinics in Haematology. Vol 13 No. 2.

Mohandas, N. Chasis, J.A. Shohet, S.B. (1983). The Influence of Membrane Skeleton on Red Cell Deformability, Membrane Material Properties and Shape. Seminars in Haematology. 20, No.3, 225-242

Moncada, S. and Korbut, R. (1978). Dipyridamole and other Phosphodiesterase Inhibitors Act as Antithrombotic Agents by Potentiating Endogenous Prostacyclin. The Lancet, June 17th, 1286-1289.

McManus, L.M. Morley, C.A. Levine, S.P. Pinckard, R.N. (1979). Platelet Activating Factor (PAF) Induces Release of Platelet Factor 4 (PF4) In Vitro during 1gE Anaphylaxis in the Rabbit. Journal of Immunology, 123, 2835-2841.

Mills, D.C.B. and Roberts. G.C.K. (1967). Membrane Active Drugs and the Aggregation of Human Blood Platelets. Nature, January 7th.

Moncada, S. Bunting, S. Mullane, K. Thorogood, P. Vane, J.R. Raz, A. and Needleman, P. (1977). A Selective Inhibitor of Thromboxane Synthetase. Prostaglandins, 13, No.4, 611-618.

Morris, D.R. and Williams, A.R. (1979). The Effects of Suspending Medium Viscosity on Erythrocyte Deformation and Haemolysis In Vitro. Biochimica et Biophysica Acta, 550, 288-296.

Needleman, P. Raz, A. Ferrendelli, J.A. Minkes, M. (1977). Application of Imidazole as a Selective Inhibitor of Thromboxane Synthetase in Human Platelets. Proceedings of National Academy of Science U.S.A., 74, No.4, 1716-1720.

Nishio, T. Hirota, S. Yamashita, J. Motohashi, Y and Kato, Y (1982). Erythrocyte Changes in Aqueous Polyethylene Glycol Solutions Containing Sodium Chloride. Journal of Pharmaceutical Sciences, 71, No. 9, 977-979.

Ogiso, T. Iwaki, M. and Mori, K. (1981). Fluidity of Human Erythrocyte Membrane and Effect of Chlorpromazine on Fluidity and Phase Separation of Membrane. Biochimica et Biophysica Acta, 649, 325-335.

Olaisen, B. and Oye, I. (1973). Interactions of Membrane Stabilising Drugs Affecting Human Erythrocyte In Vitro. European Journal of Pharmacology, 22, 112-116.

Oshida, Diegawa, Takahashi Akaishi (1979). Physico - Chemical Properties and Local Toxic Effects of Injectables. Tnhoku, Journal of Experimental Medicine., 127, 301-316.

Rao, A.K. Walsh, P.N. (1983). Acquired Qualitative Platelet Disorders. Clinics in Haematology, 12, No.1, 201-238.

Rachmilewitz, E.A. (1974). Denaturation of the Normal and Abnormal Haemoglobin Molecule. Seminars in Haematology 11, 441-462.

Reed, K.W. and Yalkowsky, S.H. (1985) Lysis of Human Red Blood Cells in the Presence of Various Cosolvents. Journal of Parenteral Science and Technology 39, No 2, 64-68

Salzman, E.A. Rosenberg, R.D. Smith, M.H. Lindon, J.N. and Favreau, L. (1980). Effect of Heparin and Heparin Fractions on Platelet Aggregation. Journal of Clinical Investigation, 65, 64-73.

Sauberman, N., Fortier, N.L. Joshi, W. (1983) Spectrin - haemoglobin Crosslinkages Associated with In Vitro Oxidant Hypersensitivity in Pathologic and Artificially Dehydrated Red Cells. British Journal of Haematology, 54, 15-28.

Seeman, P. Kwant, O.W. Sauks, T. (1969). Membrane Expansion of Erythrocyte Ghosts by Tranquillisers and Anaesthetics. Biochemica et Biophysica Acta, 183, 499-511.

Shattil, S.J. Bennett, J.S. McDonough, M and Turnbull, J. (1980). Carbenicillin and Penicillin G. Inhibit Platelet Function In Vitro by Impairing the Interaction of Agonists with the Platelet Surface. J. Clin. Invest., 65, 329-337.

Sheetz, M. (1983). Membrane Skeletal Dynamics : Role of Modulation of Red Cell Deformability, Mobility of Transmembrane Proteins and Shape. Seminars in Haematology, 20, 175-188.

Smith, R.P. and Olson, M.V. (1973). Drug-Induced Methaemoglobinaemia. Seminars in Haematology, 10, No.3, 253-268.

Siess, W. Lorenz, R. Roth, P. and Weber, P.C. (1983). Effects of Propranolol in vitro and in vivo on Platelet Function and Thromboxane Formation in Normal Volunteers. Agents and Actions, 13, No.1, 29-34.

Theus, R. and Zbinden, G. (1984). Toxicological Assessment of the Hemostatic System, Regulatory Requirements and Industry Practice. Regulatory Toxicology and Pharmacology, 4, 74-95.

Ward, P.C.J. Schwartz, B.S. and White, J.G. (1983). Heinz-Body Anaemia: "Bite Cell" Variant - A Light and Electron Microscopy Study. American Journal of Hematology 15, 135-146.
Weiss, H.J. (1980). Congenital Disorders of Platelet Function. Seminars In Haematology, 17, 228-264.
Weiss, H.J. (1972). The Pharmacology of Platelet Inhibition. Progress in Haemostasis Thrombosis, 1, 199-231.
Weiss, S.J. (1980). The Role of Superoxide in the Destruction of Erythrocyte Targets by Human Neutrophils. Journal of Biological Chemistry, 255, No.20, 9912-9917.
Winterbourn, G.C. and Carrell, R.W. (1973). The Attachment of Heinz Bodies to the Red Cell Membrane. British Journal of Haematology 25, 585-592.

General and topical toxicity

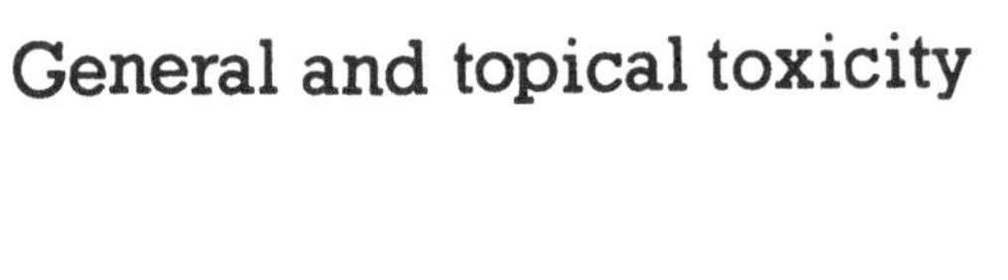

THE CHORIOALLANTOIC MEMBRANE IN IRRITANCY TESTING

R.S. Lawrence
Environmental Safety Laboratory, Colworth House, Sharnbrook, Bedford MK44 1LQ.

INTRODUCTION

There has been increasing pressure over recent years to find suitable alternative procedures to the Draize rabbit eye test (Draize *et al*., 1944). The majority of the proposed substitute tests are cell culture systems or isolated tissue preparations. As yet none of these potential alternative techniques have either been generally accepted or fully validated. Included amongst these techniques are the isolated rabbit ileum, from which results have at times been found to be inconsistent (Muir, 1984a), and bovine cornea (Muir, 1984b). The cell culture systems examined are wide ranging both in cell type and also the proposed end point which can be based on morphology or various biochemical tests. Some examples of these end points include uridine uptake (Shopsis & Sathe, 1984) histamine release (Prottey & Ferguson, 1975) and neutral red uptake (Hockley & Baxter, in press) while the different cell types include rabbit corneal cell (North-Root *et al*., 1982) and human diploid fibroblasts (Knox, in press). A system for assessing skin corrosivity has been proposed by Pemberton *et al*., (in press) which employs rat epidermal skin slices.

At our laboratories the isolated whole eye organ preparation, the *in vitro* eye corneal injury test, is used routinely to assist in assessing the potential of materials to damage the cornea (Burton *et al*., 1981; York *et al*., 1982). This system has been quite widely used and has been included in the Guidelines for the Testing of Chemicals for Toxicity (HMSO 1982) as a possible screening method. It is, however, solely a method for assessing the irritation potential of a material to the cornea and gives no indication as to effects on the ocular mucous membranes or of the eyes recovering from insult.

The response of the cornea of the eye to an irritant material, however, differs from that of the mucous membranes of the eye lids (Parish, 1985a). Thus, this area of potential eye irritation is at present without a suitable alternative model system. A possible model for assessing the irritation potential of a chemical or product to such a vascularized tissue is the chorioallantoic membrane of the embryonated hen's egg, as this is a highly vascular, thin membrane with relatively easy access for both treatment and assessment.

The chorioallantoic membrane has been used extensively for many years in various fields of biological research including virology, bacteriology and tumour research (see for example Beveridge & Burnet, 1946). More recently the chick embryo has been used for assessing the potential toxicity and teratology of materials (see for example Verrett *et al.*, 1980; Fisher & Schoenwolf, 1983). Similarly, the potential use of the chorioallantoic membrane for assessing *in vivo* eye irritation potential has only recently been described (Leighton *et al.*, 1983; Leighton *et al.*, 1985; Luepke, 1985; Parish, 1985a; Lawrence *et al*, in press).

The technique should strictly be described as an *in vivo* procedure and is likely to be a licenced procedure in the U.K. if the proposed new legislation on animal experiments becomes law. Although, at present, the chorioallantoic membrane is unlikely to be of value as a replacement procedure for the *in vivo* Draize rabbit eye test as a whole, it has a possible application to compare the tissue damaging potential of limited ranges of similar products, for example anionic based detergent actives, and may also have an application as a screening procedure for irritants.

The techniques to be described can be divided into two main areas of investigation. Firstly, those which attempt to use the procedure as a replacement for the Draize rabbit eye test as a whole and, secondly, those which use the chorioallantoic membrane as a potential model for inflammatory changes. The latter alternative would thus be of use for predicting the irritation potential of materials to the conjunctiva of the eye lids.

The first area of research can be further subdivided into two distinctly different techniques.

(1) The first of these techniques utilizes prolonged test material contact time with observation over an extended period. The main effect of such treatment is usually necrosis within a localized area (Leighton *et al.*, 1983; Leighton *et al.*, 1985).

(2) The second technique utilizes a very short contact period and the assessment of vascular changes which occur directly after treatment (Luepke, 1985; Price *et al.*, in press).

The second area of investigation is to observe possible inflammatory changes in the membrane and to correlate these with conjunctival effects *in vivo*. A prolonged contact period is used with macroscopic assessment at several time periods post treatment and also histological examination of lesions which develop as a result of treatment (Parish, 1985a; Lawrence *et al.*, in press). Acute *in vivo* skin inflammatory responses have recently been well described by Parish (1985b) together with the relevances of *in vitro* tests for this type of effect. Severe inflammation will cause damage to blood vessels supplying that tissue and this may result in cell death or necrosis. This inflammatory effect of some chemicals is in contrast to corrosion in which necrosis is produced by direct action of a chemical or a biological toxin on cells. Parish (1985b) states that "immediate acute inflammation in the dermis is manifested mainly by changes in the blood vessels, with erythema, oedema and fibrin deposition, and by infiltration and activation of leucocytes. The degree of neutrophil infiltration is influenced by the severity of the tissue damage, and the nature and persistence of the irritant. Following a simple application of an irritant inducing mild-to-moderate inflammation, the acute phase is of short duration and evidence of healing is observed within twenty four hours."

STRUCTURE OF THE CHORIOALLANTOIC MEMBRANE

The chorioallantoic membrane of the embryonated hen egg is a highly vascular extra embryonic fusion membrane. It is formed by the fusion of the mesodermic layer of the allantois, which develops rapidly between the fourth and tenth days of incubation, and the mesodermic layer of the serosa. The membrane is therefore a stratified structure with an inner endodermal layer, a central mesoderm and an outer ectodermal layer. An extensive vascular network lies within the mesoderm and this is connected to the embryonic vasculature by the allantoic arteries and veins (Patten, 1958).

A photomicrograph depicting the structure of an untreated chorioallantoic membrane is shown in Plate 1.

Plate 1 Chick chorioallantoic membrane in cross-section showing normal structure (H&E x 445)

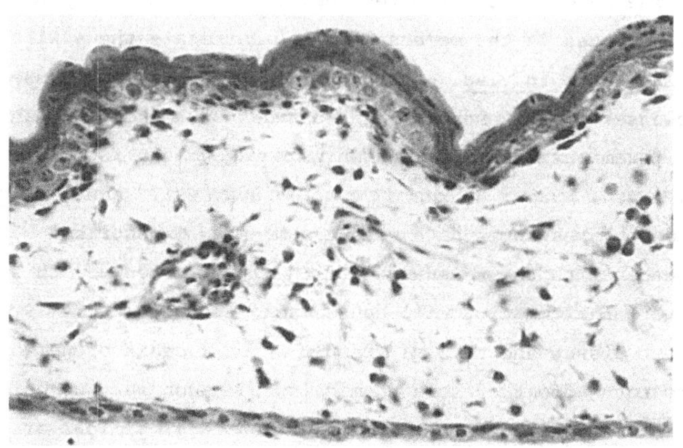

PRACTICAL ASPECTS

Eggs and incubation

Fertile hens eggs can be purchased relatively cheaply and stored prior to use if kept in a cool room (5 C to 10 C). Incubation temperature should be 100 F and a relative humidity of 56% maintained in the incubator. The eggs should be turned at least twice a day until any invasive procedures are undertaken. In our investigations (Parish, 1985a; Lawrence *et al.*, in press) we purchased eggs from ISA Poultry (ISA Poultry Services, Peterborough) and used Marsh Roll-X automatic incubators (USA manufacture, supplied by Robin Haigh Incubators, Chertsey, Surrey).

Preparation of the chorioallantoic membrane

In order to treat the chorioallantoic membrane, access must be gained and this can be either via the air space of the egg or at the equator of the egg. If entry is via the equator then the chorioallantoic membrane, which is normally in close association with the shell membrane when fully developed, must be dropped from this position to enable treatment and assessment to take place.

(i) Access via the air space (Figure 1)

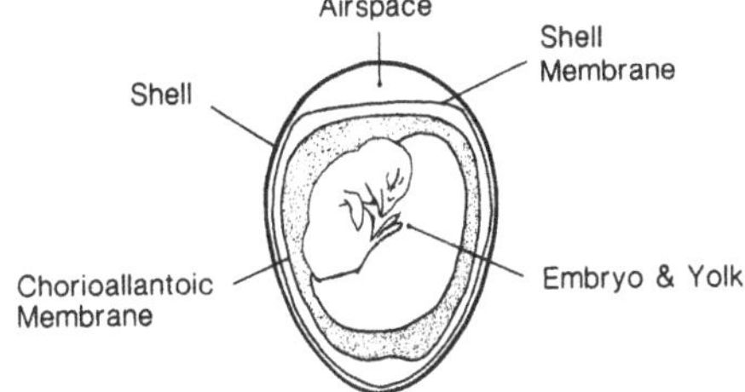

Figure 1

Diagram of procedure used by Luepke (1985) to access the chorioallantoic membrane.

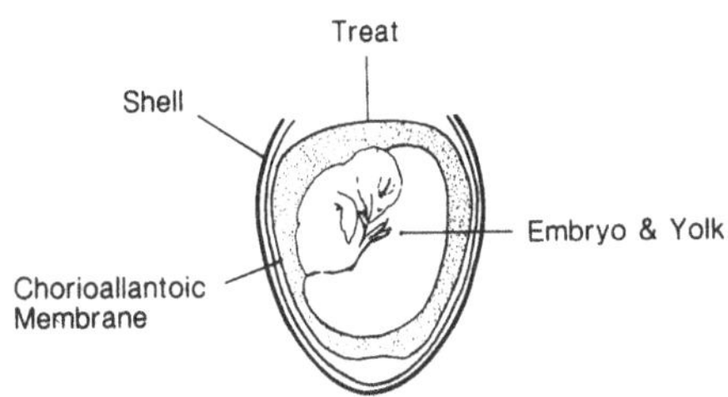

When the chorioallantoic membrane has developed, which is around the tenth day of incubation, the shell over the air space is carefully removed by using either a small circular saw or grinding tool attached to a modelling drill or a dentist's drill, (for example, Drillmaster Junior A400, Microflame (U.K.) Ltd., Norfolk). Once the area of shell has been removed from the air space the shell membrane must be carefully removed to expose the chorioallantoic membrane. (Luepke, 1985).

(ii) Access at the equator of the egg

There are two methods for gaining access via the equator. These are described overleaf:

(a) Dropped membrane procedure (Figure 2)

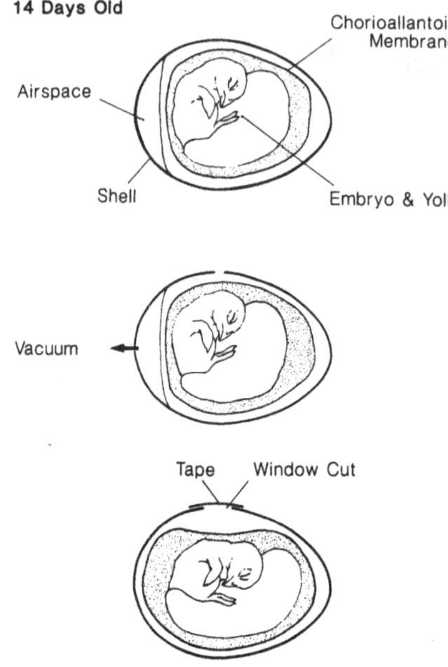

Figure 2

Diagram of procedure of the standard dropped membrane technique.

A small hole is drilled in the shell at the equator of the egg on day fourteen of incubation such that no damage is caused to the shell membrane. The shell membrane is then carefully pierced with a needle tip avoiding damage to the chorioallantoic membrane which lies directly below the shell membrane.

A second hole is then drilled through the shell into the airspace and the air withdrawn from this area by application of a vacuum. A window (approx 1cm x 1cm) is cut at the equator of the egg to allow access for treatment and assessment. The window can then be sealed by adhesive tape eg. Blenderm (3M) and the holes with collodion (Fisons Ltd.).

(b) Zwilling technique (Figure 3)

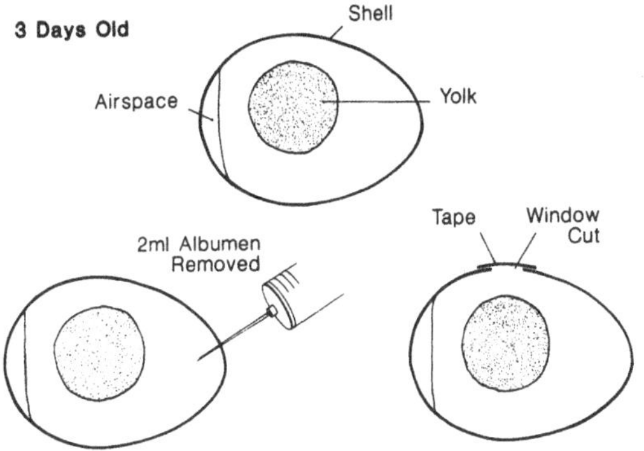

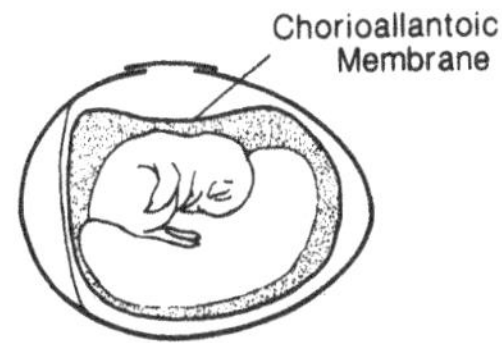

Figure 3

Diagram of procedure of the Zwilling (1959) technique.

On day three of incubation a small hole is drilled at the 'pointed end' of the egg through the eggshell but not penetrating the shell membrane. Two millilitres of albumen are then removed using a syringe and needle and the hole sealed. A window as in (a) above is then cut at the equator of the egg. This is sealed with tape and the eggs replaced in the incubator, window uppermost. The chorioallantoic membrane will then develop over the reduced level of albumen and access to the lowered membrane, for treatment and assessment, is through the window (Zwilling 1959).

Work in our laboratory has shown that the membranes prepared by the Zwilling technique are likely to be less damaged than those prepared by the dropped membrane procedure. This is because during the latter technique the chorioallantoic membrane is slightly damaged, firstly by the needle when piercing the shell membrane and, secondly, by small shell fragments falling onto the chorioallantoic membrane when the window is cut, producing small areas of haemorrhage. This does not occur when the Zwilling procedure is employed as at day three of incubation, when drilling takes place, the membrane has not yet formed.

There is however, a slight structural difference in the Zwilling membrane in that the outer ectoderm becomes keratinized. It is believed that this is due to the membrane being exposed directly to air which does not occur for any extended period when using the dropped membrane procedure and does not occur at all in normal fertile eggs.

EXPERIMENTAL EXAMPLES

Luepke (1985) treats the chorioallantoic membrane of the airspace on the tenth day of incubation with 0.2ml of the test substance or 0.1g, if the test material is a solid, and then rinses the test material from the membrane with five millilitres of warm water twenty seconds after treatment. Assessment is by grading the degree of hyperaemia, haemorrhage and coagulation which occurs in the chorioallantoic membrane, blood vessels, and albumen 0.5, 2, and 5 minutes after treatment. It is not clear from Luepke's paper if this time relates to post treatment or post rinsing.

Based upon a mean total score for four eggs Luepke then classifies these scores into four grades of irritancy from practically non-irritant to strongly irritant. These grades have then been compared with _in vivo_ eye irritation data.

An alternative procedure is described by Leighton _et al._, (1983) and Leighton _et al._, (1985) in which the authors treat the chorioallantoic membrane on day fourteen of incubation with forty microlitres of test material placed into a Teflon ring of ten millimetres diameter which rests on the membrane. The window is then resealed until day seventeen of incubation. At this time the tape is removed from the window and assessment undertaken.

Assessment of several parameters including size of lesion and general appearance of the reaction are recorded. The major assessment parameter is lesion size coupled with the amount of necrosis present. Leighton usually uses four dilutions for the test material which are; 1:8, 1:16, 1:32 and 1:64 with fifteen eggs treated at each dilution.

The reactions are graded from 0 to 3+ and those eggs with 2+ and 3+ reactions are classed as positive. The number of positive eggs in each treatment group is then expressed as a percentage of the total number of eggs in that group.

This technique has been used by Leighton on a number of unnamed household materials and these have then been ranked in order of irritancy comparing the rank order with the known ranking from *in vivo* eye data.

The studies in our laboratories (Parish, 1985a and Lawrence *et al.*, in press) have entailed a treatment with fifty microlitres of a range of dilutions of materials directly onto the chorioallantoic membrane at day fourteen of incubation.

Initially we were looking for inflammatory changes. However as our investigations proceeded it became apparent that typical inflammatory responses were not produced in the chorioallantoic membrane. Changes, as observed histologically, were generally degenerative with necrosis at the treated site. Assessment was therefore descriptive for the reactions produced, instead of a score for inflammation.

Macroscopic assessment was undertaken at 4 hours, 24 hours and 48 hours post treatment. The assessment included size, colour, and general description of any changes in the membrane. Forty eight hours post treatment the treated site was excised, fixed in formal saline and prepared for histological assessment. Groups of six eggs were used for each dilution of the test material. Macroscopic and microscopic assessment were then combined and reactions graded from no effect to severe.

The means of assessment in all the experimental examples described above are based upon morphological changes in the membrane. Some of the methods, as mentioned, employ microscopic as well as macroscopic observations but none of the methods utilize biochemical techniques for assessment.

Lesions and reactions observed

The responses assessed by Luepke (1985) are severely limited due to the very short period of observation. Capillary dilatation together with some haemorrhage and possible coagulation of the membrane and the albumen are observed. Although this method as described demands rinsing of the test substance, this type of response will be seen even if the test material is not rinsed from the membrane. However if the material is irritant to the chorioallantoic membrane and is not rinsed then a necrotic lesion will eventually develop.

Luepke considers that the results he has obtained in the hens egg test correlate well with findings in the Draize eye test for a limited number of materials which he has examined. However Price *et al*., (in press) have used an adaptation of the Luepke method in which they treat Zwilling prepared membranes with assessment for up to one hour post-treatment without rinsing. The authors consider this technique to be a useful screen for distinguishing between non-irritant and irritant materials, but that there is no significant grading of effects between these extremes (Price, personal communication).

The results of Leighton *et al*., (1985) describe the lesions observed 72 hours post treatment. Severe effects were seen as cell death throughout the thickness of the membrane or, if injury had not extended through the entire thickness, repair and proliferation was apparent. Leighton also considers that the membrane responds to injury with a complete inflammatory response.

By using a ranking procedure for results obtained in the chorioallantoic membrane procedure and comparing this with a rank order of irritation from *in vivo* data Leighton considers that a relatively good correlation has been achieved with *in vivo* eye data for twelve household preparations which are not named in the authors paper.

The second area of investigation is described by Parish (1985a) and Lawrence *et al*., (in press). In this we have attempted to use the chorioallantoic membrane as a predictive model for conjunctival inflammation. It was considered that a combination of this test with the *in vitro* corneal injury test (Burton *et al*., 1981) would lead to a better overall assessment of *in vivo* eye irritancy but as we have found no indication of a true inflammatory response being produced in the chorioallantoic membrane this has not proved possible. The major effect occuring was necrosis either full depth or virtually full depth through the membrane (Plate 2). However proliferative lesions have been observed with hyperplasia of the ectoderm and endoderm and a mesodermal response (Plate 3). This latter type of lesion, dependant upon extent, was generally classified as moderate.

Plate 2 Chick chorioallantoic membrane in cross-section showing a typical necrotic lesion 48 hr post treatment (H&E x 445).

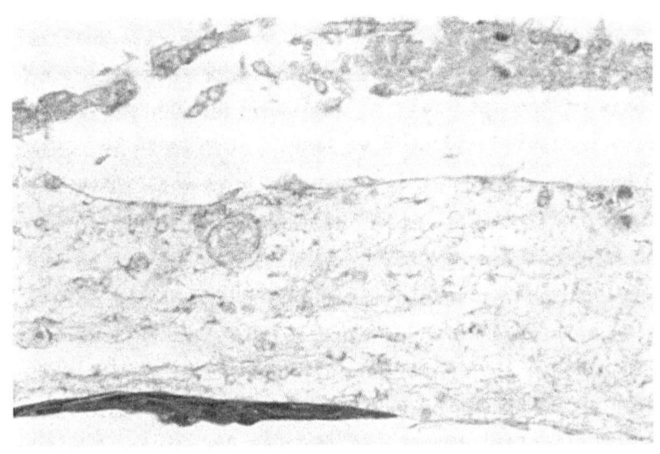

Plate 3 Chick chorioallantoic membrane in cross-section showing a proliferative lesion which were occasionally observed 48 hr post treatment (H&E x 90).

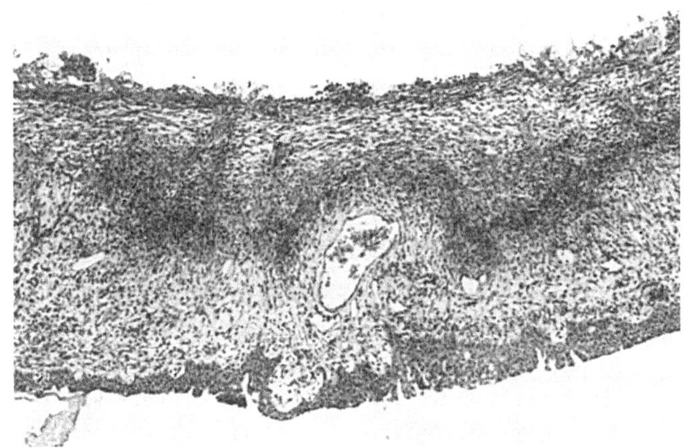

Our studies involved the selection of nine chemicals which were representative of both differing conjunctival and overall eye irritation potential. The materials were selected by reference to irritancy as reported in the literature in order to avoid an *in vivo* testing programme solely for comparitive purposes. For all the chemicals examined a dose response relationship was generally observed, and no effect levels were obtained with most materials examined.

Generally, severe effects, as shown by full depth necrosis, occurred in at least the top concentration examined. When comparing the results obtained on the chorioallantoic membrane with the data on overall *in vivo* eye irritation potential only a limited correlation was observed. At least three of the materials investigated showed embryotoxic effects, both undiluted and at 50%, these being Tween 80; polyethylene glycol 400 and glycerine. It is worthy of note that these materials are all either non-irritant or at most slight irritants in the *in vivo* eye. Tween 80 was shown to produce significant lesions on the membrane at the lowest concentration examined, 10%, while at the same concentration both ethanol and acetone produced at most very slight effects. This again is a major anomaly when *in vivo* eye irritancy data is considered as both acetone and ethanol are ranked above Tween 80 in eye irritation potential (Grant, 1974).

DISCUSSION AND CONCLUSIONS

The application of the chorioallantoic membrane procedure for replacing the *in vivo* eye test as a whole seems from data available at present rather limited. In our laboratories the investigation of nine chemicals possessing a wide range of *in vivo* eye irritancy has shown only limited correlation with *in vivo* eye data (Lawrence *et al.*, in press). There are major anomalies between the chorioallantoic membrane results and *in vivo* eye data in that non-irritant or very slightly irritant materials such as Tween 80; glycerine and polyethylene glycol 400 when tested undiluted have produced embryotoxicity in the embryonated hens egg and severe effects on the membrane.

Also the slight eye irritant, propylene glycol, produced effects in the chorioallantoic membrane test which were similar to ethanol whereas ethanol is much the more irritant material in the eye. Similarly Tween 80 ranked above both ethanol and acetone in this procedure yet Tween 80 is virtually non-irritant to the eye *in vivo* while ethanol and acetone are known eye irritants (Grant, 1974).

We have also examined shampoos in the chorioallantoic membrane test (unpublished data) and can differentiate between a typical adult shampoo and a baby shampoo which also differ in *in vivo* eye irritancy. These latter data would thus be in agreement with some of

Leighton's (1985) findings in which he has ranked twelve unnamed household products in order of eye irritancy by using the chorioallantoic membrane. It may therefore be that this procedure could be used to differentiate between products of a similar type, for example anionic surfactant based materials, but not across different product types or for chemicals with very different characteristics. However, even if the chorioallantoic membrane were to be suitable for differentiating between shampoos containing different levels of a similar active, or other materials within a similar product type, some current cell culture techniques and also the in vitro corneal injury test (York et al., 1982) can be used for this type of examination. As the chorioallantoic membrane procedure is technically an in vivo technique these other alternative procedures are probably more acceptable. The in vitro eye injury procedure also has the advantage that it can be used for a wider range of materials and comparisons between chemicals.

It should be noted that although Leighton indicates a good correlation between the results he obtained on the chorioallantoic membrane and in vivo eye data there are some discrepancies within these data. These may be occuring because the household materials are not all products of a similar type. This lack of complete correlation would further indicate that the hen's egg test is not suitable for total replacement of an in vivo procedure but may, as is the case with many alternative methods, be suitable as a screening technique.

Our investigations have also shown that the chorioallantoic membrane does not show a typical inflammatory response, in that degeneration or necrosis are the main histological changes and that no significant neutrophil and macrophage infiltration is observed. This observation is at variance with Leighton et al., (1985) who states that the chorioallantoic membrane 'responds to injury with a complete inflammatory reaction, a process similar to that induced in the conjunctival tissue of the rabbit'. We consider that the blood cellular system of the embryo at fourteen days of incubation is immature and thus unable to produce an inflammatory response. Haematological studies of blood taken from the membrane of embryos at fourteen days of incubation have shown very few leucocytes and the majority of these are in an immature state (unpublished data). Thus the chorioallantoic membrane would not at this stage appear to be a suitable model for mimicking inflammatory responses of the conjunctiva of the eye.

The essential changes which we observed in the chorioallantoic membrane were degeneration or necrosis to varying depths with well defined edges to the lesions. Proliferative healing responses were often apparent and it is likely that these are similar to the lesions reported by Leighton.

Luepke (1985) indicates good correlation between in vivo eye data and results from short treatment periods of the chorioallantoic membrane with a limited number of chemicals. However, over a wide range of materials the short term effects observed during a five minute assessment period may prove a limiting factor in correlating chorioallantoic membrane results with in vivo eye irritation data. Also data from Price et al., (in press) using a short treatment and observation period, although without rinse of test material, indicate that this particular approach may be of limited value.

Thus considering the data available to date from studies using the chorioallantoic membrane of the embryonated chicken there is, overall, little promise for this procedure to replace the Draize eye test as a whole. It is also unlikely to be of value in mimicking inflammatory responses. The chorioallantoic membrane may, therefore, have some limited application as a screen for products of a similar type and perhaps for screening out some severely irritant materials although certain cell culture systems can be used for differentiating surfactants (Scaife 1982, for example) and also the in vitro corneal injury test may give a more informed assessment of eye irritation potential with reference to corneal damage.

ACKNOWLEDGEMENTS

I thank the many persons of the Environmental Safety Laboratory who contributed to the data reported and advised on the content of this chapter, including Dr W E Parish, Dr M G Adams, Mr M H Groom, Mr T C Williams and Miss D M Ackroyd. I am also indebted to Mr A Shaw and Mr G L Dudley for the high quality of illustrations and photographs.

REFERENCES

Beveridge WIB., & Burnet FM., (1946). The cultivation of viruses and rickettsiae in the chick embryo. Medical Research Council, Special Report Series No. 256, London.

Burton ABG., York M., & Lawrence RS., (1981). The in vitro assessment of severe eye irritants. Fd. Cosmet. Toxicol. 19 471.

Draize JH., Woodard G., & Calvery HO., (1944). Methods for the study of irritation and toxicity of substances applied to the skin and mucous membranes. J. Pharmac., exp. Ther. 82 377

Fisher M., & Schoenwolf GC., (1983). The use of early chick embryos in experimental embryology and teratology: improvements in standard procedures. Teratology 27 65.

Grant WM., (1974). Toxicology of the eye. 2nd ed. Charles C. Thomas, Springfield, Illinois.

HMSO, (1982). Guidelines for the Testing of Chemicals for Toxicity. Committee on Toxicity of Chemicals in Food, Consumer Products and the Environment. DHSS Report on Health and Social Subjects No. 27.

Hockley K. & Baxter D. Use of the 3T3 cell-neutral red uptake assay for irritants as an alternative to the rabbit eye (Draize) test. In Press.

Knox P. The F.R.A.M.E. multicentre project on in vitro cytotoxicology. In Press.

Lawrence RS., Groom MH., Ackroyd DM., & Parish WE. The chorioallantoic membrane in irritation testing. In Press.

Leighton J., Nassauer J., Tchao R., & Verdone J., (1983). Development of a procedure using the chick egg as an alternative to the Draize rabbit test. Alternative Methods in Toxicology. Ed. AM. Goldberg. 1 163.

Leighton J., Nassauer J., & Tchao R., (1985). The chick embryo in toxicology : an alternative to the rabbit eye. Fd. Chem. Toxic. 23, No. 2, 293.

Luepke NP., (1985). Hen's egg chorioallantoic membrane test for irritation potential. Fd. Chem. Toxic. 23, No. 2, 287.

Muir CK., (1984a). Further investigations on the ileum model as a possible alternative to in vivo eye irritancy testing. ATLA 11 No. 129.

Muir CK., (1984b). A simple method to assess surfactant induced bovine corneal opacity in vitro. Preliminary findings. Toxicol. Lett. 22 No. 199.

North-Root H., Yackovich F., Demetrulias J., Gacula Jnr. M., & Heinze JE., (1982). Evaluation of an in vitro cell toxicity test using rabbit corneal cells to predict the eye irritation potential of surfactants. Toxicol. Lett. 14. 207.

Parish WE., (1985a). Ability of in vitro (corneal injury - eye organ - and chorioallantoic membrane) tests to represent histopathological features of acute eye inflammation. Fd. Chem. Toxic. 23, No. 2, 215.

Parish WE., (1985b). Relevance of in vitro tests to in vivo acute skin inflammation: potential in vitro applications of skin keratome slices, neutrophils, fibroblasts, mast cells and macrophages. Fd. Chem. Toxic. 23, No. 2. 275.

Patten BM., (1958). Foundations of embryology. Mcgraw-Hill Book Co. Inc., New York.

Pemberton MA., Rhodes C., & Oliver GJA. An in vitro assessment of skin corrosive potential. In Press.

Price JB., Barry MP., & Andrews IJ. The use of the chick chorioallantoic membrane to predict eye irritants. In Press.

Prottey C. & Ferguson T., (1975). Factors which determine the skin irritation potential of soaps and detergents. J. Soc. Cosmet. Chem. 26, 29.

Scaife MC., (1982). An investigation of detergent action on cell in vitro and possible correlations with in vivo data. Int. J. Cosmet. Sci. 4 179.

Shopsis C. & Sathe S., (1984). Uridine uptake inhibition as a cytotoxicity test: correlations with the Draize test. Toxicology 29 195.

Verrett MJ., Scott WF., Reynaldo EF., Alterman EK., & Thomas CA., (1980). Toxicity and teratogenicity of food additive chemicals in the developing chicken embryo. Toxicol. and App. Pharmacol. 56 265.

York M., Lawrence RS., & Gibson GB., (1982). An in vitro test for the assessment of eye irritancy in consumer products - preliminary findings. Int. J. of Cosmet. Sci. 4, 223.

Zwilling E., (1959). A modified chorioallantoic grafting procedure. Transplantation Bulletin 6, 115.

IN VITRO DERMAL IRRITANCY TESTS

P A Duffy and O P Flint
Imperial Chemical Idustries PLC
Pharmaceuticals Division
Mereside, Alderley Park
Macclesfield, Cheshire.
SK10 4TG England

INTRODUCTION

Current methods for predicting the dermal irritation potential of new compounds to man rely mostly on *in vivo* techniques. The method most commonly employed is based on that designed by Draize and co-workers (1944) using the visual assessment of oedema and erythema produced in rabbit skin after topical application of a test substance (Hood et al. 1977). Other workers have favoured the use of other species (using essentially similar methodology), such as the guinea pig and mouse (Hood et al. 1977).

One of the major disadvantages of *in vivo* predictive dermal irritancy tests is the subjectivity associated with visual assessment and interpretation of the dermal response. This is best illustrated by Weil and Scala's report (1971) of blind testing a range of dermal irritants in an interlaboratory collaborative study using a standardized Draize assay. The results from 25 laboratories revealed high inter and intralaboratory variability in scoring and rating the test compounds as irritants. In some cases this was so extreme that a compound listed as most irritating by some laboratories was listed as least irritating by others.

There have been some attempts to improve the objectivity of in vivo dermal irritant assessment. Gloxhuber and Kastner (1985) used image analysis of irritant reaction in mouse skin and Waltz (1984) attempted statistical analysis of oedema related skin fold number in mice In both cases the systems may prove useful in comparative studies with known irritants but still retain the use of animals and dubious relevance to man due to differences in species sensitivity. A further alternative *in vivo* approach is the use of human volunteers (Van Der Valk et al. 1984, Hurkmans et al. 1985, Marks and Kingston 1985). However, at the preliminary stages of testing of new compounds this would raise numerous ethical problems.

There are moral, financial and scientific reasons for developing in vitro alternatives to in vivo irritancy tests. The benefits of suitable tests would be twofold. First the number of animals used for dermal irritancy testing would be dramatically reduced and secondly the more objective design of in vitro tests should prove more reproducibly predictive of irritant hazard to man.

The majority of reports describing alternative methods of irritancy testing refer to correlations against Draize rabbit eye irritation tests, and occasionally to the skin, using either measurements of cytoxicity in in vitro cell lines (Shopsis and Sathe, 1984; Kemp et al. 1985; North-Root et al. 1985; Reinhardt et al. 1985; Scaife, 1985; Shopsis et al. 1985), lethality to chick embryos in ovo (Leighton et al. 1985), damage to the hens egg chorioallantoic membrane (Luepke, 1985) or toxicity to organ cultures for example, the explanted rabbit ileum or eye (Burton et al. 1981; Muir, 1983, 1985). Development of in vitro tests correlating with cutaneous toxicity has concentrated on methods of mouse or rat skin organ cultures (Kao et al. 1983; Oliver and Pemberton, 1985).

The methods described in this chapter illustrate an in vitro approach chosen to reflect dermal irritation in vivo. This approach looks at the effect of test compounds on components of epithelial differentiation in vitro; stratification, keratinocyte cytolethality, subcytolethal leakage of enzymes through plasma membranes and keratin production. The object is to predict irritant potential in vivo for man.

In addition to screening industrial and pharmaceutical compounds, structurally or pharmacologically related groups of compounds, for example, can be pre-screened, prior to animal testing, to select the most promising low toxicity candidate at a fraction of the cost of conventional animal studies.

PROCEDURES AND METHODS

The in vitro system that has been developed has two components. (A) A cytoxicity component using the 3T3 Swiss mouse fibroblast cell line (Todaro and Green, 1963) purchased from Flow Laboratories, Irvine, UK and (B) An in vitro model of a keratinizing and stratifying epithelium using the mouse teratoma derived XB-2 cell line (Rheinwald and Green, 1975) purchased from the American Type Culture

Collection, Maryland, U.S.A. Both cell lines are easily maintained in Dulbecco's modified Eagle medium (DMEM-Gibco) supplemented with 2mM L-glutamine (Flow), 100 units ml^{-1} penicillin, 100 ug ml^{-1} streptomycin and foetal calf serum (FCS); 10% (v/v) for 3T3 cultures and 20% for XB-2 cultures. The initial requirement of a 3T3 feeder layer for the XB-2 cells to differentiate during assay cultures (Rheinwald and Green, 1975) has been successfully replaced by the use of 3T3 conditioned medium (DMEM exposed to a 70% confluent culture of 3T3 cells for 24 hours and supplemented with FCS to increase the content from 10% (v/v) to 20% (v/v)). Specialised media used for specific procedures are described below.

Aside from standard items of equipment necessary for tissue culture (CO_2 incubators, laminar flow cabinet, inverted microscopes etc) the in vitro irritancy test system requires two further items of specialised apparatus. A majority of the assays use 96 well flat-bottomed microtitre plates (Flow) and have coloured product endpoints. For colorimetric analysis a Titertek Multiskan 96 well plate reader is essential. The remaining assays are related to the development of differentiated XB-2 cell colonies whose areas are analysed on an AMS 40-10 image analyser. Both the Multiskan and the AMS are controlled by a Commodore CBM microcomputer with twin disc drives which facilitates suitable data storage and statistical analysis.

Cytotoxicity component (Figure 1)

Mouse 3T3 fibroblast cells are established in 96 well plates, one plate for each intended assay, at a density of either 5 x 10^3 or 1 x 10^4 cells per well and incubated overnight. The subsequent assays are designed to measure the effects of test compounds on the following:

(1) Cell proliferation by colorimetric assay of neutral red uptake by fixed cells (Parish and Mullbacher, 1983).

(2) Cellular metabolism; a colorimetric measurement of a dark blue formazan product resulting from the cleavage of the tetrazolium salt MTT (3- (4,5-Dimethyl Thiazol-2-yl)-2, 5-diphenyltetrazolium bromide) by mitochondrial dehydrogenases (Mosmann, 1983).

(3) The integrity of cell membranes by measuring the levels of leakage of lysosomal hexosaminidase (HEX) and cytosolic lactate dehydrogenase (LDH) following exposure to test compound. In practical terms each assay only requires one 96 well plate. The plate incorporates

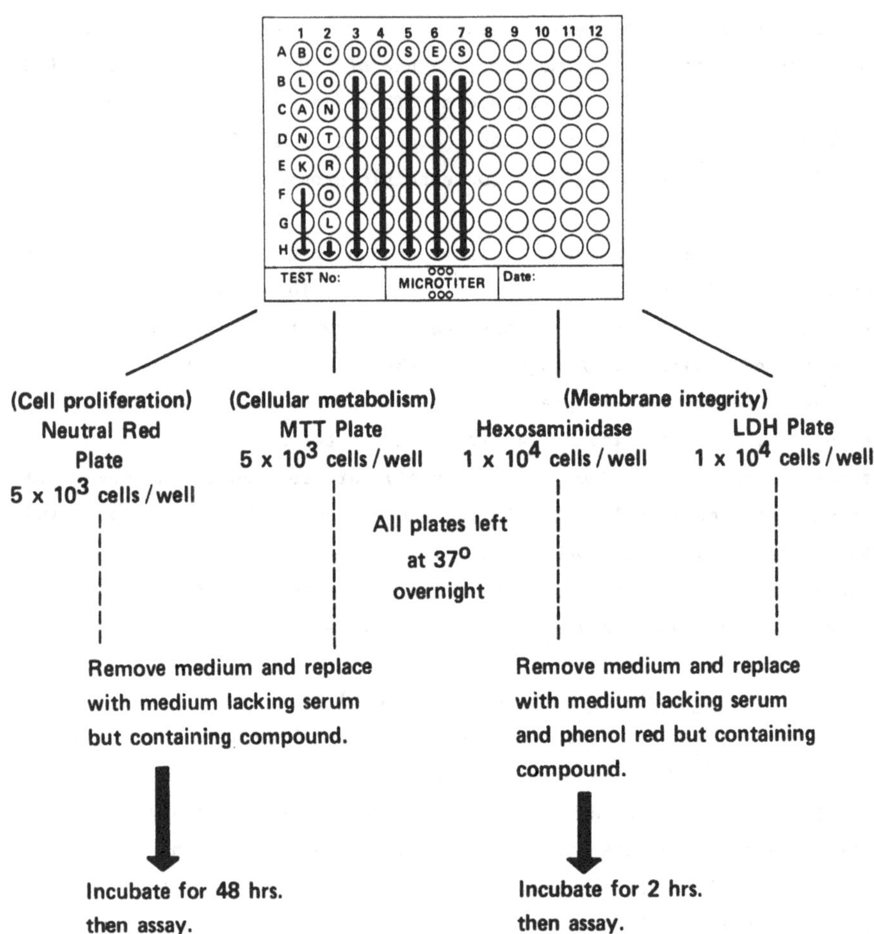

Figure 1 Summarised protocol of the 3T3 cytotoxicity component of the *in vitro* dermal irritant test.

one column used to 'blank' the Multiskan plate reader (column 1, wells A to H), a control column of cells treated with the appropriate medium and compound vehicle only (column 2 all 8 wells). The remaining columns on the plate are treated with medium containing the test compound, each column used for a different concentration. All treatments are done in serum free DMEM and, in the case of the enzyme release assays, modified Eagle's medium without glutamine, phenol red and serum.

For both the neutral red assay and the MTT assay systems the cultures are established at the density indicated (Figure 1) in 100 µl of culture medium per well and the two assays are done at the end of a 48 hour exposure to the test compound. The neutral red assay is essentially as described by Parish and Mullbacher (1983). Briefly the culture medium is removed from the 3T3 monolayers in the wells and, after washing, they are fixed with 4.5% glutaraldehyde and stained with a 0.1% solution of Neutral red. This stain is leached from the cells into 200 µl/well acid alcohol (0.5% v/v acetic acid in 50% v/v ethanol) and can be colorimetrically analysed to indicate the number of cells surviving exposure to the test compound. The MTT assay is a measure of metabolic competence based on that described by Mosmann (1983). In practical terms it is easier to perform than the neutral red assay as the reagent mix (5 mg ml^{-1} MTT in phosphate buffered saline) is added directly to medium in 10 µl aliquots to the culture wells without fixing the cells and after a 4 hour incubation at 37°C the blue formazan crystals are solubilised by 100 µl of acidified isopropanol (0.04 N HCl in isopropanol) before analysing on the Multiskan plate reader.

The two enzyme leakage assays use a slightly different procedure from the neutral red and MTT assays described above. Following a 2 hour exposure to the test compound the supernatant culture medium from each well is transferred to the corresponding well of a second microtitre plate in which the enzyme reaction is done. The hexosaminidase assay method is that described by Landegren (1984) and the reaction is shown below. The two hour time period is chosen to identify immediate subcytolethal toxicity, such as one might expect with mild irritants, causing release of inflammatory mediators.

p-Nitrophenol-N-acetyl- -D-glucosaminide <u>HEXOSAMINIDASE</u>

⟶p-Nitrophenol + Acetyl- D-glucosaminide.

Hexosaminidase in the supernatant culture medium is detected by colorimetric analysis of the yellow nitrophenol produced in the reaction.

The LDH assay is a modification of the method described by Korzeniewski and Callewaert (1983). Essentially lactate is converted to pyruvate by LDH and the electron carrier phenazine methosulphate then reduces the tetrazolium salt 2-(p-Iodophenyl)-3-p-Nitrophenyl-5-Phenyltetrazolium chloride (INT) to a red coloured product.

The reaction is shown below:

$$\text{Lactate} + {}^{*}\text{NAD}^{+} \xrightarrow{\text{LDH}} \text{Pyruvate} + \text{NADH} + \text{H}^{+}$$

then

$$\text{INT} + \text{NADH} \longrightarrow \text{Reduced INT} + \text{NAD}^{+}$$

* Nicotinamide Adenine Dinucleotide

The production of the coloured form of reduced INT is an irreversible reaction and thus is a very suitable fixed time point assay system for LDH released by cells exposed to test compound. The importance of using serum and phenol red free MEM should be stressed at this point. Obviously serum would contaminate the system with endogenous enzymes that would mask low levels of leaked enzyme and the presence of phenol red would mask the appearance of coloured products of enzyme reactions. In addition, MEM culture medium lacks added pyruvate and thus favours the lactate to pyruvate specific reaction.

Epithelial cell differentiation component (Figure 2)

The component of the test system that examines the effect of compounds on epithelial differentiation uses the stratifying and ketatinizing mouse XB-2 cell line. In order to induce the XB-2 cultures to differentiate the cells have to be seeded at a density of 50 cells per cm^2 in 3T3 conditioned DMEM (Rheinwald and Green 1975). The cultures are established in 6 well cluster tissue culture plates (NUNC) and these are most efficiently used if arranged in a group of 5 as shown in Figure 2.

The endpoint assays in this component are all performed after the cells have been exposed to the test compound for 6 days of culture, a period required to allow differentiation of the cells. The assays are

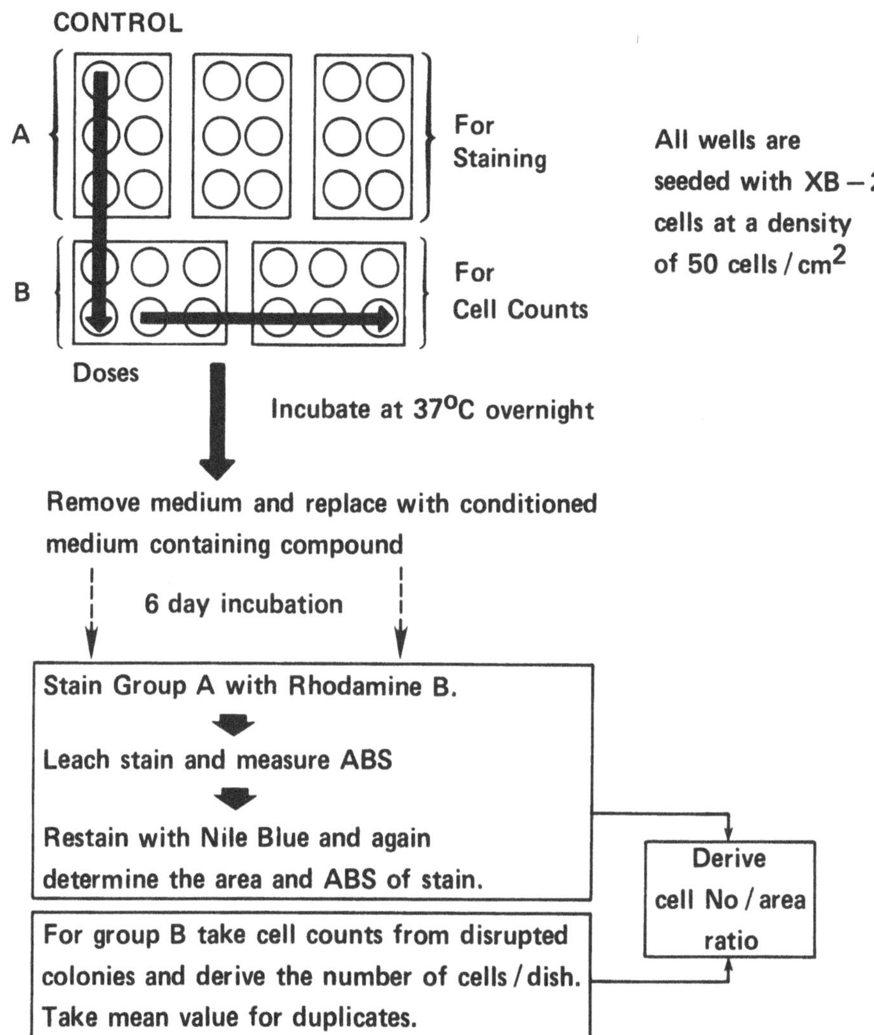

Figure 2 Summarized protocol of the XB-2 epithelial differentiation component of the in vitro dermal irritancy test.

specifically designed to measure the effect of the compound on the following features of the XB-2 cell line.

(1) The level of keratinization in XB-2 colonies using keratin specific Rhodamine B stain.

(2) Cell proliferation and cytotoxicity in the XB-2 cell line assessed by staining with Nile Blue.

(3) The degree of stratification associated with exposure to test compound and derived from the relationship of cell number to colony area.

The use of the 5 plate arrangement (Figure 2) allows the staining procedures and area analysis to be done in triplicates (group A) and cell counts to be determined from duplicate wells (group B). Following exposure to the test compound the cells in wells comprising group A are fixed with 10% formalin and stained with Rhodamine B. Excess stain is removed by washing. The stain bound to the keratin of XB-2 colonies is leached from the cells using 1 ml per well acid alcohol (0.5% v/v acetic acid, 49.5% v/v ethanol in deionised water). A 200 ul aliquot is removed from each well and transferred to the well of a 96 well plate for analysis using the Multiskan spectrophotometer. The destained cultures are then restained with Nile Blue dye and the total colony area of each culture determined with an AMS 40-10 image analyser. The Nile Blue stain is then leached from the cultures and analysed colorimetrically as described for Rhodamine B.

The cells in cultures comprising group B are enzymatically dispersed (using standard cell culture methods and trypsin (0.02% V,V)-EDTA (0.05% V/V) in saline) in DMEM and cell counts done with a standard haemocytometer.

The two staining procedures are used to compare changes in keratinization with cytotoxicity in order to ensure that any reductions observed in the former are not due simply to cell death. The stratification of XB-2 colonies can be illustrated numerically by comparing the increase in area of colonies of an XB-2 culture with the increase in cell number. Figure 3(a) clearly shows that in the early stages of colony development there is a proportional increase in both cell number and colony area. However, after 144 hours of growth there is a disproportionate increase in cell number compared to colony area and beyond 168 hours of culture there is a rapid increase in cell numbers with almost no increase in colony area. This represents the cells forming layers within the colonies rather than increasing their horizontal area. The appearance of layered XB-2 cells viewed with the electron microscope is shown in Figure 3(b).

EXPERIMENTAL EXAMPLES

Data produced from the 3T3 and XB-2 assay systems is expressed graphically and used to derive two endpoints, the maximum tolerated concentration (MTC) and the concentration that reduces a parameter by 50% of control values (IC50). Examples of graphical data for retinol (vitamin A), a known skin irritant, are shown in Figures 4-10.

The concentration response curves shown in Figures 4-10 demonstrate the effect of increasing concentrations of retinol on the test assays in both the 3T3 cell system and the XB-2 cell system

The data collected, for a given test compound, are used to determine if the test compound meets one of four criteria logically chosen to represent *in vitro* perturbations of the epidermis that would be associated with dermal irritation *in vivo*. The criteria are:

1) That a compound is more cytotoxic to the XB-2 epithelial cell line than the 3T3 fibroblast cell line. This can be determined by comparing MTC and IC50 values for Nile Blue and Neutral Red cytotoxicity curves.

2) That keratinization is affected at non cytotoxic concentrations; determined by comparing Rhodamine B keratinization and Nile Blue cytotoxicity MTC and IC50 values in XB-2 cells.

3) That an effect on stratification is observed; determined by comparing MTC and IC50 values for colony area and cell number curves. Changes in cell number, without corresponding changes in colony area, represent changes in the number of cell layers per colony.

4) That cell membrane integrity has been disrupted resulting in leakage of intracellular enzymes (LDH or HEX) to the supernatant culture medium. The MTT assay serves to confirm cytotoxicity measured with neutral red. This is required as some compounds can fix cells and thus give rise to an apparent increase in cell number with higher concentrations of test compound when using the Neutral red assay. These cell have simply been rapidly fixed by the test compound.

The variability of IC50 values between repeat experiments is approximately 20%. Thus with this level of variability the limit for

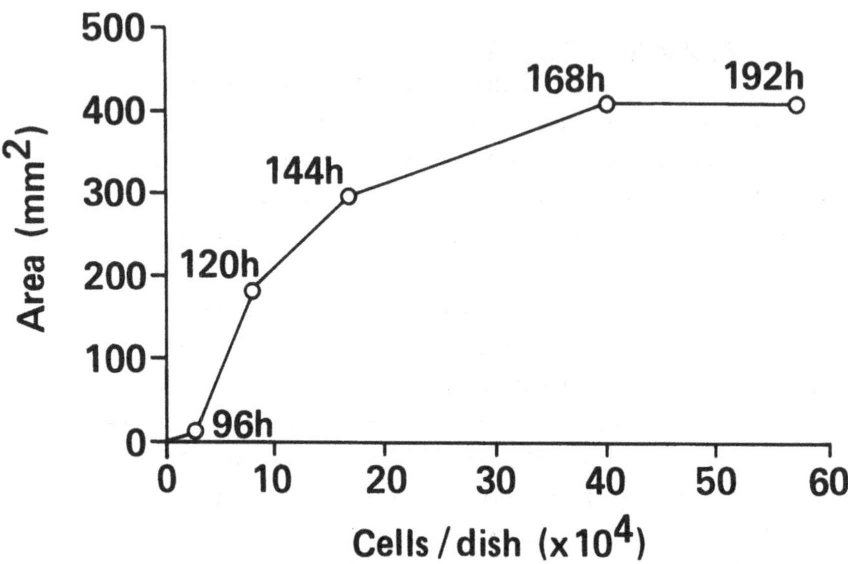

Figure 3(a) Increase in cell number and area in differentiating XB-2 colonies during 192 hours of culture.

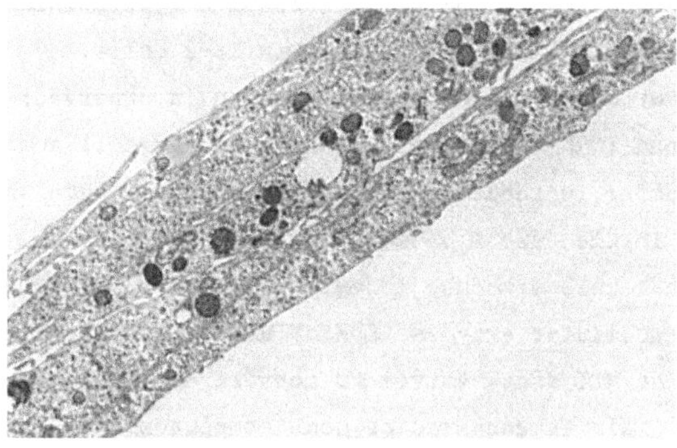

Figure 3(b) Electron micrograph of section through a stratified XB-2 colony showing 5 distinct layers (prepared according to the method of Rheinwald and Green, 1975). Magnification x 6880.

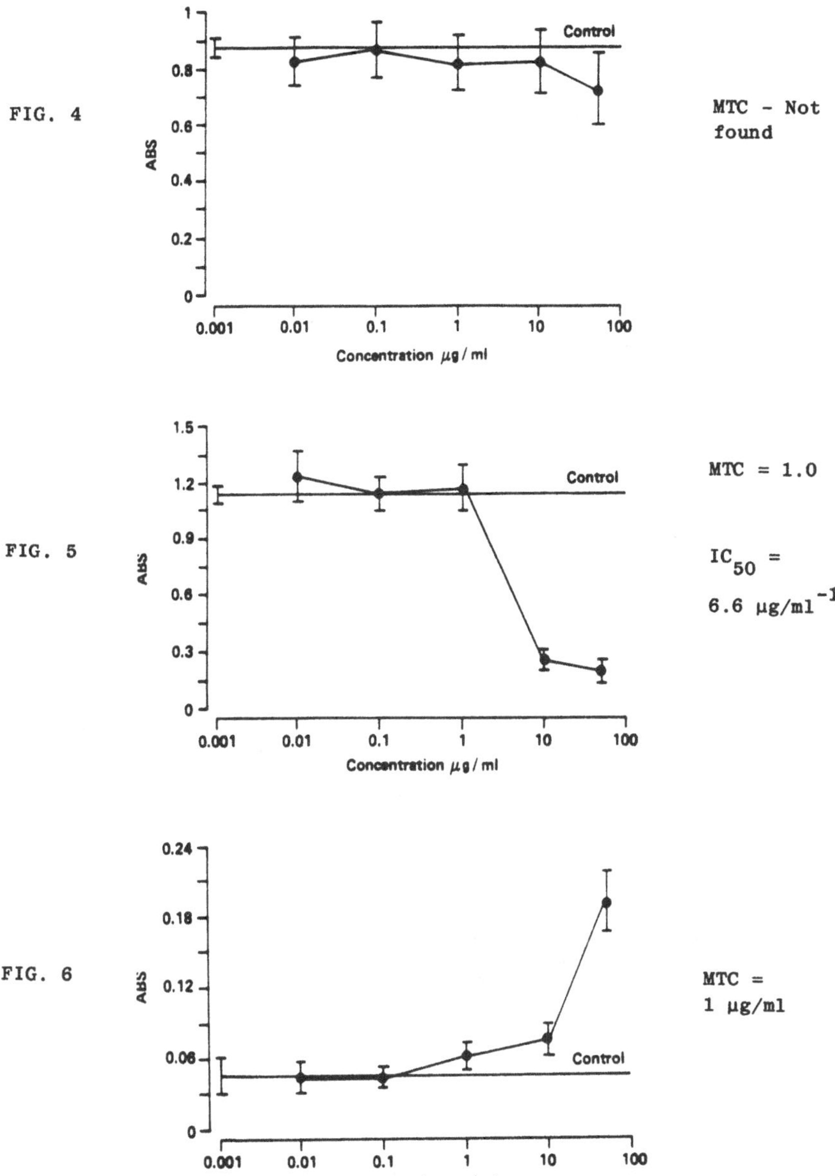

MTC - Not found

MTC = 1.0

IC_{50} = 6.6 $\mu g/ml^{-1}$

MTC = 1 $\mu g/ml$

Change in absorbance units (ABS) against concentration of retinol for Neutral red assay, representing cell survival, at 2 hours (Figure 4), Neutral red assay at 48 hours (Figure 5) and LDH release assay, indicating membrane damage (Figure 6) in 3T3 cells. Bars indicate standard deviations.

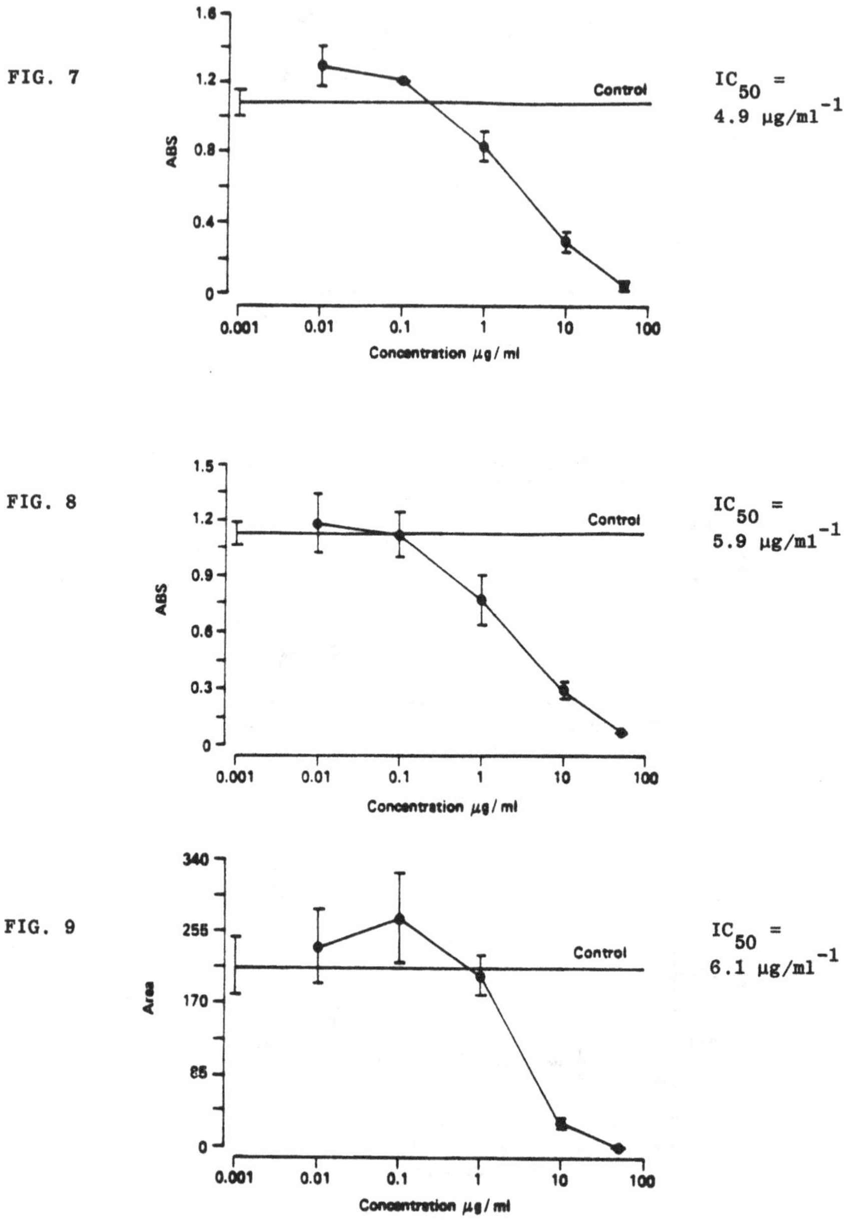

Change in absorbance units (ABS) or colony area (mm^2) against concentration of retinol for Nile blue destain assay, representing cell survival (Figure 7), Rhodamine B destain assay (Figure 8) and Nile blue stained colony area assay, indicating keratin production, (Figure 9) in XB-2 cells. Bars indicate standard deviations.

FIG. 10

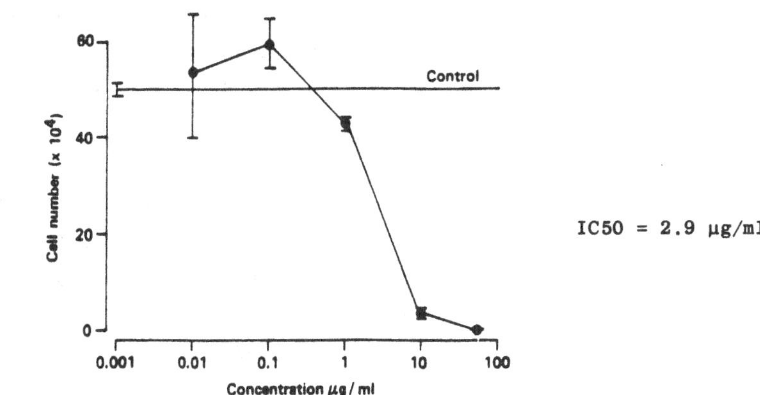

IC50 = 2.9 µg/ml

Change in counted cell number against concentration of retinol. Bars indicate standard deviations.

Table 1. <u>SUMMARY OF IN VITRO ASSAY DATA FOR RETINOL</u>

RETINOL			EFFECT	
1.	Nile blue IC50 in XB-2 cells	4.9 µg/ml	= 0	1
	Neutral red IC50 at 48h in 3T3 cells	6.6 µg/ml		
	Nile blue MTC in SB-2 cells	0.1 µg/ml	= 1	
	Neutral red MTC at 48h in 3T3 cells	1.0 µg/ml		
2.	LDH MTC in 3T3 cells	1.0 µg/ml	= 1	1
	Neutral red MTC at 2h in 3T3 cells	NF		
3.	Rhodamine B IC50 in SB-2 cells	5.9 µg/ml	= 0	0
	Nile blue IC50 in XB-2 cells	4.9 µg/ml		
	Rhodamine B MTC in SB-2 cells	0.1 µg/ml	= 0	
	Nile blue MTC in XB-2 cells	0.1 µg/ml		
4.	Nile blue stained colony area IC50 in XB-2 cells	6.1 µg/ml	= 1	1
	Counted cell number IC50 in XB-2 cells	2.9 µg/ml		
	Nile blue stained colony area MTC in XB-2 cells	1.0 µg/ml	= 1	
	Counted cell number MTC in XB-2 cells	0.1 µg/ml		

a scored as positive (1) or negative (0) by comparison of IC50 and MTC.
b combined score from comparisons of IC50 and MTC.

scoring a difference between compared IC50 values was set at 50%. Using such a high set limit, at least two standard deviations in relation to the variability, one could be sure that any difference scored as positive was highly significant. Of course when MTC values are compared the log concentration dosing regime ensures that any difference scored as positive is from values at least 10 fold apart.

Using this approach the data from the assays of retinol can be analysed and retinol scored for its effects on the four criteria of epidermal toxicity. The result of this analysis is summarised in Table 1. For criterion 1, if one compares the IC50 value for the Nile blue assay of XB-2 cells (4.9 μg/ml) with that for the Neutral red assay of 3T3 cells (6.6 μg/ml) according to the 50% difference limit no effect would be scored. However, a comparison of the respective MTC values does score a positive effect and thus for the ability to be, under these conditions, selectively cytotoxic to XB-2 epithelial cells retinol would be scored as positive.

Similarly a significant difference is observed following comparison of MTC values for LDH release (1μg/ml) and Neutral Red assay (MTC not found) of 3T3 cells, after a 2 hour exposure to the test compound. Thus retinol causes subcytolethal release of LDH in 3T3 cells.

Examination of either IC50 or MTC values in Rhodamine B and Nile blue assays in XB-2 cells shows no significant difference. Thus, retinol does not score as positive for an ability to cause a subcytolethal reduction in keratinization.

In the last criterion, looking for effects on stratification, comparison of the IC50 values for the Nile blue stained XB-2 colony area assay (6.1 μg/ml) and XB-2 counted cell number assay (2.9 μg/ml) shows a significant difference by the 50% change limit. A significant difference is also seen when comparing the MTC values (1.0 μg/ml and 0.1 μg/ml, respectively). Thus retinol scores positive against the criterion of causing subcytolethal reduced stratification.

In summary, with the example of retinol, a known irritant, assayed and analysed through the complete test, scored positive effects in three of the four set criteria. These were specific cytotoxicity to XB-2 epithelial cells, subcytolethal enzyme release and subcytolethal reduced stratification. Given these significant effects, had retinol been an unknown test compound, it would have been predicted to have a stong likelihood of being an irritant, consistent with in vivo experience of dermal exposure to retinol.

DISCUSSION AND CONCLUSIONS

The major strengths of this approach to determining skin irritancy lie in the fact that it does not use cytotoxicity alone as a measure of irritant potential, which logically one would not expect to give accurate predictions, but focuses on the effects irritants could display in relation to epithelial sensitivity, stratification and keratinization. A criticism that perhaps could be directed towards the test system described is that it is an incomplete model of the *in vivo* organ. Further research might lead to the use of lipophilicity values to predict the penetration of compounds and thus eliminate the above criticism or this test may be used in conjunction with measurements of penetration through explants of human or animal cadaver skin (Dugard, 1983).

Prelimininary results also suggest it is not possible, to rank the severity of predicted response in those compounds that are judged to have irritant potential. This could be closely related to the penetration properties of test compounds. Further work on this problem, and the incorporation of such data, as it becomes available, into the overall analysis will no doubt improve the predictions of irritancy and may provide an indication of the severity of the predicted *in vivo* response.

Other proposed alternatives to the use of animals in dermal irritancy testing have suggested the use of general non-specific cytotoxicity tests to predict irritancy. Rheinhardt and co-workers (1985) for example studied the effect of known irritants on BHK and human fibroblasts by measuring cell detachment, cloning efficiency and growth inhibition. They did not try to correlate their *in vitro* results with Draize skin and eye irritancy data but, by grouping their test compounds into the 3 crude classes of non-irritant, mild to moderate irritant and strong irritant or corrosive, they found a greater than 80% correlation with data derived from human exposure (mostly obtained from the Merck Index). Another approach is to use biochemical and biophysical measurements in organ culture as described by Oliver and Pemberton (1985) and described elsewhere in this book. These workers have developed an *in vitro* model using rat epidermal skin slices to identify corrosive and irritant potential by changes in skin resistance and the penetration of tritiated water. This test system selectively identifies corrosive agents but in its current form has not been useful in predicting mild and moderate irritants.

Dermal irritation is a complex response to an insult that has numerous mechanisms of action. General cytotoxicity assays, conducted in isolation from other tests, are too simplistic to model toxic mechanisms relating to a specific differentiated organ like the skin. Organ culture techniques are better methods than simple cell cytotoxicity for predicting the *in vivo* dermal response to irritants. They have the advantages of retaining the permeability barrier of intact skin thus giving results relevant to penetration properties and greatly reducing the number of animals required. However, since these systems do not possess a vascular blood supply they do not detect slight and mild irritants that produce inflammation by the pharmacological action of released inflammatory mediators. In addition to irritation produced by the release of inflammatory mediators more long term irritancy could result from perturbation of the stratification and/or keratinization pathways of differentiation. Sensitivity of epithelial cells to specific classes of irritant compound could also contribute to more long term effects by resulting in epidermal necrosis. The 3T3 cytotoxicity and XB-2 epithelial differentiation have the advantage of being designed as a multifactorial battery of assays designed to reflect the actual mechanisms of irritancy as they might occur in the skin *in vivo*.

In addition to dermal irritation studies the relative ease with which the *in vitro* techniques can be manipulated would permit studies of mechanistic problems in dermal and epithelial toxicology. These studies could use a biochemical approach, such as effects of compounds on XB-2 cell keratin electrophoresis profiles, or of a morphological approach by studying the modification of stratification by new compounds. One particular mechanistic problem currently under investigation in this laboratory, using the XB-2 and 3T3 techniques, is the hyperproliferative effect some compounds have specifically towards epithelial cells.

The use of *in vitro* systems to study specific mechanistic problems, although superficially appearing to be a simplistic approach, could provide valuable information that would not have been obtained from the complex interactions occurring in a whole animal study. However, with regard to regulatory toxicity testing, the system for _in vitro_ prediction of dermal irritant potential described here will not immediately replace the use of animals in the current regulatory authority requirements for safety evaluation toxicity tests. After the complete and full validation of this system of tests it has now been integrated into a predesigned tier system of safety evaluation of novel compounds (Jackson and Rutty, 1985). Further analysis of the results of the blind trial support the use of this test system to predict potential ocular irritancy and this method will be described in subsequent publications.

ACKNOWLEDGEMENTS

The authors wish to thank Mrs K Jones and Miss M J Fursey for excellent technical assistance. They would also like to thank Dr T C Orton and Dr J C Topham for advice and comments on preparation of this manuscript.

Burton, A.B.G., York, M. and Lawrence, R.S. (1981). The In Vitro Assessment of Severe Eye Irritants. Fd. Cosmet.Toxicol. 19, 471-480.

Draize, J.H., Woodard, G. and Calvery, H.O. (1944). Methods for the study of irritation and toxicity of substances applied topically to the skin and mucous membranes. J.Pharmac.exp.Ther. 82, 377-390.

Dugard, P.H. (1983). Skin permiability theory in relation to measurements of percutaneous absorption in toxicology. In Dermatotoxicology (ed. F.N. Marzulli and H.J. Mailbach) 2nd Edition Hemisphere, London, p91.

Gloxhuber, Ch. and Kastner, W.(1985). The Mouse Intradermal Tests, a Well-established and Reliable Model in Skin Tolerance Testing. Fd.Chem.Toxic. 23, N°2 195-197.

Hood, D.B. (1977). Practical and Theoretical Considerations in Evaluating Dermal Safety. In Cutaneous Toxicity, ed. V.A. Drill and P. Lazar pp. 19-21.

Hurkmans, J.F.G.M., Bodde, H.E., Van Driel, L.M.J., Van Doorne, H. and Junginger, H.E. (1985). Skin Irritation Caused by Transdermal Drug Delivery Systems During Long Term (5 Days) Application. Brit.J.Dermatol, 112, 461-467.

Jackson, J. and Rutty, D.A. (1985). Ocular Tolerance Assessment - Integrated Tier Policy. Fd. Chem. Toxic. 23, No2 309-310.

Kao, J., Hall, J. and Holland, J.M. (1983). Quantitation of Cutaneous Toxicity: An In Vitro Approach Using Skin Organ Culture. Toxicol.Appl.Pharmacol, 68, 206-217.

Kemp, R.B., Meredith, R.W.J. and Gamble, S.H. (1985. Toxicity of Commerical Products on Cells in Suspension Culture: A Possible Screen for the Draize Eye Irritation Test. Fd.Chem.Toxic. 23, N°2 267-270.

Korzeniewski, C. and Cullewaert, D.M. (1983). An Enzyme Release Assay for Natural Cytotoxicity. J.Immunol.Methods 64, 313-320.

Landegren, U. (1984). Measurement of Cell Numbers by Means of the Endogenous Enzyme Hexosaminidase. Applications to Detection of lymphokines and Cell Surface Antigens. J.Immunol.Methods 67, 379-388.

Leighton, J., Nassauer, J. and Tchao, R. (1985). The Chick Embryo in Toxicology: An Alternative to the Rabbit Eye. Fd.Chem.Toxic. 23, N°2 293-298.

Luepke, N.P. (1985). hens Egg Chorioallantoic Membrane Test for Irritation Potential. Fd.Chem.Toxic. 23 N°2 287-291.

Marks, R. and Kingston, T. (1985). Acute Skin Toxicity Reactions in Man-Tests and Mechanisms. Fd.Chem.Toxic. 23, 155-163.

Mosmann, T. (1983). Rapid Colorimetric Assay for Cellular Growth and Survival: Application to Proliferation and Cytotoxicity Assays. J.Immunol.Methods 65, 55-63.

Muir, C.K. (1985). Opacity of Bovine Cornea In Vitro Induced by Surfactants and Industrial Chemicals Compared with Ocular Irritancy In Vivo. Toxicol.Lett. 24, 157-162.

Muir, C.K. (1983). The Toxic Effect of Some Industrial Chemicals on Rabbit Ileum In Vitro Compared with Eye Irritancy In Vivo. Toxicol. Lett. 19, 309-312.

North-Root, H., Yackovich, F. Demetrulias, J, Gacula, M. and Heinze, J.E. (1985). Prediction of the Eye Irritation Potential of Shampoos Using the In Vitro SIRC Cell Toxicity Test. Fd. Chem.Toxic. 23, N°2, 271-273.

Oliver, G.J.A. and Pemberton, M.A. (1985). An In Vitro Epidermal Slice Technique for Identifying Chemicals with Potential for Severe Cutaneous Effects. Fd.Chem.Toxic. 23, No2 229-232.

Parish, C.R. and Mullbacher, A. (1983). Automated Colorimetric Assay for T Cell Cytotoxicity. J.Immunol.Methods 58, 225-237.

Rheinhardt, Ch.A., Pelli, D.A. and Zbinden, G. (1985). Interpretation of Cell Cytotoxicity Data for the Estimation of Irritant Potential. Fd.Chem.Toxic 23, No2 247-252.

Rheinwald, J.G. and Green, H. (1975). Formation of a keratinsizing Epithelium in Culture by a Cloned Cell Line Derived From a Teratoma Cell 6, 317-330.

Scaife, M.C. (1985). An In Vitro Cytotoxicity Test to Predict the Ocular Irritation Potential of Detergents and Detergent Products. Fd.Chem.Toxic. 23, No2 253-258.

Shopsis, C, Borenfreund, E., Walberg, J. and Stark, D.M. (1985). A Battery of Potential Alternatives to the Draize Test: Uridine Uptake, Morphological Cytotoxicity, Macrophage Chemotoxis and Exfoliative Cytology. Fd.Chem.Toxic. 23 No2 259-266.

Shopsis, C and Sathe, S. (1984). Uridine Uptake Inhibition as a Cytotoxicity Test: Correlations with the Draize Test. Toxicol. 29, 195-206.

Todaro, C.J. and Green, H. (1963). Quantitative Studies of the Growth of Mouse Embryo Cells in Culture and Their Development into Established Cell Lines J.Cell.Biol. 17, 299-313.

Van Der Valk, P.G.M., Nater, J.P. and Bleumink, E. (1984). Skin Irritancy of Surfactants as Assessed by Water Vapour Loss Measurements. J.Invest.Dermatol. 82, 291-293.

Walz, D. (1984). Towards an Animal-Free Assessment of topical Irritancy. Tips June 221-224.

Weil, C.S. and Scala, R.A. (1971). Study of Intra- and Interlaboratory Variability in the Results of Rabbit Eye and Skin Irritation Test. Toxicol.App.Phrmacol. 19, 276-360.

GENETIC TOXICOLOGY

Margaret Richold
Huntingdon Research Centre, Huntingdon, Cambs. England

INTRODUCTION

Genetic toxicology is the study of the effect of chemicals on DNA, the unit of heredity, and the impact of this on mutation, a permanent heritable change in DNA. Many mutations are deleterious perhaps resulting in the inactivation of an enzyme or in change of cell function, but some may prove beneficial enabling the new cell or organism to survive in a changing environment.

The detection of chemicals that may be potential mutagens (mutagenic agents) is a rapidly expanding discipline relying on a variety of *in vivo* and *in vitro* assays some of which will be described in detail below. One reason for its wide acceptance in spite of the esoteric nature of the subject is that tests to identify mutagens are now frequently used to provide an indication of carcinogenic potential. The fact that the majority of mutagens are also carcinogens revived the somatic mutation theory of cancer proposed by Bauer and Boveri in the 1930's but which had not been substantiated by earlier genetic experiments.

The hypothesis was that the induction of cancer was the consequence of a mutation arising in somatic (non-germinal) cell tissue which led, at a later date, to uncontrolled cell division of the mutated cells to produce tumours and eventually cancer.

To understand the rationale linking tests for mutagenicity and cancer induction, a knowledge of DNA and the way this unique molecule operates is helpful. DNA is a macro-molecule made up of sub-units known as deoxyribonucleotides, which themselves comprise a pentose sugar 2 deoxy ribose, a phosphate ester and a nitrogenous base which may be one of two purines or one of two pyrimidines. It is the unique sequence of bases, along the DNA molecule which provides the foundation of the genetic code in that the information contained in the code leads to the production of functional proteins. Each amino acid which helps to form the protein molecule is coded for on the DNA molecule by means of codons. Each codon is a sequence of 3 bases. Since there are 4 bases, 64 codons (4^3) can be described. There are 20 essential amino acids, so it will be apparent that the genetic code is degenerate. In fact any one amino acid can be coded for by more than one codon. This degree of degeneration is useful as it provides latitude for minor errors. Also a number of codons are used to provide simple instructions like start, stop (the synthesis of proteins) etc..

DNA is located in the nucleus but protein synthesis takes place in the cytoplasm. Thus the DNA code has to be 'transcribed' and the message carried to the cytoplasm where it is 'translated' on ribosomes to produce the new protein (a polypeptide chain).

The major consequences of DNA damage are the production of point or gene mutations, the induction of chromosome damage and a change in chromosome number. Point or gene mutations occur when nucleotides are inserted or deleted thereby changing the sequence of bases on DNA, or if they are miscoded/misread during transcription and translation. This type of damage is usually identified indirectly by screening for the production of mutant colonies, but nowadays DNA adducts may sometimes be identified, albeit with difficulty. DNA adducts are the stable chemical entities arising from covalent binding of DNA to a chemical. They can either form links between bases on the same strand of the DNA duplex or can form a link between strands of the molecule.

Chromosome damage occurs when a complete break in one or both strands of the chromosome (a DNA: protein complex) occurs, leading to chromosome deletion, translocation or even duplication. Losses or gains in chromosome number may arise after exposure to certain chemicals causing non-disjunction.

As stated above, most mutations are deleterious, and a number of disorders in humans are due to mutation. It is thought that 30-50% of spontaneous abortions are due to chromosomal aberrations or other genetic disorders. (Polani et al 1981). Examples of disease due to abnormal chromosomal number include Mongolism (Down's syndrome), Edwards syndrome, Klinefelter and Turner syndromes, whereas Huntingtons chorea and Tay Sach disease are due to point mutations. Other diseases such as muscular dystrophy and cystic fibrosis are also due to genetic disorders.

It is therefore of paramount importance to test chemicals for their mutagenic potential, but genotoxicity testing serves another purpose in aiding the identification of potential carcinogens. Tests of chemicals for these properties should occur at an early stage in the development of novel substances. Thus, if a series of analogues has been synthesised, it would be prudent to select only those which were non-genotoxic for further development. _In vitro_ tests to identify chemicals possessing transforming ability are also available and these provide a direct correlation with potential carcinogenicity. These types of assay will not be described in this chapter, but the interested reader will find the book edited by Mishra (1980), a useful reference.

METHODS

Most short-term screening tests have been designed to be rapid, relatively inexpensive, _in vitro_ and yet highly predictive for mutagenicity and potential carcinogenicity. Such expectations can only be realised, and then maybe partially, by using a range of assays to detect gene mutations, clastogens (chromosome breaking agents) changes in ploidy (chromosome number) and effects on body fluids. Tables 1 and 2 illustrate the range of tests currently available. Detailed practical methodologies will not be provided since two excellent books are already available (Kilbey et al 1984, Venitt & Parry, 1984).

In vitro assays to detect gene mutagens

The above type of assay can be undertaken using bacterial or mammalian cells. The best known bacterial mutation assay is that devised by Ames (1973/1975) and Maron & Ames (1983).

Known colloquially as the Ames test but more accurately as the Salmonella Microsome Assay, it is a reverse mutation test measuring gene mutation in strains of _Salmonella typhimurium_. A number of strains are available but at the present time the use of 4 is recommended. Two of these detect base-pair substitution mutagens (agents which cause the wrong base to be inserted into the new DNA strand), and 2 strains detect frame-shift mutagens (agents which cause the insertion or deletion of nucleotide bases). These strains are already mutants since part of the operon which codes for the bio-synthesis of the amino acid histidine is inactive. The strains are rendered even more sensitive by possessing excision repair deficiencies, alterations in the cell wall affecting permeability of chemicals and in addition two of them contain extra genetic material (plasmids) which induces "error-prone" repair

Table 1 - Non mammalian tests for mutagenesis
*indicates the end point measured by the test organism.

Organism	Gene mutation		DNA Repair	Chromosome damage
	forward °	reverse +		
Bacteria, e.g.				
S. typhimurium	*	*		
E. coli		*	*	
Yeast, e.g.				
S. cerevisiae	*	*	*	*
S. pombe	*	*		*
Fungi, e.g.				
A. Nidulans	*	*		*
N. crassa	*	*		*
Plants, e.g.				
T. paludosa	*	*		
V. faba				*
Insects, e.g.				
D. melanogaster	*	*		*

° change of state from parental to altered (mutant) form

+ change of state from altered to original (parental) form.

Table 2 - Tests for mutagenesis in Mammals or mammalian cells
*indicates the end point measured by the test organism

Animal	In vitro	In vivo	Gene mutation	DNA repair	Chromosome damage	Ploidy
Chinese hamster	V79(lung)		*	*	*	*
	CHO (ovary)		*	*	*	*
		Micro-nucleus			*	
Mouse	Lymphoma L5178Y		*		*	
	Lymphoma P388F		*	*		
		Lympho-cytes			*	*
	Urine		*			
Mouse & Rat		Micro-nucleus			*	*
		Metaphase			*	*
		Dominant-lethal			*	
		Host-mediated-assay	*			
		Specific-locus	*			
		Spot test	*			
		Heritable translo-cation			*	
Human	Lymphocytes		*		*	*
	HeLa		*	*		

synthesis. The end point studied is that of reversion or back-mutation of the histidine auxotrophic mutants to the wild type prototrophic form which is then able to synthesize histidine. After exposure of approximately 2 x 10^8 bacteria to the test agent either in the presence or absence of a metabolic activation system, they are plated in soft agar which is essentially deficient in histidine. Only mutated bacteria will be able to grow and form colonies which are then counted after three days incubation at 37°C. A positive response is claimed when a reproducible increase, of at least 2.5 times the control, in the number of mutant colonies is obtained. The introduction of a metabolic activation system (S-9 mix) is important, as it is known that a number of carcinogens need to be metabolised to a reactive form before tumour induction occurs such as nitrosamines, dimethylbenzanthracene and benzαpyrene. Bacteria and many mammalian cells used in tissue culture do not possess any metabolising activity, so the addition of one is necessary if indirect acting mutagens are to be detected. The metabolic system most frequently used in _in vitro_ experiments is a liver postmitochondrial supernatant. It is preferable to increase the mixed function oxidase enzyme activity in the liver supernatant to be used, so the animals are induced using either a mixture of polychlorinated biphenyls (Arochlor 1254) or with a combination of phenobarbitol and B napthoflavone (Matsushima et al, 1976).

In the original validation of 300 chemicals, the assay was less effective in detecting certain classes of chemical carcinogens such as halogenated hydrocarbons, hormones and antibiotics. The detection rate can now be improved by using some of the new tester strains such as TA 102, TA 97 and TA 92 (Maron & Ames 1983). It is also claimed by some (Ashby 1986) that the use of a pre-incubation phase in which the bacteria, test substance and, if required, S-9 mix are incubated together for 20-30 minutes at 30°C before adding to the soft agar, makes the assay more reliable. Table 3 provides some data illustrating how this procedure has helped to clarify weak responses obtained in the standard plate assay (Jones and Richold, unpublished data). In addition the original effects can sometimes be enhanced by varying the % S-9 mix used in the assay or by using primary hepatocytes as the metabolising source. Choice of solvent may also have a modifying effect, the most frequently used being water, ethanol or DMSO.

Table 3 - Effect of Pre-incubation on bacterial mutation test with Salmonella typhimurium strain TA 100

Conc. ug/ plate	Assay S9 10%	Plate						Preincub.			
		-			+			-		+	
Test		1	2	3	1	2	3	1	2	1	2
10000		-	164	135	-	108	148	490	595	965	988
5000		88	91	129	203	124	131	390	333	497	343
2500		-	101	119	-	109	127	162	160	170	185
1000		92	-	110	102	-	124	-	-	107	126
500		88	-	-	109	-	-	-	-	-	-
100		99	-	-	95	-	-	-	-	-	-
50		70	-	-	92	-	-	-	-	-	-
10		66	-	-	106	-	-	-	-	-	-
0		82	80	121	88	89	120	80	85	121	120

- = not tested

Following on from bacterial gene mutation tests of which the Ames assay is just one example, the test substance may also be examined in a mammalian cell gene mutation test. Such tests are technically more difficult to conduct and the data more difficult to interpret, largely because of the variation in response seen in untreated cultures. The selection of cell lines which may be of mouse, Chinese hamster or human origin depends largely on personal preference. For routine screening purposes it is probably inadvisable to use the less well validated human cell lines at this time. A forward mutation assay is generally conducted since mutation induction from the normal parental, or Wild Type, form to a mutant form is easier to detect. Thus, one could look for the inactivation of a gene (locus) by forward mutation as expressed by the ability of cells with this deficiency to grow in selective medium. If Chinese hamster V79 or CHO cells were used, inactivation of the HGPRT locus (hypoxanthine guanine phosphoribosyl transferase) is detected by assessing the colony forming ability of treated cells following challenge with 6-thioguanine (Jensen, 1984). HGPRT converts hypoxanthine and guanine to the corresponding nucleoside 5 monophosphate, on reaction with phosphoribosyl pyrophosphate. The purine analogues 8-Azaguanine and 6-thioguanine are also converted, but to toxic ribonucleotide, and thereby kill cells with normal activity of the enzyme. Mutated cells with an inactive HGPRT gene product survive in growth medium containing one of these purine analogues. Since HGPRT is needed only as a salvage pathway, the mutant cells grow to produce colonies due to their ability to synthesize the required purines by a *de novo* pathway.

Unlike the Ames test, results are usually expressed as induced mutation frequency, therefore it is essential to know the effect of a test substance on cell viability. The normal practice is to treat cells over a concentration range which kills up to 90% of the cell population. This may seem drastic but a study could be criticised if sufficient toxicity had not been induced, unless hindered by practical limitations. A positive response would be claimed in this assay if:

(a) the increase in mutation frequency was approximately 3 times the spontaneous control frequency or double the maximum response seen in the normal laboratory range.

b) the response is dose related and reproducible.

There are a number of pitfalls to beware of when attempting to interpret the data. One of the more problematical areas is that of weak positive responses occurring at highly toxic concentrations. Sometimes the test concentration may be so high as to cause acidity in spite of the buffering system present in the culture medium. Under such conditions the data would be considered invalid. Responses of this type have been described elsewhere (Cifone et al, 1984) and the writer can confirm observing this phenomenon in her own laboratory.

In Vitro assays to detect clastogens

The more frequently used cell lines for this type of assay are primary human lymphocytes or established animal cell lines, frequently of Chinese hamster origin and chosen because of their low, relatively stable chromosome number. The tests involve the examination of individual contracted chromosomes at the metaphase stage of mitosis.

At this stage DNA duplication has already occurred and the replicated chromosomes are joined together by a single centromere.

When human lymphocytes are used they must be stimulated into division, usually by addition of a mitogen such as phytohaemagluttinin (PHA). Once in division, cells are exposed to the test substance either in the presence or absence of S-9 mix. The period of exposure is usually the length of one cell division cycle. With Chinese hamster cells the principle of the assay is the same except that stimulation of cells into division is not required.

Cells are arrested in the metaphase stage of cell division using a spindle poison (colchicine or colcemid) made hypotonic to allow cell swelling, fixed, stained and examined under the light microscope for structural abnormalities, including gaps, breaks, fragments, exchange configurations and translocations. A number of classification schemes for identifying and recording types of damage are available (Savage 1976).

In vitro assays to detect ploidy.

Chromosomal numerical aberrations are probably the most serious change that can occur in a genotype. Higher organisms are diploid, having two sets of chromosomes. Changes in ploidy can give rise to fewer chromosomes (aneuploidy), or to 3 or 4 sets of chromosomes (tetraploidy). Change in chromosome number can occur to the euploid state, in which the chromosome number is an exact multiple of the haploid number, or to the aneuploid state in which the abnormal chromosome number is not an exact multiple of the haploid number. Aneuploidy is frequently caused during the breakdown of the mitotic spindle, a collection of protein fibres, which locate the contracted chromosome in the centre of the cells and later aids their segregation to opposite poles of the cell during the final phases of cell division.

Tests for ploidy are frequently carried out in Yeast. Strain D6 of Saccharomyces cerevisiae is often used (Parry and Zimmerman 1976). It allows detection of aneuploidy during mitotic cell division. Other strains are available which enable the event to be monitored during meiosis. Because of the unique genotype of strain D6 it forms red colonies when grown in complete growth medium due to a block in the adenine synthesis pathway. The strain is also sensitive to cycloheximide. Aneuploid mutants, able to synthesize adenine, form white colonies and they are resistant to cycloheximide. Thus, it is possible to test for aneuploidy without possessing a detailed knowledge of the complex genetics of the system.

The performance of Yeast assays in general in interlaboratory trials has sometimes been less than impressive (de Serres 1981) and therefore the identification of aneuploid inducing agents in a mammalian cell assay is desirable. One such method has been developed by Danford (1984) which appears promising although has not yet undergone extensive validation. Briefly, the method involves a reduced hypotonic regime whereby chromosomes can be counted accurately yet retained within the cell membrane.

In vitro indicator tests.

Assays placed in this category are those in which a mutational end point such as chromosome damage or point mutation is not clearly defined. Data from such assays, sometimes thought of as supplementary assays, provide a suggestion that an agent may be mutagenic based on the demonstration that it reacts with DNA in some way. DNA repair, sister chromatid exchange and mitotic recombination assays in lower eukaryotes are just 3 types of indicator test available.

The failure of DNA to replicate faithfully may occur sporadically in cells and is not always a result of physical or chemical damage. Fortunately, living cells possess repair processes whereby DNA is monitored for errors which are then repaired. This process is under the control of at least four enzyme systems involving the recognition of damaged sites, the excision of such lesions, the insertion of undamaged nucleotides using the opposite strand of DNA as a template, and the final rejoining of newly synthesized DNA to the pre-existing strand. These repair systems are vitally important and it is their failure which can lead to a variety of disorders, one of which may be cancer.

In bacteria, DNA repair can be monitored fairly simply by estimating differential killing rates after exposure to mutagens in bacterial strains which have been rendered defective in their repair capacity. In established mammalian cell lines or in hepatocytes DNA repair is measured by the uptake of labelled nucleotides into damaged DNA using either autoradiographic or scintillation counting techniques (Williams 1976, Martin et al 1978). Other tests are available which quite simply monitor the reaction of a test agent with DNA to determine whether strand breakage occurs. The successful repair of DNA damage is important and it has been proposed that one cause of mutation is the mis-repair of damaged DNA.

Sister Chromatid Exchanges (SCE) are due to exchanges between sister chromatids of the same chromosome in the mitotic cell and should be distinguished from the exchange and recombination of genetic material which frequently occurs between chromatids of paired homologous chromosome at meiosis. Human lymphocytes or mammalian cell lines can be used. The detection of SCE is based on the principle that when cells have undergone two replication cycles in the presence of the thymidine analogue,5-bromodeoxyuridine (BrdU), one chromatid will have both polynucleotide chains of the DNA helix substituted with the analogue, while its sister will have only one chain substituted. The chromatids can then be distinguished by differential staining (Perry & Evans, 1975). At present there is no clear evidence that the cause of SCE induction is the same event which causes chromosome breakage, so a direct link between SCE and conventional chromosome damage cannot be made. SCE events are believed by some to represent that degree of DNA damage which is capable of repair by normal enzymic repair processes present in mammalian cells. Other attempts to correlate SCE with mutation and cancer have been made, but the correlation is not constant (Parodi 1983).

In vivo assays

In vivo assays are mainly used in the context of genetic toxicology to determine whether the potential to induce mutation seen *in vitro* is expressed *in vivo* (Richold 1982, Ashby 1986). The more standard *in vivo* assays measure chromosome damage as the end point in either somatic or germinal tissue. Well validated *in vivo* assays to assess gene mutation are uncommon but will also be briefly discussed.

The micronucleus assay is one of the most rapid tests for estimation of gross chromosomal damage (Schmid 1975, Salamone et al 1983). Rodents, usually rats or mice, are treated with the test substance by the most appropriate route. Animals are killed 24, 48 or 72 hours after dosing, bone marrow smears obtained, fixed and stained are erythrocytes are examined. Immature polychromatic erythrocytes stain blue with Giemsa and it is this population of cells which are scored for chromosome damage. If damage has occurred, fragments of nuclear material known as Howell-Jolly bodies or micronuclei will be left behind in the cell after the nucleus has been expelled. Mature erythrocytes, normochromatic cells, are also examined since the ratio of mature : immature cells provides an index of toxicity and an increase of micronuclei in normochromatic cells suggests a test agent may have delayed effects. The mouse has traditionally been used in preference to the rat because with the rat the presence of mast cell granules made the Giemsa staining technique less reliable for the identification of micronuclei. This can be conveniently overcome by staining with haematoxylin and eosin (Pascoe & Gatehouse, 1986).

The intraperitoneal route is frequently used so as to establish the hazard associated with a test substance, but for the assessment of risk the route of administration of the test substance should be related to the most likely route of human exposure. Possible routes include oral, dermal, inhalation, intravenous or intraperitoneal injection. A particularly useful extension of this test is to collect the urine from treated groups of animals and to test it using the Ames test procedure. This can provide valuable information on the presence of mutagenic metabolites in the urine either conjugated or unconjugated.

Rodent bone marrow and germinal cell tissue can also be used to assess more complex types of chromosome damage, the type of damage being the same as that looked for in _in vitro_ tests.

In germinal cells dominant lethal mutation effects can be monitored (Bateman, 1984). A dominant lethal mutation is one occurring in the germ cell usually as a consequence of chromosome damage which may result in the immediate death of a fertilised egg or in the later death of the young embryo. Study designs vary but that most frequently practised is to treat male rodents with the test substance and then to mate males with successive batches of females throughout the spermatogonial cycle. A dominant lethal mutation may be expressed by the failure of mated dams to fertilise and/or produce the usual litter size. The defective embryo may not implant, or, if it does so, may die shortly thereafter leaving a mole or deciduoma. Not all mutagens give positive responses in the dominant lethal assay even though they may cause chromosome damage in the bone marrow. One possible reason for this lack of agreement may be that germ cells are protected by the blood-testis barrier so that the chemical, or its metablolite, cannot reach the target tissue in sufficiently high concentrations.

Because of target organ specificity of a chemical some mutagens may not give positive responses if the bone marrow is the only site examined. The nuclear anomaly assay (Proudlock & Allen 1986, Wargovich et al, 1983) provides one attempt to overcome this inadequacy. Other sites such as colon, intestine, liver, kidney and lung have been examined for the induction of aberrant nuclei with an encouraging profile of results being obtained so far. However, this assay is not yet sufficiently validated to become a routine screening test.

In vivo tests for gene mutation are generally less widely used than are those for chromosome damage. The mouse spot test is however becoming more widely used following the extensive validation by Russell et al (1981). The test is performed in mice in which developing embryos are exposed to the test substance. The target cells are the melanoblasts which affect pigmentation and hence, eventually, coat colour. The strain of mice used are heterozygous for some of the coat colour genes. A mutation in the dominant allele will allow the expression of the recessive phenotype so that the mouse will have spots of changed coat colour. The frequency of such spots in treatment groups is compared with that in the control groups. The mice are usually treated during days 8-10 of gestation and the pelts of surviving offspring examined between 3 and 4 weeks after parturition.

Perhaps because of the paucity of reliable and inexpensive *in vivo* gene mutation assays a few hybrid *in vivo*/*in vitro* assays have been developed. One of these, the intra-sanguinous host mediated assay (Mohn et al 1984) involves treating mice with the test substance followed by injection into the tail vein of 2 strains of the bacterium *Escherichia coli*, one of which is repair deficient and one repair proficient. After a few hours the recovery of bacteria in organs such as liver, spleen, kidney and lung are monitored. Since the test measure relative survival of the repair deficient and proficient strains, a differential killing index (DKI) can be defined which expresses the genotoxic effect. The theoretical advantage of this type of assay is that it allows for metabolism and detoxification of the test substance by the host. Furthermore, with a very limited range of chemicals, it has been possible to correlate data from this assay with DNA adduct formation. However, it must be stressed that this assay requires extensive validation before it could be used as a routine screen.

Legator first proposed the use of a host mediated assay in which the indicator organism was injected into the peritoneal cavity and recovered after a few hours to determine mutagenic effects. The method enabled the detection of indirect acting mutagens suggesting that diffusion of the metabolite into the peritoneal cavity occurred from either the gastrointestinal tract or the blood stream, depending on the route of administration. In a review of the published data on this assay (Rinkus & Legator 1980), it became clear that its value was dependent on factors such as host species, indicator strain and route of administration of test substance. Thus, to be useful as a predictive screen it may be necessary to use various permutations of the above three parameters.

Another _in vivo_/_in vitro_ assay has been described by Mirsalis and Butterworth (1980) in which rats are treated with the test substance followed, a few hours later, by perfusion of the liver. The isolated hepatocytes are then examined microscopically for evidence of induced DNA repair synthesis. This assay appears promising for the early detection of hepatocarcinogens.

Finally, a non mammalian _in vivo_ assay which is proving particularly useful is the sex linked recessive lethal assay in the fruit fly Drosophila melanogaster (Vogel & Sobels, 1976). Although the test involves treating the male parental generation with the test substance and examining the second filial generation for signs of genetically induced lethality initiated in the parental line, it is still a relatively rapid test as the generation time in Drosophila is 10-12 days. The induced lethality may be caused by both chromosomal and gene mutations, although it is not usually possible to discriminate between the different types of genetic damage. Indirect acting mammalian carcinogens can also be detected with this organism since insect microsomes are capable of enzyme reactions remarkably similar to those occurring in mammalian liver.

Test substances are normally added to the food consumed by adult flies although other routes including inhalation and injection are occasionally used. Ideally a negative response in this assay with adult flies should be confirmed by assessing the response at other stages of development. The end point measured is the absence in the F2 generation of a class of male flies with normal red eyes. The genetics of the system will not be described here, but excellent reviews can be found in (Lee et al 1983).

DISCUSSION

One of the problems confronting genetic toxicologists who use _in vitro_ and _in vivo_ assays to predict carcinogenic potential is that most carcinogens are not direct acting but require metabolism to produce the reactive electrophilic intermediate. The usefulness of extrinsic metabolic activation systems has already been frequently alluded to, as also has the use of freshly isolated hepatocytes. For general screening purposes there is no great advantage in selecting Aroclor induced S-9 over phenobarbitone/benzoflavone S-9, over hepatocytes, except that liver post mitochondrial systems are easier to prepare than are hepatocyte cultures. More specifically, there are instances where S-9 from a different species or different organ appears beneficial in demonstrating mutagenic activity (Malaveille & Bartsch 1984). Thus, if one is interested in the response of a particular chemical class, great attention should be paid to the choice of exogenous metabolic activation system.

The biotransformation of most chemical carcinogens/mutagens is usually a multistep process. The first step is to create or modify functional groups whilst the second step involves conjugations that add various groups to the parent compound or to a metabolite of the parent compound, thereby providing a detoxifying role. When added extrinsically, any metabolic activation system has to be considered to provide both functions.

Cofactors are usually added to exogenous activation systems. In the S-9 mix described by Ames et al (1975), NADPH or an NADPH generating system is used. Other cofactors or modifying agents preferred by others include EDTA, riboflavin, glutathione, norharman, vitamins and others (Malaveille & Bartsch 1984). At present there is still insufficient information on the value of some of the above additives to be able to recommend their use in standard screening protocols, but should be helpful on a case-by-case basis to explain the underlying mechanism of action of a test substance.

When attempting to assess the carcinogenic potential of a test substance based on mutagenicity data, the predictive accuracy of any one particular assay should be appreciated. When validating a new assay it is standard practice to include known carcinogens and non carcinogens from a wide range of chemical classes (Purchase et al 1978, Purchase 1982). To see how effective a new assay is one can determine sensitivity and specificity values (Cooper et al 1979).

Sensitivity is the proportion of carcinogens tested that give a positive response and this represents the true positive fraction; specificity is the proportion of non carcinogens tested that give a negative response, this representing the true negative fraction. The accuracy of the assay is determined by assessing the proportion of chemicals correctly identified (as carcinogenic or non carcinogenic) by the assay. One important assumption that must be made is that the chemicals included in the validation have been correctly identified as carcinogenic or non carcinogenic, based on the adequate performance of long term carcinogenicity studies. Also, it is important to realise that the predictive value of an assay can be influenced by the proportion of carcinogens included in the validation and the chemical classes from which they were selected. In general, the greater the number of carcinogens that are included the higher the accuracy (predictive value) of the assay, assuming the same specificity and sensitivity.

Although short term mutagenicity tests are widely used to predict the carcinogenic potential of a test substance, the main reason for conducting such assays should be to obtain information concerning the mutagenic activity of a chemical. Apart from radiation, a human germ cell mutagen has not yet been identified (Polani 1981). There is indirect evidence suggesting that certain categories of work place activities may be associated with a high incidence of spontaneous abortions. but these are not clearly proven.

If a compound gives positive responses after carrying out a battery of short term tests in well conducted assays, the next step would be to evaluate the risk to man either by conducting _in vivo_ germ cell tests such as the specific locus or heritable translocation assays, or to attempt to extrapolate the animal data to man. In doing this, it may be helpful to measure the absorbed dose preferably in a range of key target organs including the germinal organs. It has been demonstrated that the dose to the germ cells is frequently far less than that to other organs. The kind of approach described above is sometimes referred to as the parallelogram method (Sobels, 1982).

An example of the kind of decision making processes involved in the rejection or acceptance of a test substance for which genotoxicity data are available is outlined schematically below.

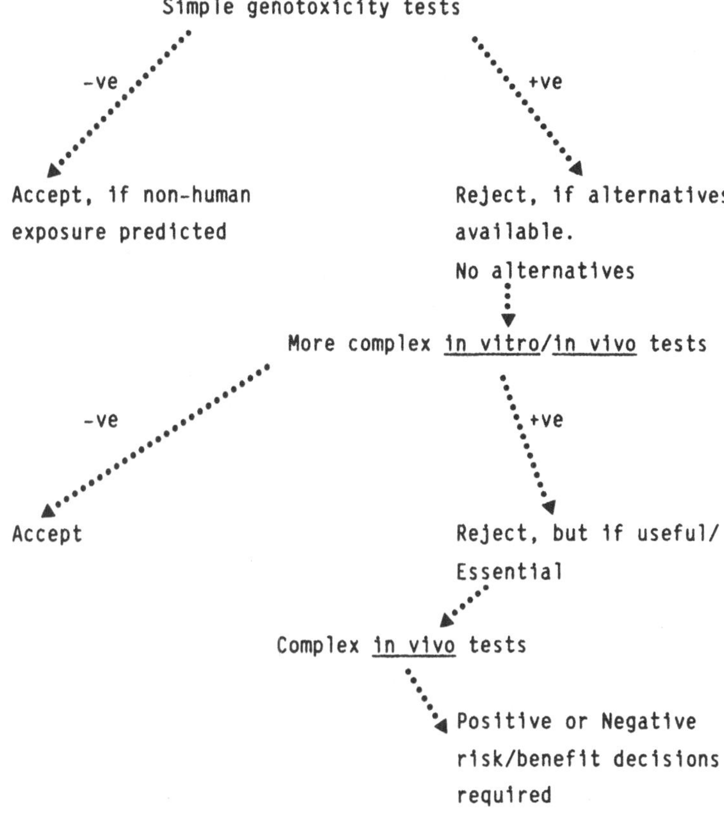

Whichever approach is taken, at some stage decisions must be made which frequently involve a risk/benefit analysis. Clearly mutagenicity data would not be reviewed in isolation as this forms only a very small part in the overall toxicological profile of a test substance.

Genotoxicity testing has become, within 10 years, an integral part of toxicology. Its wide use is largely because of the practice of including *in vitro* tests at the early stages of chemical safety evaluation. Such practices will hopefully extend to other aspects of toxicology as new techniques are developed and validated.

REFERENCES

Ames, B.N., Lee, F.D. & Dunston W.E. (1973). An improved bacterial test system for the detection and classification of mutagens and carcinogens. Proc. Natl. Acad. Sci. (USA), 70, 782-786.

Ames, B.N., McCann & Yamasaki E. (1975). Methods for detecting carcinogens and mutagens with the Salmonella/mammalian-microsome mutagenicity test. Mutation Res. 31 347-364.

Ashby, J. (1986) The prospects for a simplified and internationally harmonized approach to the detection of possible human carcinogens and mutagens. Mutagenesis 1 No.1, 3-16.

Bateman, A.J. (1984). The dominant lethal assay in the male mouse. IN Handbook of Mutagenicity test procedures, eds. B.J. Kilbey, M. Legator, W. Nichols & C. Ramel pp 471-483, Elsevier.

Cifone, M.A., Fisher, J & Myhr, B. Evidence for pH effects in the LS178Y TA+/- Mouse lymphoma forward mutation assay. EMS Abstracts, 15th Annual Meeting 1984, Quebec, Canada p.107.

Cooper, J.A., Saracci, R. & Cole P. (1979). Describing the validity of carcinogen screening tests. Br. J. Cancer, 39, 87-89.

Danford, N. (1984). Measurements of aneuploidy in mammalian cells using a hypotonic treatment, Mutation Res., 139, 127-132.

de Serres, F.H. and Hoffman, C.R. (1981). Summary Report on the performance of Yeast assays IN Progress in Mutation Research Vol. 1, eds F.J. de Serres & J. Ashby pp 68-76, Elsevier.

Jensen. D. (1984). A quantitative test for mutagenicity in V79 Chinese hamster cells, IN Handbook of Mutagenicity test procedures, eds B.J. Kilbey, M. Legator, W. Nichols & C. Ramel, pp 269-270, Elsevier.

Kilbey B.J., Legator M., Nichols W, and Ramel C. (1984). Eds. Handbook of Mutagenicity test procedures, Elsevier.

Lee, W.R., Abrahamson, S., Valencia, R., von Halle, E.S., Wurgler, F.E. and Zimmering, S. (1983). The sex linked recessive lethal assay test for mutagenesis in Drosophila melanogaster. Mutation. Res. 123, 183-279.

Maron, D.M., and Ames, B.N. (1983). Revised methods for the Salmonella mutagenicity test. Mutation Res. 113 173-215.

Martin, C.N., McDermid, A.C. & Garner R.C. (1978). Testing of known carcinogens and non-carcinogens for their ability to induce unscheduled DNA synthesis in the Hela cells. Cancer Res. 38, 2621-2627.

Malaveille, C., & Bartsch, H. (1984). Metabolic activation systems in short term in vitro tests IN Handbook of Mutagenicity test procedures eds. B.J. Kilbey, M. Legator, W. Nichols & C. Ramel pp 615-641, Elsevier.

Matsushima, T., Sawamura, M., Hara, K., and Sugimura, T. (1976). A safe substitute for polychlorinated biphenyls as an inducer of melabolic activation system IN In vitro Metabolic activation in Mutagenesis testing eds. F.J. de Serres, J.R. Fouts, J.R. Bend and R.M. Philpot pp 85-85, Elsevier.

Mirsalis, J.C. and Butterworth, B.E. (1980). Detection of unscheduled DNA synthesis in hepatocytes isolated from Rats treated with genotoxic agents: an in vivo - in vitro assay for potential carcinogens and mutagens. Carcinogenesis 1, 621-625.

Mishra, D., (1981). Ed. Mammalian Cell Transformation by Chemical Carcinogens, Senate Press.

Mohn, G., Kerklaan, P. and Ellenberger, J. (1984). Methodologies for the direct and animal-mediated determination of various genetic effects in derivatives of strain 343/113 of Escherichia coli K-12 in Handbook of Mutagenicity Procedures, eds B.J. Kilbey, M. Legator, W. Nichols & C. Ramel pp 189-214, Elsevier.

Pascoe, S. and Gatehouse, D. (1986). The use of a simple haematoxylin and eosin staining procedure to demonstrate micronuclei within rodent bone marrow. Mutation Res. 164, No. 4, 237-243.

Parodi, S., Zunino, A., Ottaggio, L., De Ferrari, M., and Santi, L. (1983). Lack of correlation between the capability of inducing sister chromatid exchanges in vivo and carcinogenic potency, for 16 aromatic amines and azo derivatives. Mutation Res, 108 225-238.

Parry, J.M. and Zimmerman, F.K. (1976). Detection of monosomic colonies, produced by mitotic non disjunction in the yeast Saccharomyces cerevisiae. Mutation Res., 36, 49-66.

Perry, P.E. and Evans, H.J., (1975). Cytological detection of mutagen/carcinogen exposure by sister chromatid exchange. Nature 258, 121-125.

Polani, P.E. (1981). Guidelines for the testing of chemicals for mutagenicity. DHSS Report on Health and Social Subjects 24, HMSO.

Proudlock, R.J. and Allen, J.A. (1986). Micronuclei and other nuclear anomalies induced in various organs by diethylnitrosamine and 7,12-dimethyl benz [a] anthracene. Mutation Res., 174, 141-143.

Purchase, I.F.H., Longstaff, E., Ashby, J., Styles, J.A., Anderson, D., Lefevre, P.A. and Westwood, F.R. (1978). An evaluation of 6 short-term tests for detecting organic chemical carcinogens. Br. J. Cancer 37, 873-959.

Purchase, I.F.H., (1982). An appraisal of predictive tests for carcinogenicity. Mutation Res. 99, 53-71.

Richold, M. (1982). Assessing potential mutagenic and carcinogenic risks. Biologist 29 (5), 263-267.

Russell, L.B., Selby, P.B., von Halle, E., Sheridan, W and Valcovic, L. (1981). Use of the mouse spot test in chemical mutagenesis: interpretation of past data and recommendations for future work. Mutation Res. 86, 355-379.

Salamone, M.F., Heddle, J.A., Stuart, E and Katz. M. (1980). Towards an improved micronucleus test - studies on three model agents, mitomycin C, cyclophosphamide and dimethyl benzanthracene. Mutation Res. 74, 347-356.

Savage, J.R.K. (1976). Annotation: Classification and relationships of induced chromosomal structural changes. J. Med. Genet 13, 103-122.

Schmid, W. (1975). The micronucleus test. Mutation Res. 31, 9-15.

Sobels, F.H. (1982). The parallelogram. An indirect approach for the assessment of genetic risks from chemical mutagens. IN K.C. Bora, E.R. Douglas and E.R. Nestmann (Eds.) Progress in Mutation Res. Vol. 3, pp 323-327. Elsevier.

Venitt, S., and Parry, J.M. (Eds) (1984). Mutagenicity testing, a practical approach. IRL press.

Vogel, E. and Sobels, F.H. (1976). The function of Drosophila in genetic toxicology testing. IN Chemical Mutagens, Principles and Methods for their detection, Vol. 4. ed. A. Hollaender, Plenum Press.

Wargovich, M.J., Goldberg, M.T., Newmark, H.L. and Bruce, W.R. (1983). Nuclear aberrations as a short term test for genotoxicity to the colon: evaluation of nineteen agents in mice. J. Natl. Cancer Inst. 71, 133-137.

Williams, G.M. (1976). Carcinogen-induced DNA repair in primary rat liver cell cultures: a possible screen for chemical carcinogens. Cancer Lett. 1, 231-236.

IN VITRO IMMUNOTOXICOLOGY

Klara Miller, S. Nicklin and S.G. Volsen

Immunotoxicology Department

The British Industrial Biological Research Association
Woodmansterne Road, Carshalton, Surrey. SM5 4DS.

INTRODUCTION

Increasing concern that certain environmental agents may be directly responsible for adverse changes in immune competence has resulted in immunotoxicology becoming established as an important sub-discipline of toxicological studies.

Whilst traditional pathological methods have implicated various lymphoid organs as possible targets for toxic insult, it is only relatively recently that the complexity and far-reaching consequences associated with local and/or systemic immunotoxic interactions have become fully appreciated. This increasing awareness stems in part from recent advances in immunology and molecular biology which have provided new and precise techniques for the detection and evaluation of immune associated toxic lesions. These novel approaches to toxicity study have not only increased our understanding of the regulatory mechanisms which govern the normal functions of the immune system but have also emphasised the importance of the immune system as a sensitive and perhaps early indicator of cellular toxicity.

THE IMMUNE SYSTEM : STRUCTURE AND FUNCTION

The unique sensitivity of the immune system is without doubt a consequence of its inherent complexity. Analysis of the immune repertoire of man and a variety of experimental animals has revealed the mammalian immune system to be a finely tuned and precisely regulated mechanism involving multiple interactions between numerous subsets of T cells (thymus-matured lymphocytes), B cells (bone marrow-matured lymphocytes) and a variety of antigen processing accessory cells of macrophage origin (Figure 1). These cellular elements are seen to act either independently or in concert with a spectrum of other cell types including polymorphonuclear leukocytes, natural killer cells, null cells, basophils, eosinophils and mast cells. Together these cells maintain an integrated surveillance network that not only functions as an effective and versatile defence against invasion by parasitic or pathogenic microorganisms but also provides a mechanism whereby the hosts own tissues may be continously monitored for neoplastic changes (immunosurveillance).

In most instances the macrophage is the first cell to encounter antigen entering the tissues. This is usually phagocytosed, processed and the antigenic components presented to antigen receptive lymphocytes. These cells are in their turn triggered to undergo clonal expansion; T cells differentiate into a variety of antigen specific effector cells, while B cells undergo a limited series of divisions which terminate in antibody secreting plasma cells. In both situations a proportion of these cells, although triggered remain as a population

Figure 1

Cellular Organisation within a Lymph Node

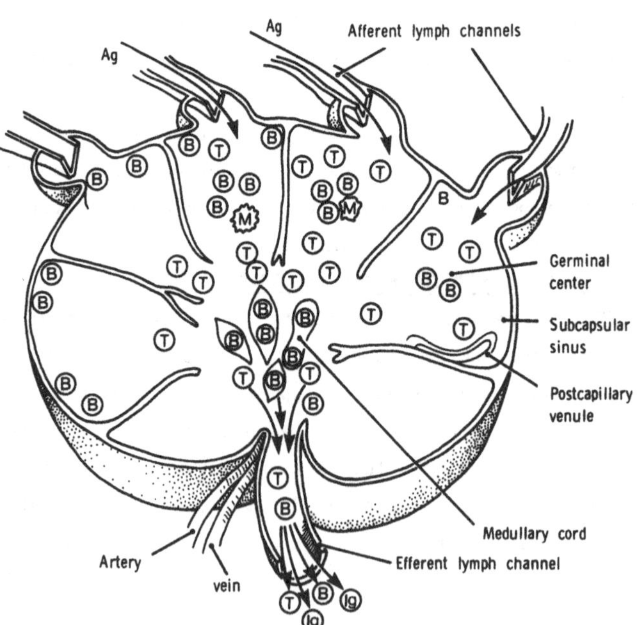

of long lived memory cells which are capable of an anamnestic reaction following subsequent re-exposure to antigen (see Miller, 1978; Katz & Benecaaraf, 1972 for general review). Activation, regulation and feed back control of immune responses clearly depends on precise cell-cell communications, this occurs either by direct contact between the relevant cells or via the release of biological mediators either locally into the cellular microenvironment or systemically into the circulation (Figure 2). Many of these secreted cell products have been isolated and characterised and include prostaglandins, leukotriene products of lipoxygenase metabolism, cytokines such as the interferons and interleukins, and a variety of less well defined thymic hormones (Bloom, 1980; Rumjanek, Hanson & Morley, 1982; Nicklin & Shand, 1982). The facility for co-operative cellular interaction between the various components of the immune system provides a complex homeostatic mechanism which can both direct and regulate the immune mechanism. In addition to this network of intercellular communication, the integrity of the system may be further modified both via the endocrine/neurological axis and by nutritional/environmental factors (Dean <u>et al</u>. 1982).

Figure 2

Development of the Cellular Immune Response

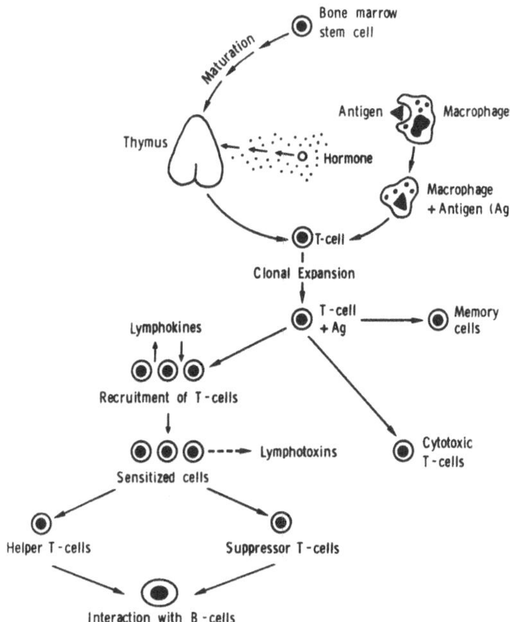

Immune competence is therefore the result of a series of adaptive cellular and biochemical changes which are designed to ensure the survival of a species in a changing and hostile environment. The inherent complexity of this system, however is also its Achilles heel, since even minor perturbations within the immune network can produce drastic changes in immune reactivity. This imbalance can be manifested in a variety of ways including the induction of an aberrant or inappropriate response to self determinants resulting in autoimmune disease, or an exaggerated response to antigen which may lead to a hypersensitivity response becoming established. Suppression of some of the effector arms of the immune response may also increase susceptibility to infectious agents or even increase tumour incidence following the loss of immune surveillance.

IMMUNOTOXICOLOGY : GENERAL CONCEPTS

Interest in the immune system as an important parameter in the evaluation of the toxicity of chemicals is a result of the increasing number of compounds that have been shown to produce distinct effects on the immune competence of laboratory animals (Dean, Luster, Boorman & Lauer, 1982; Faith, Lustar & Vos, 1980; Koller, 1979; Vos, 1977). Studies have also shown that low level exposure of humans to certain environmental chemicals may induce immunological alterations similar to those that occur in experimental animals (Bekesi, Holland, Anderson *et al*., 1978; Miller *et al*., 1979). The importance of immunotoxicological testing and the role of the immune system as a very sensitive and perhaps early indicator of cellular toxicity has been emphasised at several recent symposia (International Symposium on Immune Toxicology, Guildford, 1982; International Seminar on the Immunonological System as a target for Toxic damage, Luxembourg, 1984).

It is not feasible with the confines of a short text to review fully all current immunotoxicity assessment regimens. Discussion will therefore be restricted to presenting details of agents and methods which have most attracted the attention of immunotoxicologists in recent years. At present there are three principal approaches to studying alterations in immune parameters as indicators of toxicological damage: 1) Animals may be exposed to a compound *in vivo* and immune functions tested *in vivo*, 2) the functional integrity of the immune system may be assessed *in vitro* following *in vivo* exposure and 3) cells may be exposed to a compound *in vitro* and examined *in vitro*. *In vitro* assays utilising more recent molecular biological techniques will also be discussed under a separate heading.

PRACTICAL ASPECTS

1) *In vivo* Approaches

A number of *in vivo* methods have been used to assess cell mediated immunity in laboratory animals including skin graft assays and delayed type hypersensitivity (DHR) (Vos, 1977). Delayed hypersensitivity responses are initiated by specifically sensitized lymphocytes and manifested by cellular infiltration at the site of antigen administration. In the clinical situation DHR is assessed 24 and 48 hours after intradermal challenge. In experimental animals, where skin tests are sometimes difficult to assess, more sensitive radiometric assays in which ^{3}H-thymidine is administered before antigen challenge, are often employed (Lefford, 1974; Luster *et al*., 1982).

Humoral immune competence can be assessed in treated animals by determination of serum immunoglobulin levels, by enumeration of B lymphocytes in the spleen, or by detection of antibody-forming cells. Determination of the level of the main immunoglobulin classes present in the serum may also provide valuable information about alterations in humoral immune responses.

The presence of antibodies can only be assessed by methods which evaluate the primary function of antibodies, that is their ability to combine with specific antigens. Techniques in use for determining antibody titres include extremely sensitive assays such as radioimmunoassay and enzyme-linked absorbent assay (ELISA). In the ELISA assay, antigen is coupled to a solid phase, incubated with serum from control or treated animals, and the amount of serum antibody bound to the solid phase quantified by peroxidase-labelled class specific anti-immunoglobulin. Immunoglobulin M (IgM), IgG and IgE titres have been measured by ELISA after immunisation with ovalbumin (Vos, Kreijne & Beeklof, 1982). Less sensitive but reliable methods for measuring antibody titres include immunodiffusion, haemagglutination, passive haemagglutination and immunoelectrophoresis. The commonest practical method for the detection of antigen-antibody precipitation is to allow them to diffuse towards each other in agar gel, usually from wells or holes cut into the gel (Ouchterlony technique). Where the antigen is insoluble because it is an intrinsic antigenic determinant of a sheep red blood cell membrane, or bound firmly to the surface of a cell addition of serum will cross-link the antigenic determinants on individual cells causing them to agglutinate. Immuno-electrophoresis allows the identification of several antibodies in serum by combining immunochemical specificity with characteristic differences in electrophoretic mobility.

Single cells secreting antibody molecules can be identified by a haemolytic technique termed the Jerne plaque assay (Jerne & Nordin, 1963; Cunningham, 1965). Splenic lymphoid cells obtained from an animal sensitised for sheep red blood cells (SRBC) are incubated in agar together with the red blood cells. The addition of complement causes the haemolysis of the SRBC that are coated with specific antibody and plaques of lysis will be seen around each antibody-producing cell. The Jerne technique can also be applied to other antigens by binding them to the surface of SRBC so that both T lymphocyte dependent and independent antibody responses by splenic lymphocytes can be assessed following exposure to a compound.

During the past few years development of systems to assess host resistance in animals after exposure to chemicals or drugs have also received much attention. This interest has been generated by observations that exposure of experimental animals to certain chemicals can result in altered host resistance to bacteria (Thigpen, Faith, McCovell & Moore, 1975), viruses (Gainer & Pry, 1972) and parasites (Loose, 1982), as well as to transplantable tumour cells (Dean, Luster, Boorman _et al_. 1980a). Methods to assess the altered host susceptibility in experimental mice have been described in detail (Dean, Luster, Boorman, _et al_. 1980b). The effect of exposure to compounds on normal surveillance and immunological mechanisms are assessed by observing the incidence of tumours after injection of a fixed concentration of tumour cells. Competence of murine lymphocytes and macrophages _in vivo_ are investigated by their ability to control the intracellular replication and destruction of _Listeria monocytogenes_ or after infection with parasites (Loose, 1982) and mortality frequencies compared with control groups.

2) In vitro Approaches

A widely used approach in immunotoxicity studies is the *in vitro* testing of cell populations involved in immune responses obtained from animals during safety evaluation studies. Methods include the enumeration of cell populations, the evaluation of cell-mediated immunity, humoral immunity, macrophage function and, in certain laboratories, bone marrow progenitor cells.

One of the most commonly used assays is the induction of lymphocyte proliferation with mitogens or specific proteins, known also as the transformation or blastogenic assay (see Oppenheim, Mizel & Meltzer 1978; Rosenstreich, 1976). Lectins such as concanavalin A (ConA) and phytohaemagglutinin (PHA) selectively stimulate T lymphocytes whilst bacterial products such as lipopolysaccharide (LPS) stimulate B lymphocytes. In contrast to specific antigens, mitogens activate a relatively high percentage of lymphocytes to undergo DNA synthesis in a polyclonal fashion. The *in vitro* responses of lymphocytes to antigens and mitogens provide important information about the functional capabilities of these cells *in vivo*. Depressed lymphocyte proliferative responses in experimental animals are generally interpreted as being due to non-responsive lymphocytes. Decreased proliferative responses may be caused by a chemically induced lymphocytotoxicity, an aleration in lymphocyte subpopulations, or regulatory factors effecting lymphocyte proliferation or macrophage function. Specific antigens or alloantigenic stimulation (mixed leukocyte reaction) are also utilised to examine proliferative function in lymphocyte populations.

Cell-mediated cytotoxicity (CML) can also be assayed *in vitro* by several techniques including radioactive labelling of target cells an then measuring ^{51}chromium release. Direct cytotoxicity is primarily mediated by the T lymphocyte and contact of lymphocytes with target cells results in target cell destruction within 3 to 24 hours. *In vitro* functional cytotoxic impairment cannot, however, clearly implicate the T cell, as modificatiion of the response by macrophages or B lymphocytes may occur.

The graft-versus-host (GVH) reaction in which lymphoid cells from a donor animal are injected into a histo-incompatible recipient is a combined *in vivo* and *in vitro* assay of cell-mediated immunity.

Donor cells from a parental strain are tolerated by F_1 hydrid recipients because they do not possess any antigens which are foreign to the hybrid whereas immunocompetent donor cells induce a reaction against the foreign antigen. Donor animals or cells in vitro are exposed to the test compound, after which lymphocytes are injected into the foot pad of recipient animals and the enlargement of the draining popliteal lymph node determined (Ford, Burr & Simensen, 1970), thus providing a means for assessing the immune competence of the donor cells.

3)In vitro exposure followed by in vitro testing

One advantage of in vitro assays is that a population of cells involved in a particular phase of the immune response can be isolated, and a number of functions examined separately on the same population. Effects of various compounds on mononuclear phagocytes, in particular, have been evaluated by in vitro exposure followed by in vitro assessment of phagocytosis and intracellular killing of bacteria (van Furth et al., 1978). Functional alterations in alveolar macrophages exposed to the plasticizer di-(2-ethylhexyl) phthalate have been demonstrated by in vitro assays (Bally, Opheim & Shertzer, 1980) whilst many studies have been concerned with evaluating the toxic properties of mineral dusts on these cells (Miller & Harington, 1972). In vitro exposures of macrophages to cadmium and zinc have demonstrated that cadmium causes an inhibition of macrophage motility (Kiremidjian- Schumacher, Stotzky, Kickstein & Schwertz, 1981) as well as interfering with macrophage capacity to destroy tumour cells (Nelson et al., 1982).

In vitro effects of compounds on mitogen-induced lymphocyte blastogenesis have also proved valuable in investigating both dose-response relationships and suppression of lymphocyte responses (Masuda, Takemoto, Tatsumo & O'Hara, 1981). The determination of mitogen induced lymphocyte proliferation in these systems can assess the lymphocytotoxic potential of the compound, or its potential inhibitory or over-stimulatory effect on lymphocyte activation. It is clearly advantageous that lymphocyte populations of either animal or human origin can be used in such studies.

GENERAL DISCUSSION AND FUTURE DEVELOPMENTS

Recent advances in cellular and molecular biological techniques can vastly improve the potential of _in vitro_ assays to evaluate the ability of compounds to interact with the immune system. In this respect the ability to produce homogeneous T cell clones and immortal T cell hybrids may be particularly useful. Long-term clonal cultures of normal, antigen specific T cells of either T helper (Th) or T cytotoxic (Tc) sub-class can be established by the use of repeated _in vitro_ antigen stimulation (Fathman & Fritch, 1982). T cell hybrids are generated by physically fusing cells of a specific T cell subpopulation with a transformed cell line (analagous to monoclonal antibody production) to produce an immortalized T cell hybridoma which retains functional attributes of the parent T cell (Kappler _et al_., 1981). Using either of these systems pertinent studies can be undertaken. For example, IL-2 is a T-cell proliferation factor which is produced predominantly by Th cells. Since IL-2 is essential for the development of Tc cells then any agent which could down regulate its production would have severe effects on the immune system. Such screening methods may be performed _in vitro_ by treating a human Th cell clone with appropriate concentrations of a xenobiotic and then assaying the IL-2 produced in the culture supernatant with an IL-2 dependent cell line. Should an agent cause significant depression of IL-2 synthesis then further studies would be performed to assess its activity _in vivo_. It is worthy of note that Schleimer _et al_., (1984), using an _in vivo_ system, demonstrated that glucocorticoids compromise IL-2 production which leads to a loss of T-cell mediated cytotoxicity.

Successful communication and interaction between the various cellular components of the immune system is of paramount importance in mounting any immune response. Molecules of fundamental importance in cellular communication are those which are dispersed on the outer cell surface, these include for example MHC antigens and immunoglobulin receptors. A high proportion of these molecules have been found to be glycoprotein in nature (Williams, 1982) and therefore _in vitro_ methods which could detect specific changes in the glycoprotein make up of the cytoplasmic membrane may thus consitute pertinent immunotoxicological screening techniques. The ideal probes with which to study cell surface glycoproteins are monoclonal antibodies (Köhler & Milstein, 1975). Using these reagents, molecules specific for cells of differing lineage and at different stages of differentiation have been described (Beverley, 1984). Qualitative changes in the glycoprotein makeup of the cell membrane can be assessed using a variety of immunohistochemical techniques and methods have been developed for their evaluation by light microscopy (Polak & Van Noorden, 1983), transmission electron microscopy (Volsen, 1984) and scanning electron microscopy (Molday & Moher, 1982). Quantitative changes in the expression of a particular molecule may be evaluated using the Fluorescence Activated Cell Sorter (Hoffman & Hansen, 1981) or radioactive binding assays (Mason & Williams, 1980). An example of the potential importance of studying the expression of membrane molecules was that provided by Britton and Palacios (1982) who, using an *in vitro* system demonstrated that CsA inhibited the expression of both the IL-1 and IL-2 membrane receptors on T cells which exerted profound effect on their proliferative abilities.

In order to activate specific effector mechanisms in response to an immunological stimulus, cells of the immune system can undergo dramatic changes in characteristic. For example, upon binding antigen, sessile memory B lymphocytes undergo terminal differentiation to plasma cells whose primary function is the large scale production of specific immunoglobulin. These patent physiological changes clearly reflect an alteration in the expression of specific genes. Should a xenobiotic compromise the expression of an immunologically important gene product, then the functioning of the entire immune system is at risk. *In vitro* methods which could detect such changes are thus of great potential.

The most accurate approach with which to assess changes in gene expression directly is to analyse messenger RNA (m-RNA) with specific gene probes. This can be accomplished efficiently using RNA blotting techniques. In the "Northern" blotting system, m-RNA is prepared from target cells (Maniatis, Fritsch & Sambrook, 1982) and the various transcripts size fractioned by electrophoresis in an agarose gel. The m-RNA bands are then blotted onto a membrane and probed with a radioactive gene probe specific for the gene of interest. Dot blotting methods can also be used, which work on an identical principle to that described above, but differ in that the m-RNA is not size fractioned but dot blotted in a heterogeneous nature onto a membrane (White & Bancroft, 1982). Using systems pertinent *in vitro*, screening tests may be performed with which to assess xenobiotic induced changes in the level of expression of any immunologically important molecule e.g. IL-1, IL-2 (and their receptors), the interferons, T cell receptor, or immunoglobins. Clearly, the above manipulations rely fundamentally on the availability of suitable gene probes. The rate at which molecular biologists are producing these reagents will clearly assist the development of such *in vitro* investigations in the future.

CONCLUSIONS

It appears unlikely that *in vitro* systems will replace laboratory animals completely in immunotoxicological investigations. However, the application of new experimental techniques in cell and molecular biology will improve *in vitro* screening techniques in the future.

REFERENCES

Bally, M.B., Opheim, D,J. & Shertzer, H.G. (1980). Di-(2-ethylhexyl) phthalate enhances the release of lysosomal enzymes from alveolar macrophages during phagocytosis. *Toxicology* *18*, 49-60.

Bekesi, J.G., Holland, J.F., Andersen, H.A., Fischbein, A.S., Rom, W., Wolff, M.S. & Selikoff, I.J. (1978). Lymphocyte function of Michigan dairy farmers exposed to polybrominated biphenyls. *Science*, *N.Y.* *199*, 1207-1209.

Beverley, P.C. (1984). Hybridomas, Monoclonal Cells and Analysis of the Immune System. *Br. Med. Bull. 40*, 213-217.

Bloom, B.R. (1980). Interferons and the immune system. *Nature*, *284*, 593-595.

Britton, S. & Palacios, R. (1982). Cyclosporin A. Usefulness, Risks and Mechanism of Action. *Immunol. Rev. 65*, 5-22.

Cunningham, A.J. (1985). A method of increased sensitivity for detecting single antibody-forming cells. *Nature, Lond.* *207*, 1106-1107.

Dean, J.H., Luster, M.I., Boorman, G.A., Luebke, R.W. & Lauer, L.D.(1980). The effect of adult exposure to diethylstilbestrol in the mouse: alterations in tumour susceptibility and host resistance parameters. *J. Reticuloendothel. Soc.* *28*, 571-583.

Dean, J.H., Luster, M.I., Boorman, G.A., Padarathsingh, M.L., Luebke, R.W. & Clements, M.E. (1980). Host resistance models for assessing immune alterations following chemical exposure: studies with deithylstilbestrol, cyclophosphamide and 2,3,7,8-tetrachlorodibenzo-p-dioxin. In Biological Relevance of Immune Suppression Induced by Therapeutic and Environmental Agents. Edited by J.H. Dean & M.L. Padarathsingh pp 145-189. Van Nostrand and Reinhold, New York.

Dean, J.H., Luster, M.I., Boorman, G.A. and Lauer, L.D. (1982). Procedures available to examine the immunotoxicity of chemicals and drugs. Pharmacol. Revs., 34, 137-148.

Faith, R.E., Luster, M.I. & Vos, J.G. (1980). Effects of immunocompetence by chemicals of environmental concern. In Reviews in Biochemical Toxicology. 2. Edited by E. Hodgson, J.R. Bend & R.M. Philpot. pp. 173-211. Elsevier, Oxford.

Fathman, C.G. & Fitch, F.W. (1982). Isolation, Characterization and Utilization of T Lymphocyte Clones. pp. 21-43. Academic Press, New York.

Ford, W.L., Burr, W. & Simensen, H. (1970). A lymph node weight assay for the graft-versus-host activity of rat lymphoid cells. Transplantation, 10, 258-266.

Gainer, I.J. & Pry, T.W. (1972). Effect of arsenicals on viral infections in mice. Am. J Vet. Res. 33, 2299-2307.

Hoffman, R.A. & Hansen, W.P. (1981). Immunofluorescent Analysis of Blood Cells by Flow Cytometry. Int. J. Immunopharmacol. 3, 249-254.

International Symposium on Immunotoxicology. University of Surrey, Guildford, 13-17 September 1982.

International Seminar on the immunological system as a Target organ for toxic damage. Luxembourg, 6-9 November 1984.

Jerne, N.K. & Nordin, A.A. (1963). Plaque formation in agar by single antibody-producing cells. Science, 140, 405-407.

Kappler, J.W., Skidmore, B., White, J. & Marrack, P. (1981). Antigen-inducible, H-2 resticted, interleukin 2 producing T cell hybridomas. J. Exp. Med., 153, 1198-1214.

Katz, D.H. & Benacerraf, B. (1972). The regulatory influence of activated T cells on B cell responses to antigen, Adv. Immunol., 15, 1-11.

Kiremidjian-Schumacher, L., Stotzky, G., Dickstein, R.A. & Schwartz, J. (1981). Influence of cadmium, lead and zinc on the ability of guinea pig macrophages to interact with macrophage migration inhibitory factor. Envir. Res. 24, 106-116.

Köhler, G. & Milstein, C. (1975). Continuous cultures of fused cells secreting antibody of predefined specificity. Nature, 256, 495-497.

Koller, L.D. (1979). Some immunological effects of lead, cadmium and methyl mercury. Drug Chem. Toxicol. 2, 99-110.

Lefford, M.J. (1974). The measurement of tuberculin hypersensitivity in rats. Int. Archs Allergy Appl. Immunol. 47, 570-585.

Loose, L.D. (1982). Macrophage induction of T-suppressor cells in pesticide-exposed and protozoan-infected mice. Envir. Hlth. Perspect. 43, 89-97.

Luster, M.I. Dean, J.H. & Boorman, G.A. (1982). Cell-mediated immunity and its application in toxicology. Envir. Hlth. Perspect. 43, 31-36.

Miller, J.F.A.P. (1978). The cellular basis of immune responses. In Samter M. (ed) Immunological Diseases pp. 35-48 (New York; Little Brown & Co).

Miller, K., Weintraub, Z. & Kagan, E. (1979). Manifestations of cellular immunity in the rat after prolonged asbestos inhalation. Physical interactions between alveolar macrophages and splenic lymphocytes. J. Immunol. 123, 1029-1038.

Miller, K. & Harington, J.S. (1972). Some biochemical effects of asbestos on macrophages. Br. J. Exp. Path. 53, 397-405.

Molday, R. & Moher, P. (1980). A review of cell surface markers and labelling techniques for scanning electron microscopy. Histochem. J. 12, 273-315.

Maniatis, T., Fritsch, E.F. & Sambrook, J. (1982). Molecular Cloning, a Laboratory Manual 2nd ed, p 188-193, Cold Spring Harbour Laboratory Pub.

Mason, D.W. & Williams, A.F. (1980). The Kinetics of antibody binding to membrane antigens in solution and at the cell surface. Biochem. J. 187, 1-20.

Masuda, E., Takemoto, T., Tatsuno, T. & OBara, T. (1982). Immunosuppressive effect of a trichothecene mycotoxin, Fusarenon-x in mice. Immunology, 45, 743-749.

Nelson, D.S., Kiremidjian-Schumacher, L. & Stotzky, G. (1982). Effects of cadmium, lead and zinc on macrophage-mediated cytotoxicity toward tumor cells. Envir. Res. 28, 154-163.

Nicklin, S. and Shand, F.L. (1982). Abrogation of suppression cell function by inhibitors of prostaglandin synthesis. Int. J. Immunopharmac, 4, 407-414.

Oppenheim, J.J., Mizel, S.B. & Meltzer, M.S. (1978). In Biology of the Lymphokines. Edited by S. Cohen, E. Pick & J.J. Oppenheim. p 291. Academic Press, New York.

Polak, J. Van Noorden, S. (1983). Immunocytochemistry, Practical Applications in Pathology and Biology. Ist ed. pll-43. Pub. Wright.

Rosenstreich, O.L., Farrar. J.J. & Dougherty, S. (1976). Absolute macrophage dependency of T lymphocyte activation by mitogens. J. Immunol. 116, 131-139.

Rumjanek, V.M., Hanson, J.M. and Morley, J. (1982). Lymphokines and Monokines. In Sirois, P. and Rola-Pleszczynski, M. (eds) Immunopharmacology pp 267-286.

Schlemier, R.P., Jacques, A., Shin, H.S., Lichtenstein, L.M. & Plant, M. (1984). Inhibition of T cell mediated cytotoxicity by Anti-inflammatory steroids. J. Immunol. 132, 266-271.

Thigpen, J.E., Faith, R.E., McConnell, E.E. & Moore, J.A. (1975). Increased susceptibility to bacterial infection as a sequala to exposure to 2,3,7,8,-tetrachlorodibenzo-p-dioxin. Infect. Immun. 12, 1319-1324.

van Furth, R., van Zwet, T.L. & Leijh, P.C.J. (1978). In vitro determination of phagocytosis and intracellular killing in polymorphonuclear and mononuclear phagocytes. In Handbook of Experimental Immunology. Edited by D.M. Weir. pp. 32.1-32.19. Blackwell, Oxford.

Volsen, S.G. (1984). A biotin-avidin technique for the localisation of membrane-bound monoclonal antibodies by low power transmission electron microscopy. J. Immunol. Methods, 72, 119-126.

Vos, J.G. (1977). Immune suppression as related to toxicology. CRC Crit. Rev. Toxicol. 5, 67-101.

Vos, J.G., Krajnc, E.I. & Beekhof, P. (1982). Use of the enzyme-linked immunosorbent assay (ELISA) in immunotoxicity testing. Envir. Hlth Perspect. 43, 115-121.

Williams, A.F. (1982). Surface molecules and cell interactions. J. Theor. Biol. 98, 221-236.

White, B.A. & Bancroft, F.C. (1982). Cytoplasmic dot hybridization. Simple analysis of relative m-RNA levels in multiple small cell or tissue samples. J. Biol. Chem. 257, 8569-8572.

Williams, A.F. (1982). Surface molecules and cell interactions. J. Theor. Biol. 98, 221-236.

White, B.A. & Bancroft, F.C. (1982). Cytoplasmic dot hybridization. Simple analysis of relative m-RNA levels in multiple small cell or tissue samples. J. Biol. Chem. 257, 8569-8572.

GLOSSARY OF TERMS

Alloantigen	Different (Allelic) form of an antigen coded for at the same gene locus in all individuals of a species. Directive in mixed lymphocyte responses.
Anamnestic reaction	Memory response in antigen primed cells following subsequent stimulation by the priming antigen.
Antibody	An immunoglobulin molecule capable of specific combination with antigen.
Antigen	A substance that elicits a specific immune response when introduced into the tissues of man or animals.
Antiserum	Serum from any animal which contains antibodies against the antigen used to immunise the donor.
Atopy	A constitutional or heredary tendency to develop immediate hypersensitivity states e.g. allergic asthma and hay fever.
Autoimmune disease	Specific immune response to constitutents of the body's own tissues.
B-cells	Lymphocytes derived from bone marrow without passing through the thymus. Mature B cells produce antibody.
Cell mediated Immunity	Specific immunity which is dependent upon the presence of T lymphocytes.
Delayed hypersensitivity	Hypersensitivity state mediated by primed T-cells. Can be transferred to a syngeneic recipient by T-cells but not serum.

GLOSSARY OF TERMS

Hapten	A substance that cannot initiate an immune response unless bound to a carrier (e.g. protein) before introduction into the body.
Humoral Immunity	Specific immunity mediated by antibody.
Hypersensitivity	A hightened immune response often associated with allergic reactions.
Immunoglobulin (Ig)	Serum protein responsible for antibody activity. 5 classes exist.
IgA	Major immunoglobulin of the external secretions e.g. Lungs, Gastro-intestinal tract.
IgD	Present in low concentration in serum. Function not fully understood, but apparently involved in maturation of the immune system.
IgE	Present in serum at low concentration but found bound to mast cells. Important in allergic reactions.
IgG	The major immunoglobulin found in serum, agglutinates antigen and fixes complement.
IgM	Large molecular weight immunoglobulin important in primary immune responses. It is very efficient at agglutinating particulate antigens and also fixes complement.

GLOSSARY OF TERMS

Immunological response	The development of specifically altered reactivity following exposure to an antigen. This may take a number of forms e.g. antibody production, cell-mediated immunity, immunological tolerance.
Interleukins	Generic name for immunoregulatory soluble factors released by macrophages and T lymphocytes.
Lymphocyte	White blood cells originating in the bone marrow and involved in the immune response (see T/B cells).
Macrophage	Cell of mononuclear phagocyte system, bone barrow derived. Characterised by capacity to phagocytose, to present antigen to T and B cells and to modulate lymphocyte function.
Mitogen	Any agent which induces mitosis in cells. Used in immunology to refer to any substances capable of inducing polyclonal lymphocyte transformation in either T cells and/or B cells.
Plasma Cell	Antibody secreting B-cell. End of the line in B-cell lineage.
Self determinant	All antigens expressed on individuals own cells.
Syngeneic	Pertaining to self. Genetically identical as within an inbred strain.
T-cells	Lymphocytes that are matured in the thymus and are mainly involved in cell mediated immunity. Several sub-classes exist including cytotoxic T cells (Tc), T cells associated with delayed type hypersensitivity responses (T dth), immunoregulatory helper (Th) and suppressor (Ts) T cells.

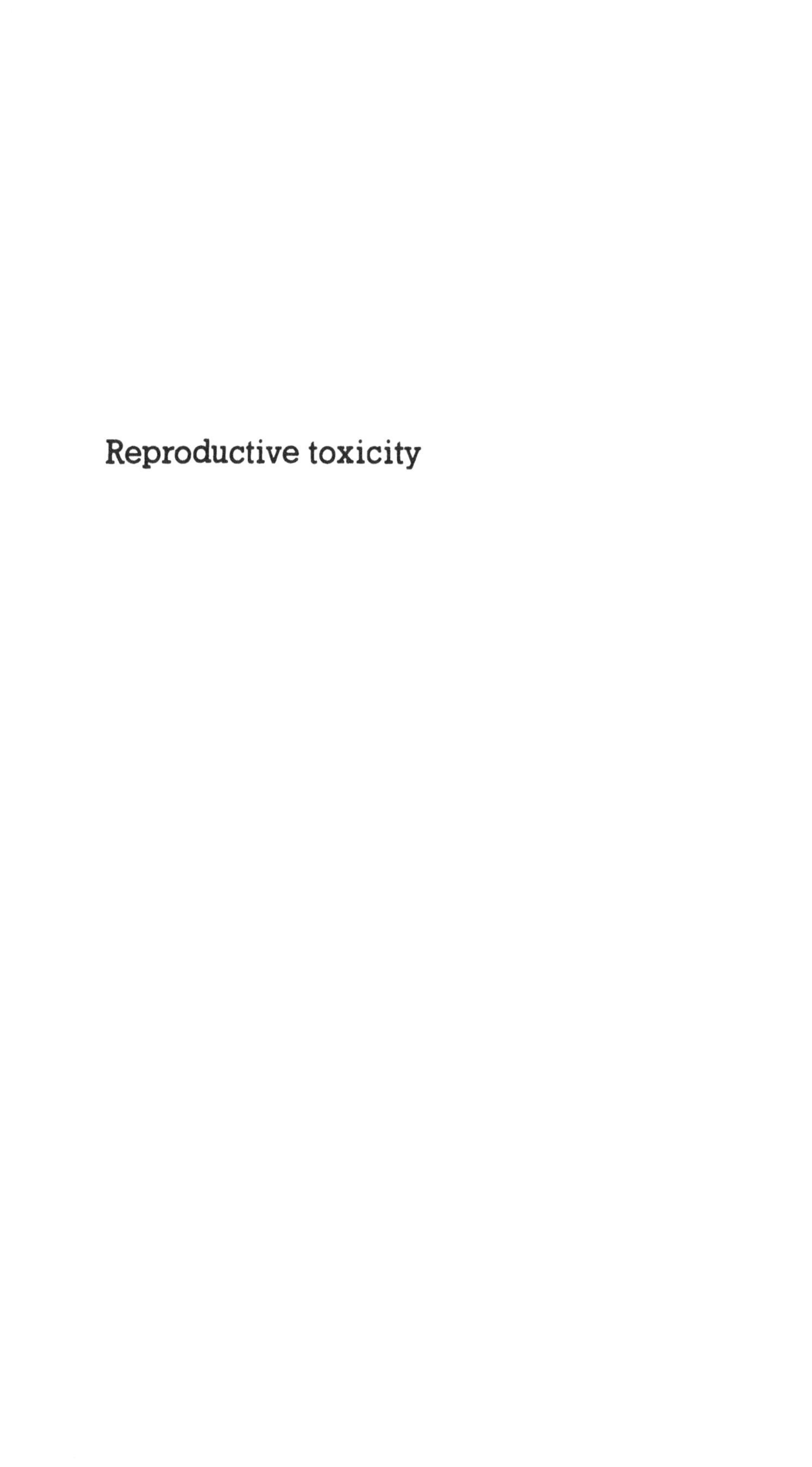

Reproductive toxicity

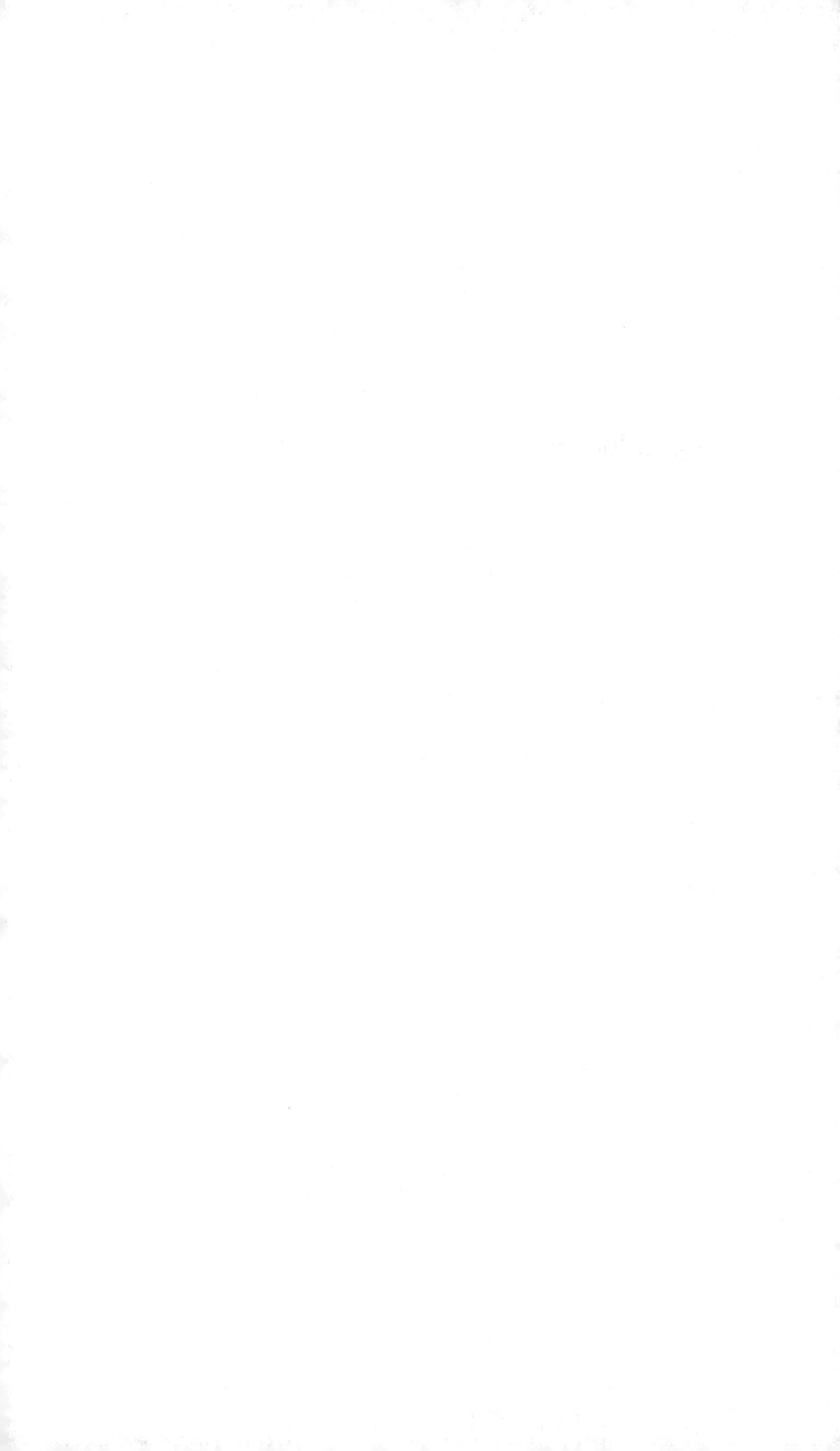

AN IN VITRO TEST FOR TERATOGENS USING CULTURES OF RAT EMBRYO CELLS

Dr O P Flint, Imperial Chemical Industries PLC,
Pharmaceuticals Division, Mereside, Alderley Park,
Macclesfield, Cheshire. SK10 4TG

INTRODUCTION

The embryo, during its phase of organogenesis, may be uniquely sensitive to toxic insult from certain drugs and other xenobiotics. Chemicals that cause irreversible abnormalities of structure and function are defined as teratogens. The mechanisms by which teratogens cause abormalities of development must be considered before designing in vitro tests for teratogens so that methods which have an inbuilt tendency to false negative or positive classification may be avoided. Thus a test which measures inhibition of cell adhesion alone should not (and does not) detect teratogens such as 5 fluorouracil or actinomycin D which are specific inhibitors of the cell cycle (Braun et al, 1979).

A significant obstacle to determining the precise mechanism of teratogenesis is our incomplete understanding of the fundamental mechanisms of embryogenesis. Thus the typical thalidomide embryopathy remains without explanation after more than twenty years, though at least twelve different modes of action have been proposed (reviewed by Helm et al, 1981). One approach to the problem of modelling embryogenesis in vitro has been to assume that certain aspects of cell behaviour which can be observed during morphogenesis are of such paramount and overriding importance that the majority of teratogens must work by inhibition of these processes. Thus tests for inhibition of cell adhesion (Braun et al, 1979; Braun and Dailey, 1981; Braun and Weinreb, 1984) or cell communication (Trosko et al, 1982; Welsch and Stedman, 1984) have been proposed as in vitro tests for teratogens. There is no convincing proof, as yet, that the majority of teratogens act by altering the cell surface in such a way as to inhibit either cell adhesion or communication.

The mammalian embryo itself (normally the rat embryo) can be cultured for limited periods and the effects of teratogens observed, thus avoiding the problem of identifying the specific mechanisms of embryogenesis affected by teratogens; effectively classical teratology but in vitro (Sadler et al, 1982 and this volume, Cockroft and Steele). The short developmental window available for toxic insult (the 24 to 48 hours prior to appearance of the limb buds) when mainly CNS structures differentiate is a source of special problems of interpretation for this technique. For example, is an unclosed posterior neuropore to be considered a sign of teratogenesis or is it simply delayed growth in culture, or, is an unclosed posterior neuropore a false positive if the test compound, though a teratogen, has never caused spina bifida in vivo? It should be noted that at least one meticulous study (vitamin A, cultured rat embryos) has demonstrated close similarities between developmental abnormalties arising in vitro and those occuring in vivo (Steele et al, 1983).

Submammalian systems have also been proposed (see Chapter by Freeman and Brown, this book). Examples are cultures of Drosphila embryo cells (Bournias-Vardiabasis and Teplitz, 1982), planarian regeneration (Best and Morita, 1982) or hydra attenuata regeneration (Johnson et al, 1982). The assumption is made that the basic mechanisms controlling embryogenesis are conserved throughout evolution. The only good evidence is that certain highly conserved cellular oncogenes appear to be developmentally regulated (Murphy et al, 1983; Slamon and Cline, 1984). No good biochemical evidence is available for comparison of the control mechanisms themselves. The function of the controlling genes is ultimately to determine when certain biochemical pathways will be switched on or amplified. It is certainly not the case that similar biochemical pathways are switched on during the morphogenesis of a rat or a Drosophila embryo. It may be assumed that some, if not many, teratogens, act by direct inhibition of these biochemical pathways and are therefore specific mammalian (or Drosophila teratogens). It also goes without saying that partitioning and metabolism of xenobiotics by the mammalian maternal-placental-embryo unit are not in any sense available to these submammalian test systems.

The test described in this chapter focuses on two aspects of mammalian (rat) embryo development, neurogenesis and chondrogenesis (Flint et al, 1980; Flint, 1983; Flint and Orton, 1984; Flint et al, 1984). These events are isolated in vitro by culturing cells from the embryo midbrain or limb, and the sequence from undifferentiated to differentiated cell followed during five days of culture. Some of the most important aspects of cell behaviour involved in embryogenesis (cell adhesion, movement, communication, division and differentiation) are retained by the cultures, though full pattern formation is not achieved. The technique permits the limited involvement of drug metabolising systems in vitro or transplacental exposure of the embryos in vivo prior to culture. The technique also permits the identification of those subtle teratogens (for example, thalidomide, Flint et al, 1985) which specifically inhibit cell differentiation with no other adverse effect on cell survival. The method has been assessed in a blind trial with 46 compounds; 93% teratogens (25/27) and 89% non teratogens (17/19) were correctly identified (Flint and Orton, 1984).

PRACTICAL ASPECTS

Equipment and solutions for the micromass teratogen test

Removal of uterus:

Equipment: Sterilised blunt and sharp ended scissors.
Pair of forceps.
4" sterile glass or plastic petri dishes.

Dissection of limb and mid brain from embryos

Equipment: Laminar flow cabinet. Zoom stereo dissecting microscope with transmitted and incident illumination.
1 pair of MC19 Pascheff Wolff micro-scissors. (Moria-Dugast, Paris).
1 MC17 drilled spatula (Moria-Dugast, Paris).
2 pairs of sharpened No 5 Watchmakers forceps.
4" glass or plastic petri dishes.

Solutions: Earl's Balanced Salt Solution (Eagles modification - EBSS).
50% v/v horse serum and EBSS (HS-EBSS).

Tissue processing for culture

Equipment: Sterile glass pasteur pipettes.
Sterile glass pipettes with 0.7 mm internal tip diameter, produced by drawing conventional pasteur pipettes in a bunsen flame.

Sterile capped plastic test tubes, conical bottom.
Sterile Universal Containers.
Sterile disposable 10 ml syringes with removable plungers.
Sterile stainless steel Swinney filter holders (Millipore) with 10 um mesh nylon filter (Simon) in place.
Modified Fuchs-Rosenthal Haemocytometer.
Benchtop centrifuge (capable of 1000 rpm).

Solutions

Calcium and magnesium-free Earl's Balanced Salt Solution (CMF).
1% solution of Trypsin (Difco, 1:250) prepared by stirring for 30-60 minutes in CMF and then filtering through a Millex (Millipore) GS 0.2 um pore filter.
Hams F12 culture medium with supplements of 10% fetal calf serum, L-glutamine (584.6 mg/l), penicillin (10^6 iu per litre) and streptomycin (100 mg/l). All solutions are used within twelve months.

Culture preparation

Equipment

Eppendorf "Multipette" 4780.
Eppendorf 'Combitips' (sterilised) 500 ul size).
Falcon Primaria (3801) sterile plastic petri dishes (35 mm diameter).

Assay of cell differentiation

Equipment

Image analyster. AMS 40-10. (Analytical Measuring Systems Ltd., Saffron Walden, Essex, UK).

Experimental procedures

Wholly in vitro test (Figure 1)

Animals. Sufficient virgin Alderley Park albino rats are mated to provide six successful pregnancies per experiment. Conception is determined by the vaginal smear technique (Short and Woodnott, 1969). The pregnant animals are maintained until the 13th day after noting a positive vaginal smear. The animals weigh 250-350 g on this day. Animals are sacrificed by CO_2 euthanasia.

Aseptic removal of the uterus. The dead animal is immersed in a bath of diluted Savlon* (approximately 10 ml concentrate in 500 ml water) prior to dissection. The animal is laid on a clean surface covered with absorbent paper and an incision made with blunt scissors through the body wall, but not entering the peritoneum. The hole is expanded by retraction. A further incision is made in the peritoneum using sharp scissors and forceps. The uterus is then located in the lower abdomen and removed using scissors and forceps with as little adherent fat as possible. It is then transferred rapidly to a dry sterile petri dish.

Embryo dissection. All procedures take place in a laminar flow cabinet, the surfaces of which are sterilised by wiping down with tissues soaked in 70% alcohol. Uteri are washed through three changes of EBSS in petri dishes. Using the dissecting microscope each conceptus consisting of the embryo plus extra-embryonic membrane is removed to EBSS by tearing a small hole in the wall of the uterus with Watchmakers forceps. After all the conceptuses are removed from a uterus, the remaining tissue is discarded. Conceptuses pooled from all six animals are transferred using the drilled spatula to fresh HS/EBSS in a petri dish. HS/EBSS should be warmed in a water bath, to approximately 37°C. Extra-embryonic membranes are removed with Watchmakers forceps and discarded. The embryos are now collected to one side of the petri dish. Approximately 10 -12 embryos are found per uterus. At this stage of development, embryos have 34 - 36 somites. Small embryos having less than 34 somites and large embryos having more than 36 somites are rejected. The mesencephalon and fore-limb bud are removed from the acceptable embryos using microdissection scissors and Watchmakers forceps, and maintained separately throughout the preparation and culture procedures.

Processing of tissues

Equipment. Tissues are transferred by pasteur pipette to separate labelled test tubes. The HS/EBSS is aspirated off with a pasteur pipette and tissues washed three times with CMF. The tubes are incubated for 20

* Savlon is a trademark, the property of Imperial Chemical Industries PLC.

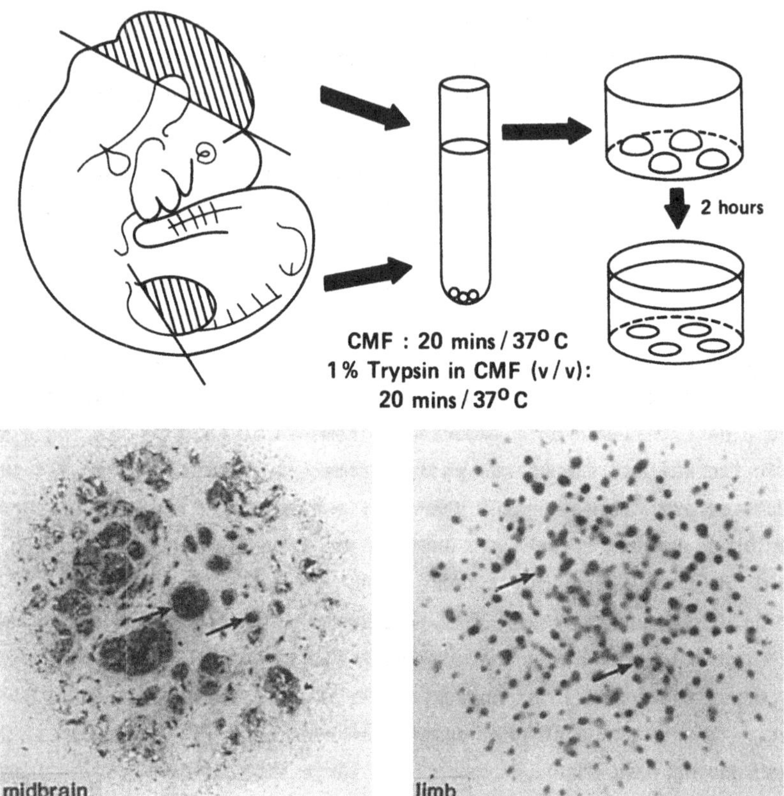

Figure 1 Micromass culture technique. Midbrain and limbs (hatched areas) are dissected free and after dissociation of the cells are cultured (separately) as described in the text. After five days of culture cells are fixed and stained (limb by alcian blue, midbrain by haematoxylin) to reveal foci of differentiated cells (arrowed).

minutes at 37°C. CMF is then exchanged for 1% trypsin in CMF and the tubes are incubated for a further 20 minutes at 37°C followed by a brief wash in CMF which is immediately replaced by 1.3 ml of the complete Ham's medium (CM). Tissue fragments are then disaggregated into their component cells by repeated aspirations through the 0.7 mm internal tip diameter Pasteur pipette (15 - 20 times). Care is taken not to make a froth. The resulting cell suspension is then poured into a 10 ml disposable syringe with a Swinney filter holder attached. Replacing the plunger forces the suspension through the 10 um mesh nylon filter and into a fresh test tube. A suspension of single cells is thus obtained. 1 ml of this suspension is transferred to a fresh test tube. The small amount of remaining suspension is diluted 1:9 with CM and counted with the Fuchs-Rosenthal Haemocytometer.

The estimated cell concentration is used to calculate the amount of medium required to produce in the case of midbrain, 5×10^6 cells per ml, and in the case of limb, 2×10^7 cells per ml. If these final concentrations can only be achieved in volumes of less than 1 ml culture medium, the 1 ml of suspended cells is centrifuged at 1000 rpm for five minutes, the supernatant removed and the cells re-suspended in the calculated volume of fresh medium. Otherwise, excess fresh medium is added to the original 1 ml to give the appropriate final cell concentration.

Culture preparation. The cell suspension is drawn up into a 500 ul 'Combitip' fitted to the 'Multipette' and delivered in 10 ul aliquots to 35 mm sterile plastic disposable petri dishes.

Cells are allowed to settle for two hours at 37°C, forming circular cell islands (6-8 mm) then culture dishes are filled to a final volume of 2 ml with CM and other supplements described below. Five (10 ul) aliquots of midbrain and at least three (10 ul) aliquots of limb cell suspension are delivered to each dish.

Sufficient dishes are prepared for assessment of a concentration response curve to the tested compound, (usually 7 dishes of each cell type).

Cultures are treated with compound alone or with compound in the presence of a rat liver metabolising system (S9-mix), with or without cofactors. The preparation of S9-mix is described below.

Six serial stock dilutions of test compound (see below) are prepared in the appropriate vehicle (see below) giving a range of concentrations (each not differing from the next by more than a factor of ten) below the maximum concentration. The maximum concentration of compound in culture medium does not exceed 500 ug per ml or the maximum solubility if this is less than 500 ug per ml. One midbrain and one limb dish receive vehicle control and each concentration of the compound in 2 ml culture medium. The medium is not changed for the following five days of culture.

Equivalent series of dishes containing 50 ul of S9-mix (with or without cofactors) per ml culture medium are prepared in the same way. Medium plus S9-mix is changed after two hours for 2 ml of fresh CM (to limit cytotoxic effect of S9) and the dishes are returned to the incubator for five days.

Formulation of stock solutions of test compounds. Compound is formulated initially as a concentrated stock solution in either dimethyl sulphoxide (DMSO), ethanol (EtOH) or Earle's Balanced Salt solution (EBSS) according to solubility. The final concentration of these vehicles in culture medium are: DMSO, 0.5% v/v and EtOH or EBSS, 1.0% v/v. The maximum solubility of compound in culture medium is then assessed by adding 10 ul stock solution in DMSO or 20 ul in EtOH or EBSS to 35 mm petri dishes (Falcon) containing 2 ml of culture medium followed by agitation. If the compound is insoluble (i.e. precipitates out) the concentrated stock is diluted until solubility in culture medium is achieved. A series of dilutions of the stock solutions are then prepared to give the desired final concentration range in culture medium.

Culture medium is brought to 37°C and gassed with 5% CO_2, 95% air in sterile beakers in a Flow CO_2 Incubator (Flow Laboratories, Irvine, Scotland). Sufficient medium and beakers are made ready to include the range of concentrations of compound plus a beaker of control medium containing vehicle only. A sterile magnetic follower is introduced into each beaker. The appropriately concentrated stock solutions are added to each beaker in a sterile laminar flow cabinet and medium is stirred on a magnetic stirrer.

Fixation and staining of midbrain cultures. Medium is removed from culture dishes by aspiration and replaced with about 1 ml of 10% formaldehyde solution per dish. Fixative is removed with running tap water after a minimum of twenty minutes fixation. Cells are then stained for one to three minutes with haematoxylin followed by washing with tap water. All the cultures are air dried.

Fixation and staining of limb cultures. After aspiration of the medium, cultures are fixed with 10% formaldehyde containing 1% cetylpyridinium chloride for a minimum of twenty minutes. Cultures are then left for one hour in 3% acetic acid and stained with 1% Alcian blue in 0.1 N hydrochloric acid (pH 1.0) for a minimum of two hours. After washing with tap water, the cultures are air dried.

Measurement of cell differentiation. Possibly the simplest method is to count the differentiated foci (Fig. 1) using an automated colony counter (Table 1). Each cell island is positioned under the lens of the television camera so that its image is presented on the TV monitor. The colony counter is then set to count the number of foci of darkly staining cells which correspond in midbrain cultures to neurons and in limb cultures to chondrocytes. These differentiated cell types were not present in the initial cell suspension prepared from the embryo but have differentiated in culture (Flint, 1983; Flint and Orton, 1984).

By counting the number of darkly staining foci an estimate is made of the total population of cells which have differentiated during the period of culture (Flint et al, 1984).

A second method using monoclonal antibodies has also been used (Girling and Flint, 1984). Cultures are grown in 96-well culture dishes on a collagen substrate and assayed by the ELISA (enzyme linked immunosorbent assay) method with a neuron specific monoclonal antibody for midbrain or with protein A (binds specifically to chondrocytes) for limb cultures.

A third endpoint is the incorporation of cell differentiation specific radio isotope labelled precursors; [^{3}H]-gamma amino butyric acid for midbrain cultures and [^{35}S]-sulphate for limb cultures (Flint et al, 1984). A comparison should be made of incorporation with total protein (Lowry et al, 1951) or the neutral red assay to determine cytotoxicity. [^{3}H] thymidine incorporation is an alternative estimate of cytotoxicity (Flint, 1980; Guntakatta et al, 1984).

Small differences of IC50 are observed, depending on the endpoint used, but the prediction of teratogenic hazard is largely unchanged. Thus if an automated colony counter of the type described is not available, it is equally possible to use scintillation counting and radio-isotopically labelled precursor incorporation.

Analysis of results. The mean and standard deviation of the number of differentiated foci per cell island is calculated for controls and each concentration of compound. Results are plotted and the concentration (IC_{50}) of compound inhibiting differentiation to 50% control level is calculated by interpolation. All data analyses comparing treatment groups with their concurrent controls are performed using Student's t-test (Sokal and Rohlf, 1969).

Cytotoxicity assay

Cultures. Preparation of cell suspensions and culture medium is as described above. Cells are plated out into 96-well (10 ul per well) microtitre dishes (Nunclon - Gibco Europe, Paisley, Scotland) which have been pre-coated with 10 μl 0.05% w/v collagen in 0.01% v/v acetic acid. The collagen layer is air dried in a laminar flow cabinet prior to addition of cells. The first column of wells is left free of cells, to be used later as a blank in the assay. After two hours settling at 37°C (5% CO_2 : 95% air) the volume of culture medium in each well is increased to 200 ul (supplemented with test compound or vehicle). Cultures are left in the incubator for five days at 37°C under an atmosphere of 5% CO_2 : 95% air.

Culture fixation and staining. Cells are fixed for 20 minutes with glutaraldehyde made approximately isosmotic with culture medium (4.5 ml glutaraldehyde : 95.5 ml water), then washed three times with phosphate buffered saline (PBS : Dulbecco's phosphate buffered saline, GIBCO; pH 7.4). PBS is replaced with 200 ul neutral red stain (0.1% w/v neutral red in PBS, Fluorochem Ltd, Glossop, England). The blank column is also filled with neutral red stain. Cells are stained for 90 minutes at room temperature, the neutral red stain is removed, and the wells are washed with PBS. Stain is then eluted from the cells into 200 ul acid alcohol (0.5% v/v acetic acid in 50% alcohol) per well for a minimum of two hours. Stain intensity (optical density) is measured colorimetrically with a Multiskan spectrophotometer (Flow Laboratories, Irvine, Scotland) at 550 nm. Cell number is directly related to the absorbance of the eluted stain.

Analysis of results. The mean optical density (and standard deviation) is calculated for the neutral red stain eluted from each group of cells. A graph is then drawn to illustrate any dose related change. Significant differences from the control (vehicle exposed) group are assessed by Student's t-test. The concentration (IC50) inhibiting cell survival by 50% control values is estimated from the graph.

Preparation of S9-mix

S-9 mix is a centrifuged rat liver post- mitochondrial supernatant with cofactors. it is used as a model in vitro drug metabolising system (Flint and Orton, 1984).

Animals. One male (Alpk/AP) rat (180-220 g). Aroclor 1254 (500 mg/kg) is dosed intraperitoneally once 4 - 6 days prior to euthanasia. Aroclor 1254 is a broad spectrum inducer of cytochrome P450.

Cofactor solution. Magnesium chloride (162.6 mg). Potassium chloride (246 mg). Glucose - 6 phosphate (disodium salt) (152 mg). Nicotinamide adenine dinucleotide phosphate (disodium salt) (336 mg). Phosphate buffer (0.2 mol/l pH 7.4) (50 ml). Distilled water (40 ml).

Method. The animal is killed by CO_2 anaesthesia and exsanguinated by opening the carotid artery. The ventral surface of the animal is swabbed with Savlon. An abdominal incision is made and the liver exposed. A portion of liver is removed and transferred to a preweighed container of ice cold 0.15 mol/l potassium chloride. A known weight of liver is homogenised in 1 : 3 w/v 0.15 mol/l sterile potassium chloride at $4^{o}C$, in a sterile cold ($4^{o}C$) Potter Elvehjem homogeniser with a teflon pestle, rotated by an electric motor at approximately 2,600 rpm. The homogenate is centrifuged at 9,000 g for ten minutes at $4^{o}C$ and the supernatant (the S-9 fraction) is withdrawn.

The S-9 fraction is mixed with the sterile cofactor solution (filtration through Millex GS 0.2 um pore filter) in the ratio 3 : 7 and the resulting S-9 mix is kept on ice for up to six hours.

This preparation is toxic to the cultured cells if exposure is extended beyond 2 hours. Toxicity resides in both the cofactor and the S9 preparation. However, the cofactor solution is less toxic than the complete actively metabolising S9 prepratation (Figure 2). The reason for the toxicity of S9-mix to the cells remains so far unclear. The need to change medium plus S9-mix after two hours has two obvious consequences. First the medium change may disturb the cell cultures and thus unevenly affect the experimental outcome. With care and experience this need not necessarily be a problem (Figure 2). Secondly exposure to compound alone and any toxic metabolites formed is for two hours only and is not strictly comparable with the more routine 5 day exposure without S9-mix. Thus cultures with the active S9-mix plus cofactors must be compared to additional cultures exposed to compound plus S-9 mix without the necessary cofactors.

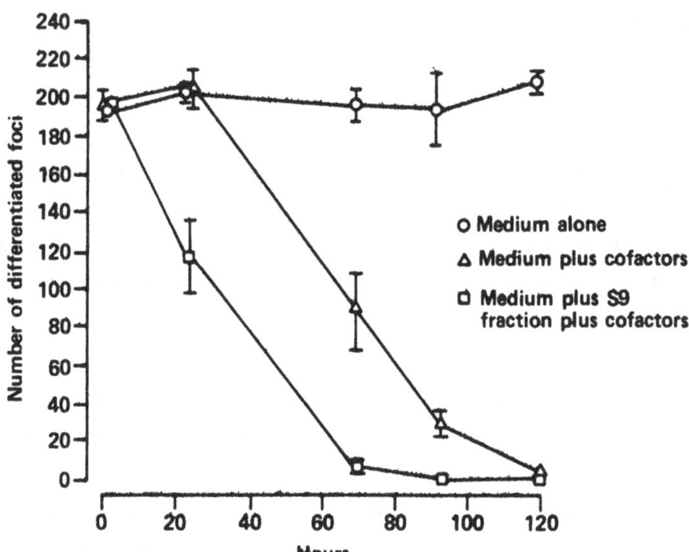

Figure 2. Effect of increasing exposure time to S9-mix (50 ul/ml) on differentiation in rat embryo LB cultures. The S9 preparation and the constitution of the cofactor solution is described in the methods section. There is essentially no difference of toxicity between midbrain and limb cultures.

In vivo/in vitro test

The following modifications to the wholly in vitro technique described above are undertaken when embryos are exposed to compound while still in utero.

Animals and treatment. Six pregnant animals are selected. On the 12th day of pregnancy, between 4 and 5 p.m. two control animals receive an intraperitoneal injection of 0.5% v/v aqueous Polysorbate 80 or EBSS (1 ml/200 g body weight) and two animals per selected dose receive compound formulated in 0.5% aqueous Polysorbate 80 for four hours prior to administration. Soluble compounds are administered in EBSS. Doses are selected from a sighting study with non pregnant rats in which the acute maximum tolerated dose (MTD) is determined. The top dose is normally just below the MTD. The lower dose is half way between the upper dose and the vehicle control.

Preparation of cultures. Cultures are prepared as described previously. Cells from embryos of each control or treated rat are cultured separately as individual groups. At least two replicate dishes per tissue (midbrain or limb) containing three cell islands are prepared for determination of the number of differentiated foci with the 40-10 colony counter as described. At least 5 cell islands per group are cultured in 96-well dishes for the determination of cytotoxicity by neutral red uptake as described above.

Analysis of results. The mean and standard deviation of the number of differentiated foci and the neutral red optical density are calculated for each treatment group. A graph is then drawn to illustrate any dose related change. Results are analysed by two way analysis of variance (Sokal and Rohlf, 1969).

EXPERIMENTAL EXAMPLES

Culture response to the direct addition of test compound

The in vitro toxicity to limb cultures of two structurally similar compounds, the teratogen 5-fluorouracil and the non teratogen 6 methyluracil, is compared in Figure 3.

First, it is clear that the non teratogen, 6 methyluracil is without inhibitory effect up to its maximum solubility in culture medium (500 ug/ml) and 5 fluorouracil is strongly inhibitory from 0.1 ug/ml. The culture system is thus exquisitely sensitive to small changes of chemical structure (6-methyl as opposed to 5-fluoro- substitution). Secondly the concentration of 5 fluorouracil inhibiting differentiation by 50% of control values (IC50: 1.5 ug/ml) is approximately five and half times smaller than the IC50 for cell survival (8.5 ug/ml). The teratogen, 5 fluorouracil thus inhibits cell differentiation at concentrations which are not cytolethal.

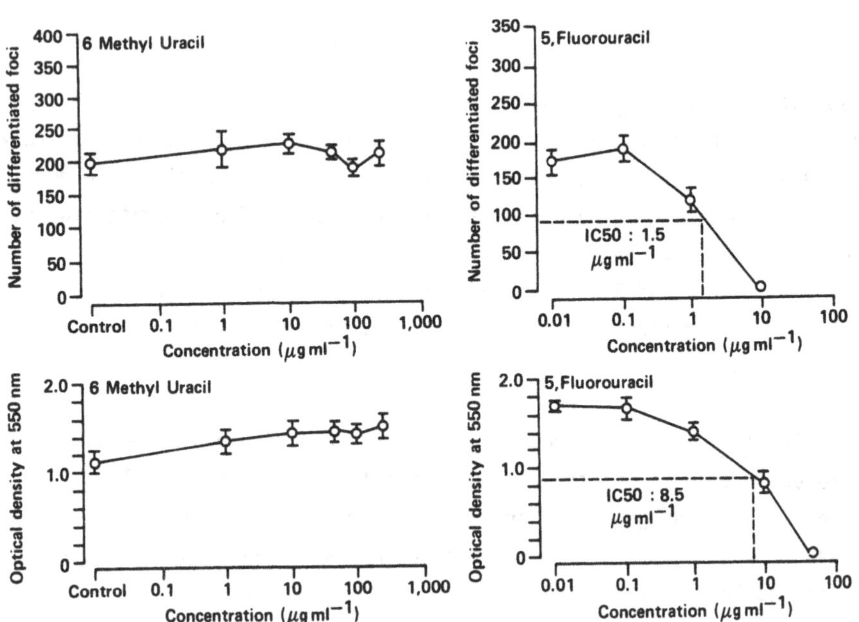

Figure 3. Effect of 5-fluorouracil and 6 methyluracil on differentiation (number of differentiated foci) and cell survival (cytotoxicity by neutral red uptake) in rat embryo limb cultures. Examples are taken from limb cultures because there was no significant difference of response between these and midbrain cultures.

The IC50 for cell differentiation of the teratogen diphenylhydantoin is 29.5 ug/ml (Figure 4) in midbrain cultures by the ELISA method. The value is half that for cell survival (65 ug/ml) so that cell differentiation is again inhibited at relatively non cytolethal concentrations.

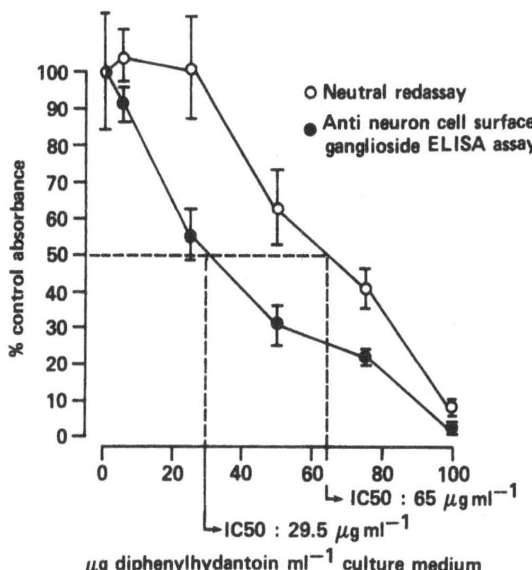

Figure 4. Effect of diphenylhydantoin on differentiation (ELISA assay) and cell survival (neutral red assay) in rat embryo midbrain cultures.

Prediction of teratogenic hazard in vitro

We have found the following guidelines useful for the interpretation of IC50 values whenever a concentration response curve indicates toxicity of the test compound.

1. Potent teratogens (e.g. aldrin, azaguanine, colchicine, cycloheximide, diethylstilbestrol, 5 fluorouracil - see Flint and Orton 1984) all inhibit differentiation with an IC50 below 10 ug/ml. Weak or poorly substantiated teratogens (e.g. aspirin, diazepam, sulfisoxazole) have IC50's greater than 50 ug/ml. As a general rule IC50's less than 50 ug/ml are indicative of teratogenic hazard and strongly indicative if less than 10 ug/ml.

2. The IC50 of vitamin A in limb cultures for cell survival (3.5 ug/ml) is 500 fold higher than the IC50 for cell differentiation (0.007 ug/ml) suggesting highly selective toxicity for cell differentiation (Table 2). In the teratogen examples described in this chapter (diphenylhydantoin, 5-fluorouracil, vitamin A) differentiation was inhibited at relatively non cytolethal concentrations. This sign of teratogenic hazard may be particularly indicative of those teratogens which will cause fetal abnormalities at doses which may not be significantly toxic to the mother.

3. Teratogens are characterised by their selective toxicity for different organs (e.g. hydrocortisone and diphenylhydantoin - orofacial clefts; thalidomide - limb reduction). Therefore a difference of IC50 between midbrain and limb cultures may be taken as a further indication of teratogenic hazard. The IC50 for cell differentiation following exposure of limb cells to vitamin A (alcohol) is 1000 fold less than in midbrain cultures (Table 3).

Metabolism of xenobiotics

The culture system models in vivo exposure to test compound in a very limited way. In vivo, the mother might detoxify the compound before significantly toxic concentrations are achieved in utero. Conversely the compound itself may not be toxic and only its metabolites cause teratogenicity.

In vitro preparations of metabolising enzymes. Preparations of xenobiotic metabolising enzymes can be added to the cultures as a substitute for in vivo metabolism. The 50 ul S9-mix per ml culture medium/2 hour exposure protocol described under the practical aspects of the test is capable of activating cyclophosphamide to its toxic metabolite(s) (Figure 5). The maximum concentration of S9-mix which is non toxic to cultures over 5 days exposure is 3 ul/ml culture medium. This concentration is still capable of activating cyclophosphamide but as a consequence of the reduced metabolising activity the IC50 is approximately 10 fold higher (2 hour IC50 : 1.3 ug/ml; 5 day IC50 : 15.5 ug/ml). The disadvantage of lowered "sensitivity" may be outweighed by the possibility of 5 days exposure to any long lived toxic metabolites; S9-mix itself is not considered to be actively metabolising beyond 2-4 hours.

The need for such metabolising systems must be seen in context. In a study of 27 teratogens Flint and Orton (1984) found that most, with the single clear exception of cyclophosphamide, appeared to be directly acting in vitro (no liver subfraction required). Brown et al (1985) have recently shown by the use of antibodies that the embryo cells themselves (especially limb cells) have constitutive levels of cytochromes P450. It thus appears that embryo cells may well be capable of metabolising compounds per se.

Culture response to transplacental exposure of the embryo. Transplacental exposure (Flint et al, 1984) clearly involves the possibility of metabolism and partitioning by mother, placenta and embryo. Normally a single (intraperitoneal) exposure is given 16 hours prior to laparotomy.

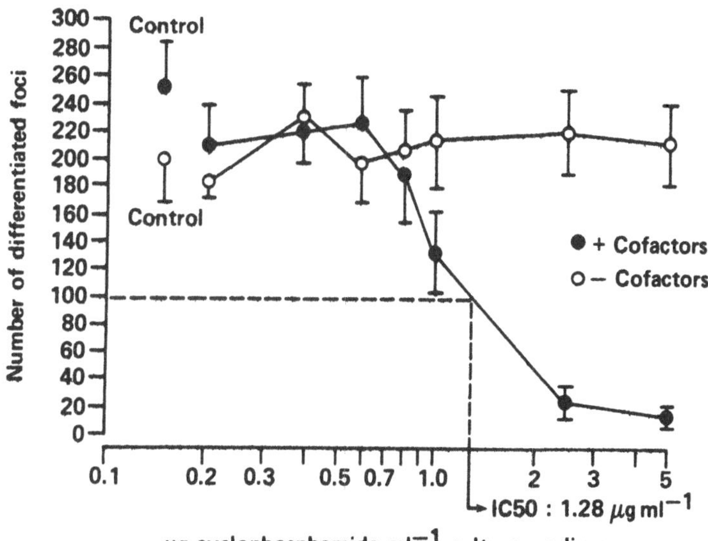

Figure 5 Concentration response of a 2 hour exposure of CNS cultures to cyclophosphamide and S9-mix (50 ul/ml culture medium) in the presence and absence of cofactors.

Two doses are selected, one just below the maternal maximum tolerated dose and the other at half this dose. In many cases the range of doses which inhibit differentiation of the subsequently cultured embryo cells is roughly equivalent to that causing teratogenicity in vivo.

The teratogen Vitamin A, for example, inhibits midbrain differentiation from approximately 100 mg/kg and limb differentiation above 100 mg/kg (Figure 6). Vitamin A is teratogenic in the rat from between 40 and 100 mg/kg (see review by Geelen, 1979).

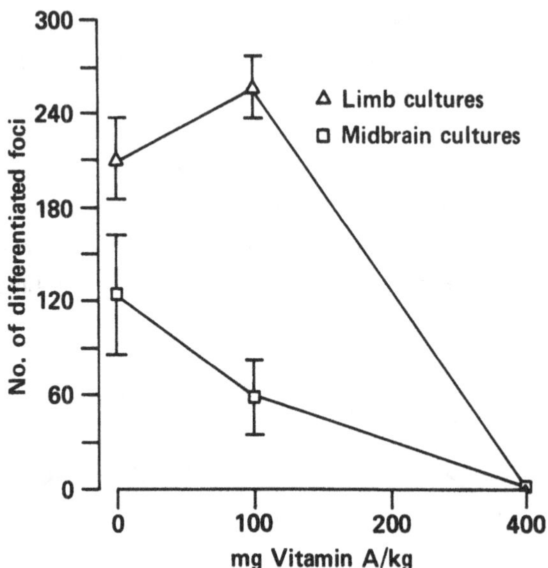

Figure 6 Differentiation of limb and midbrain cultures following transplacental exposure of the embryo to vitamin A. Controls were treated with the vehicle (Tween 80).

DISCUSSION AND CONCLUSIONS

Scope of the test

One technician can test between 250 and 300 compounds per year. In practice the use of the test must be adapted to each particular need. For example in the pharmaceutical industry the test should be used as soon as there is a reasonable degree of interest in the pharmacological activity of a new chemical structure. The initial testing should include as many as possible of the in vitro tests outlined in Figure 7. This will need between 10 and 20 mg of test compound though preferably 100 mg should be supplied in case repeat tests are required. Repeat tests are usually done when a border line (IC50 : 40 - 60 ug/ml) or positive result is obtained. The range of 40-60 ug/ml given for a border line result takes into consideration repeat studies (Flint and Orton, 1984) where the coefficient of variation for the IC50 was found to lie between 10 and 20 per cent. Should there be an indication of teratogenic hazard at this stage the next step would be to test more chemicals of similar structure and intended pharmacological activity.

Only those tests outlined in Figure 7 which appear to be most relevant need be used at this stage. For example there may be no indication of metabolic activation so that cultures with S9 mix can be omitted. The objective is to see whether teratogenicity is related to the compound's pharmacological activity or, if not, whether simple structural changes eliminate the teratogenic hazard. Such a quantitative structure activity study has been described for triazole antifungals by Flint and Boyle (1985). Finally, absence of teratogenicity can be confirmed in the few chemicals chosen for development by an in vivo/in vitro study, or if the resources are available by a sighting teratology study.

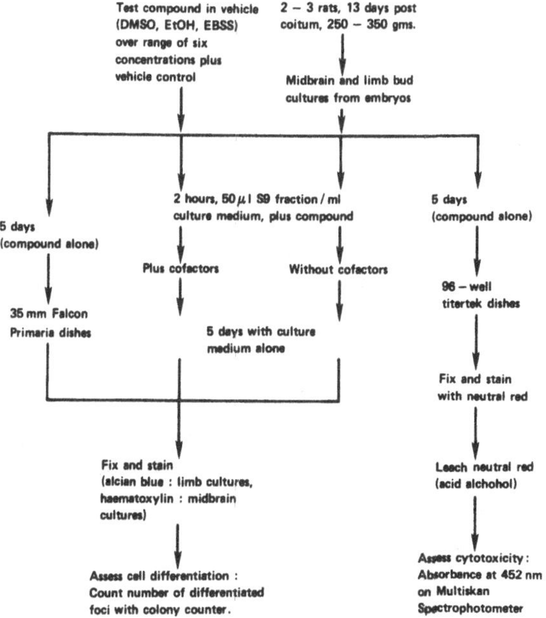

Figure 7 In vitro test system for primary screening of test compounds.

Quantitative structure activity relationships, vitamin A and related retinoids

Synthetic retinoids related to vitamin A (e.g. tretinoin, isotretinoin) have recently been successfully used for the treatment of non-neoplastic dermatological diseases in man, including acne, psoriasis and other keratinising dermatoses (Peck, 1981, 1983). Their use has also highlighted the toxicity and in particular the teratogenicity of vitamin A (Geelen, 1979, Benke, 1984). Vitamin A is an essential vitamin. At least half of the nutritional requirement is supplied in the form of carotenes (Table 2, 3) depending on diet.

Only 1% of total body carotene circulates in the blood (serum concentration: 0.85 ug/ml approximately). 80% of the remainder is stored in the fat and 10% in the liver (Olson, 84). Carotenes (e.g. beta-carotene) are without embryotoxic or teratological effect in the rat and rabbit (Heywood et al, 1985). They are also without effect on cell differentiation and are not cytotoxic in the teratogen test (Table 3). The carotenes are converted to vitamin A (aldehyde, alcohol, acid, palmitate) in the liver where 80% is stored (as palmitate). One per cent (approximately 0.32 ug/ml) circulates in the serum (90% alcohol, 10% aldehyde, ester and acid). The stored palmitate is without cytotoxicity or effect on cell differentiation in vitro (Table 3) but is teratogenic in the mouse. The explanation for this teratogenicity which is unexpected from the in vitro result is that the palmitate is metabolised to the retinol in vivo which strongly inhibits cell differentiation in vitro (Table 3) (Newall and Edwards, 1981). An experiment with S9-mix and vitamin A palmitate confirms that a toxic metabolite (presumably the alcohol) and not the parent compound inhibits cell differentiation. After only 2 hours exposure in the presence of active S9-mix and the palmitate, limb chondrogenesis is inhibited (IC50 : 45 ug/ml).

Retinol, retinoic acid and retinyl aldehyde per se are very cytotoxic and strongly inhibit cell differentiation (Table 3). In each case limb differentiation is inhibited at relatively non cytolethal concentrations and there are large differences of IC50 between midbrain and limb cultures. The in vitro test correlates with known teratogenicity of these compounds in vivo (Geelen, 1979). In each case the circulating concentration in man (0.32 ug/ml) is greater than that which inhibits differentiation of the rat embryo limb cells in vitro

(Table 3), suggesting that either there are differences of sensitivity between rat and man or that not all the vitamin A crosses the placenta. Vitamin A (as retinoic acid or retinol) easily crosses the placenta (at least in the mouse) as shown by Kocchar (1976) and Newall and Edwards (1981) and a species difference of sensitivity to vitamin A (retinoic acid) teratogenicity has been shown by Zbinden (1975). The rhesus monkey appears to be 10-20 fold less sensitive to single acute doses of retinoic acid than the rat. That rat embryo cells in vitro appear to be sensitive to concentrations of vitamin A two to three orders of magnitude lower than the circulating concentrations in man suggests that there is certainly room for further work on the pharmacokinetics of vitamin A during pregnancy. In conclusion vitamin A and congeners (Table 2) are

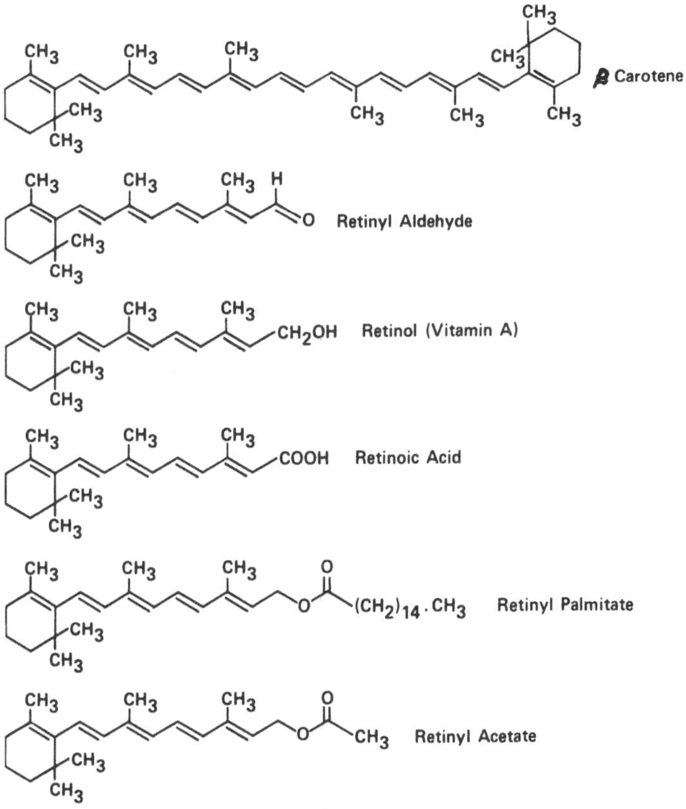

β Carotene

Retinyl Aldehyde

Retinol (Vitamin A)

Retinoic Acid

Retinyl Palmitate

Retinyl Acetate

Table 2 Chemical structure of carotenes (only β carotene given) and vitamin A metabolites tested in Table 2 and referred to in the text.

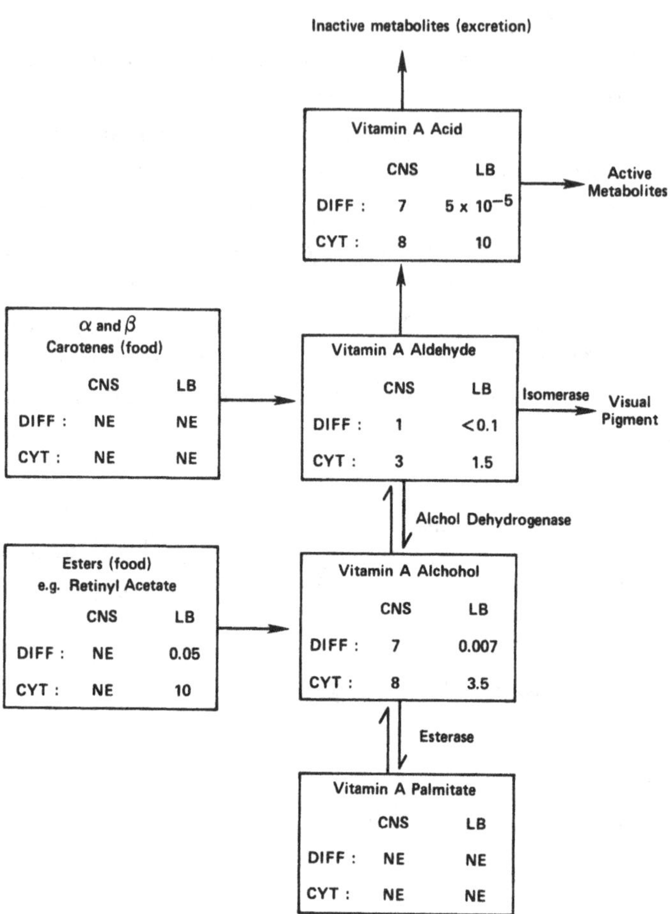

Table 3 Metabolic pathway of vitamin A in vivo. For each compound the concentration (IC50, ug/ml) reducing cell number (CYT) or cell differentiation (DIFF) by 50% control values is given for rat embryo midbrain (CNS) and limb (LB) cells in the absence of S9-mix.
NE = no effect to maximum soluble concentration in culture medium.

model compounds for the in vitro teratogen test. Large differences of toxicity have been demonstrated between compounds which have relatively small differences of structure, and there is agreement between in vitro prediction of teratogenic hazard and in vivo teratogenicity. This and a quantitative structure activity study with triazole antifungals (Flint and Boyle, 1985) suggest that the test will prove a powerful tool in the selection of non teratogenic but pharmacologically active compounds at the earliest stages of compound selection.

Comparison with other techniques. The usefulness of the technique for predicting teratogenic hazard is amply demonstrated. Whether or not other in vitro test systems for detecting teratogens will prove as useful remains to be seen and this will only be determined by interlaboratory trials. Techniques such as the test described here which aim to identify teratogens that are not simply cytolethal will probably have most success. Simple, one end point in vitro cytotoxicity tests are unlikely to be highly predictive of teratogenic hazard. Pratt and Willis (1985) for example describe the effect of 35 teratogens and 20 non teratogens on the growth of a cell line derived from human embryonic palatal mesenchyme. The criterion for teratogenic hazard was growth inhibition below 1 mM concentration. Below this concentration as many as 34% of the teratogens were non inhibitory and 40% of the non teratogens were inhibitory. This is however not yet the time or place for an extended comparison with other proposed techniques. It should be emphasised that the micromass teratogen test is the only test which has been extensively applied in an industrial environment to the problem of predicting teratogenicity and in three years of use it has proved to be a robust and valuable method.

The author wishes to thank Dr T C Orton, Dr P Duffy and Miss L P Brown for reviewing this manuscript and Mrs K Jones for her invaluable assistance towards perfecting the technique.

REFERENCES

Benke, P.J. (1984). The isotretinoin teratogen syndrome. J.Am.Med.Ass., 251, 3267-3269.

Best, J.B. and Morita, M. (1982). Planarians as a model system for in vitro teratogenesis studies. Terato. Carcino. Mutagen. 2, 277-291.

Bournias-Vardiabasis, N. and Teplitz, R.L. (1982). Use of Drosophila embryo cultures as an in vitro teratogen assay. Terato. Carcino. Mutagen. 2, 333-342.

Brown, L.P., Flint, O.P., Orton, T.C., and Gibson, G.G., (1986). In vitro metabolism of teratogens by differentiating rat embryo cells. In the Proceedings of a Conference on 'Practical in vitro toxicology', held at Reading, September, 1985. To be published.

Braun, A.G., Emerson, D.J. and Nichinson, B.B. (1979). Teratogenic drugs inhibit tumour cell attachment to lectin-coated surfaces. Nature, 282, 507-509.

Braun, A.G. and Dailey, J.P. (1981). Thalidomide metabolite inhibits tumour cell attachment to concanavalin A coated surfaces. Biochem. and Biophys. Res. Comm. 98, 1029-1034.

Braun, A.G. and Weinreb, S. (1984). Teratogen metabolism: activation of thalidomide and thalidomide analogues to products that inhibit the attachment of cells to concanavalin A coated plastic surfaces. Biochem. Pharmacol. 33, 1471-1477.

Flint, O.P. (1980). The effects of sodium salicylate, cytosine arabinoside, and eserine sulphate on rat limb buds in culture. In 'Teratology of the Limbs'. Ed. Merker, H.J., Nau, H. and Neubert, D. pp. 325-338. Pub. by Walter de Gruyter and Co., Berlin.

Flint, O.P. (1983). A micromass culture method for rat embryonic neural cells. J.Cell.Sci. 61, 247-262.

Flint, O.P. and Orton, T.C. (1984). An in vitro assay for teratogens with cultures of rat embryo midbrain and limb bud cells. Tox.Appl. Pharmacol. 76, 383-395.

Flint, O.P. and Boyle, F.T. (1985). An in vitro test for teratogens: its application in the selection of non-teratogenic triazole antifungals. Concepts. Toxicol. 3, 29-35.

Flint, O.P., Orton, T.C. and Ferguson, R.A. (1984). Differentiation of rat embryo cells in culture: response following acute maternal exposure to teratogens and non teratogens. J.Appl.Toxicol. 4, 109-116.

Flint, O.P., Orton, T.C. and Girling, L.R. (1985' In vitro inhibition of chondrogenesis in cultured rat embryo limb cells by thalidomide. Brit. J. Pharmacol. 84, 122P.

Geelen, J.A. (1979). Hypervitaminosis A induced teratogenesis. Crit.Rev. Toxicol. 6, 351-375.

Girling, L. and Flint, O.P. (1984). Inhibition of embryonic cell differentiaiton by teratogens in vitro: quantification using ELISA (Enzyme Linked Immunoabsorbent Assay). Human Toxicology 3, 155-156.

Guntakatta, M., Mattews, E.J. and Rundell, J.O. (1984). Development of a mouse embryo limb bud cell culture system for the estimation of chemical teratogenic potential. Terato.Carcino.Mutagen. 4, 349-364.

Helm, F.- Ch. Frankus, E., Friderichs, E., Graudums, I. and Flohe, L. (1981). Comparative teratological investigation of compounds structurally and pharmacologically related to thalidomide. Arzneim-Forsch. 31, 941-949.
Heywood, R., Palmer, A.K., Gregson, R.L. and Hummler, H. (1985). The toxicity of beta-carotene. Toxicology 36, 91-100.
Johnson, E.M., Gorman, R.M., Gabel, B.E.G. and George, M.E. (1982). The hydra attenuata system for detection of teratogenic hazards. Terato. Carcino. Mutagen. 2, 263-276.
Kocchar, D.M. (1976). Transplacental passage of label after administration of [^{3}H] retinoic acid (vitamin A acid) to pregnant mice. Teratology 14, 53-63.
Lowry, O.H., Rosenbrough, N.F., Farn, A.L., Randell, R.J., (1951). Protein measurement with folin phenol reagent. J. Biol. Chem., 193, 265-275.
Murphy, D. Brickell, P.M. Latchman, D.S. Willison, K. and Rigby, P.W. (1983). Transcripts regulated during normal embryonic development and oncogenic transformation share a repetitive element. Cell 35, 865-871.
Newall, D.R. and Edwards, J.R.G. (1981). The effect of vitamin A on fusion of mouse palates. Retinyl palmitate amd retinoic acid in vivo. Teratology 23, 115-124.
Olson, J.A. (1984). Serum levels of vitamin A and carotenoids as reflectors of nutritional status. J.Nat.Cancer Inst. 73, 1439-1444.
Peck, G.L. (1983). Retinoids: therapeutic use in dermatology. Curr.Ther. 24, 103-112.
Pratt, R.M. and Willis, W.D. (1985). In vitro screening for teratogens using growth inhibition of human embryonic cells. Proc.Natl.Acad.Sci. USA 82, 5791-5794.
Sadler, T.W., Horton, W.E. and Warner, C.W. (1982). Whole embryo culture: a screening technique for teratogens? Terato. Carcino. Mutagen. 2, 243-255.
Slaman, D.J. and Cline, M.J. (1984). Expression of cellular oncogenes during embryonic and fetal development of the mouse. Proc. Natl. Acad. Sci. USA 81, 7141-7145.
Sokal, R.R. and Rohlf, E.J. (1969). Biometry. The principles and practice of statistics in biological research. Pub. W.H. Freeman and Company, San Francisco.
Steele, C.E., Trasler, D.G. and New, D.A.T. (1983). An in vivo/in vitro evaluation of the teratogenic action of excess vitamin A. Teratology 28, 209-214.
Trosko, J.E., Chang, C.-C. and Netzloff, M. (1982). The role of inhibited cell-cell communication in teratogenesis. Terato. Carcino. Mutagen 2, 31-45.
Welsch, F. and Stedman, D.B. (1984). Inhibition of metabolic cooperation between Chinese hamster V79 cells by structurally diverse teratogens. Terato. Carcino. Mutagen. 4, 285-301.
Zbinden, G. (1975). Investigations on the toxicity of tretinoin administered systemically to animals. Acta Dermatovener (Stockholm), Suppl. 74, 36-40.

POSTIMPLANTATION EMBRYO CULTURE AND ITS APPLICATION TO PROBLEMS IN TERATOLOGY

D.L. Cockroft,
ICRF Developmental Biology Unit, Zoology Department,
South Parks Road, Oxford, OX1 3PS, England.

C.E. Steele,
SK&F Research Ltd., Welwyn, AL6 9AR, England.

INTRODUCTION

Techniques for the culture of postimplantation mammalian embryos have been developed for embryos explanted between the early primitive-streak stage (8th day of gestation in the rat - Buckley et al 1978) and 55 somite stage (14th day in the rat - Cockroft 1973), though the best results are obtained with embryos explanted at the head-fold or early somite stage (New et al 1976 a, b; Sadler 1979; Sadler & New 1981). These techniques are now widely used in academic research, and increasingly in contract laboratories and pharmaceutical toxicology departments.

Static culture systems may be used for the younger embryos, but will only support limited development (Tam & Snow 1980). Systems in which oxygenated medium is made to flow past embryos anchored in a culture chamber give better results (e.g. New 1967), but are relatively costly and time consuming. In much teratological testing, it is desirable to be able to culture large numbers of embryos through the major period of organogenesis with minimum fuss, and for this purpose rotating bottle cultures, which may be intermittently or continuously gassed, are most suitable.

The area of teratological testing for which *in vitro* methods may be of greatest potential benefit is for the further investigation of substances which *in vivo* tests have shown to be of toxicological interest. Growing embryos outside the mother provides opportunities to study the direct action of a teratogen or its metabolites free of the mediating effects of maternal pharmacokinetics. A degree of control is afforded over the embryo's environment - both chemical and physical - that would be impossible *in vivo*. Furthermore, an embryo may be sensitive to a particular agent for only a short critical period, and *in vivo* the variability within and between litters is such that anomalous or confusing results may be obtained. Embryos *in vitro* may be treated according to their precise developmental stage, and the facility to observe the embryos during organogenesis makes it possible to record, for example, the heart rate and its response to drugs (Robkin et al 1974) or to monitor the generation of an abnormality such as a neural tube defect. It is also possible, by culturing embryos from mutant strains, to study the interaction of an embryo's genotype with the controlled *in vitro* environment (Copp et al 1982) and thus to throw further light on teratological and normal developmental mechanisms.

In this review we shall attempt to give a brief outline of what is involved in the culture of postimplantation mammalian embryos, and to highlight some technical and analytical aspects which may be relevant to a broad range of *in vitro* teratological investigations.

PRACTICAL ASPECTS

Species

Postimplantation embryo culture techniques have been applied to several species (see New 1978 for review) but for teratological testing purposes the early head-fold (10th day) rat embryo (New et al 1976 a,b) and pre- or early somite (8th or 9th day) mouse embryo (Sadler 1979; Sadler & New 1981) have proved most valuable. For the rat the normality and extent of development obtained during at least 48 hours in culture is closely comparable with that obtained during the corresponding period *in vivo* (New et al 1976 b). The extent of development that may routinely be obtained with the head-fold rat embryo is illustrated in Fig. 1.

Results for the mouse are not quite so consistently good and both inter- and intra-litter variability are greater, but it may be the preferred species for certain studies because of its lower cost and the availability of a wide range of genetic variants. An example of the latter is the curly-tail mouse which has been used to study the ontogeny of neural tube defects (Copp et al. 1982).

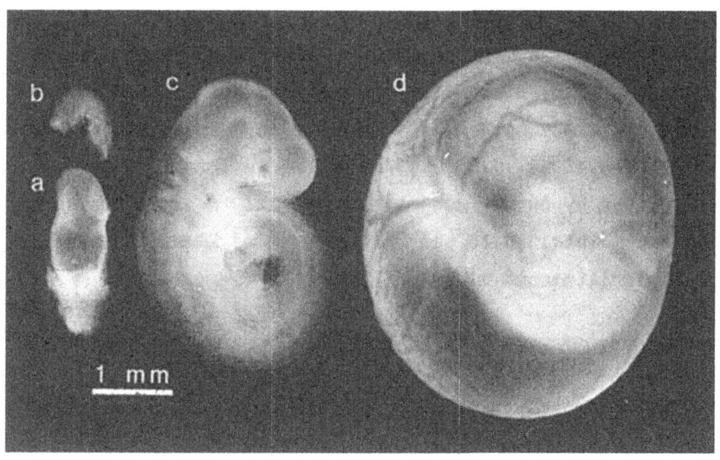

Figure 1. Development of head-fold (tenth day) rat embryos in culture. a) tenth day conceptus as placed in culture. b) dissection of tenth day conceptus to show embryonic portion. c) embryo explanted at stage shown in a,b, and cultured for 48h, followed by dissection from embryonic membranes. d) as c), but with membranes intact (i.e. as removed from culture). All embryos were littermates.

Preparation of Embryos for Culture

The explantation procedure for pre- or early somite embryos to be grown in culture has been described in detail previously (New 1971, Cockroft 1977). The uterus is opened in sterile saline (e.g. Tyrode's or Hanks') and the conceptuses separated from it. Working under a dissecting microscope the decidua surrounding each embryo is removed with watchmaker's forceps, and the parietal yolk sac (Reichert's membrane with adherent trophoblast and parietal endoderm cells) is opened, leaving the underlying visceral yolk sac intact. The ectoplacental cone (chorioallantoic placenta in older embryos) is not removed. The embryo is then ready to be placed in a culture bottle.

Culture Apparatus

The basic equipment for postimplantation embryo culture is quite simple. The main requirement is an incubator in which the embryos may be maintained at 37°C in bottles rotating at about 30 rpm. This may be achieved with sealed, gassed bottles placed on rollers (New et al 1973, Fig 2a) which are satisfactory for most purposes, or by one of a number of systems in which a constant supply of gas is maintained to the culture bottles (New & Cockroft 1979, Fig 2b; Tarlatzis et al 1984).

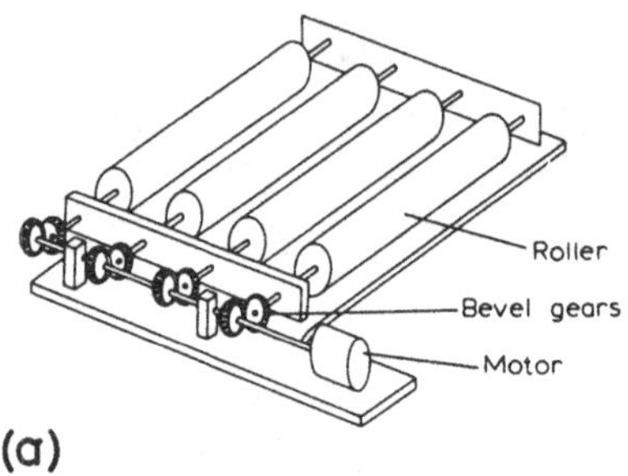

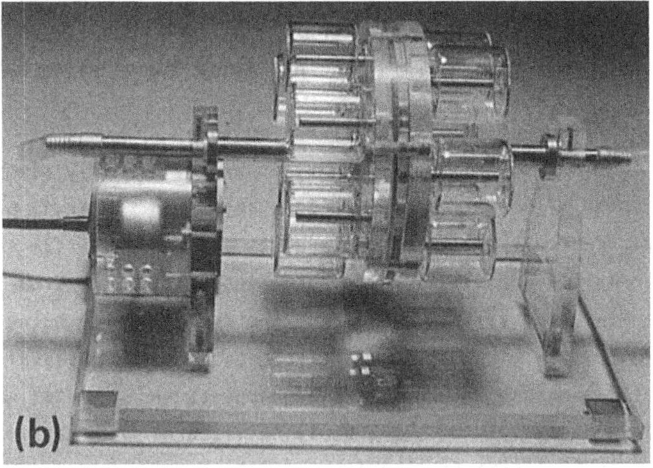

Figure 2. a) Schematic diagram of set of rollers for rotating sealed culture bottles. The rollers rotate at 30 rpm. b) Rotator apparatus which permits continuous gassing of culture bottles during rotation.

The latter systems are particularly advantageous for older embryos (12th day or more in the rat) because their greater oxygen requirements may thus be more readily met than with sealed culture vessels. Both roller and rotator systems suitable for postimplantation embryo culture are manufactured by BTC Engineering, Cambridge.

Two types of culture bottle suitable for intermittent gassing are illustrated in Fig. 3; with such glass bottles, very thorough cleaning is essential for good results. Disposable plastic vessels of suitable dimensions may also be used, though care should be taken that they are made of non toxic material and that they are gas tight.

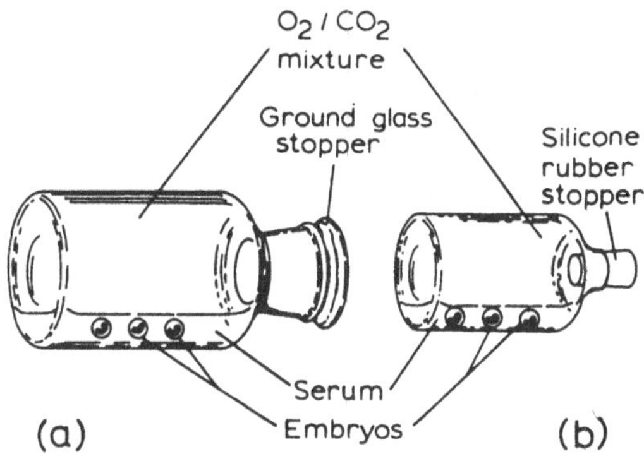

Figure 3. Two types of culture bottle containing embryos and culture medium.
a) 60 ml Pyrex bottle with glass stopper.
b) 30 ml bottle with silicone rubber stopper.

As a general guide, one tenth of the culture-vessel volume should be filled with culture medium, with the air in the remaining space being replaced with an appropriate gas mixture, and about 1 ml of culture medium should be allowed for each embryo of pre- or early somite stage. Hence, a 30 ml bottle would contain 3 ml of medium and 3 embryos.

Primitive-streak, head-fold, or early somite embryos are gassed initially with 5% O_2, 5% CO_2, 90% N_2, which is increased to 20% O_2, 5% CO_2, 75% N_2 when the embryo has around 15 somites (11th day in the rat, 10th day in the mouse). Cultures will often not be maintained for more than a further day, but if they are, 40% or 95% O_2 will be necessary. Detailed gassing schedules for the rat may be found in New et al 1976 a; Cockroft 1977, and for the mouse in Sadler 1979; Sadler and New 1981.

Media and Reagents

Although various combinations of human serum and human cord serum have been used as culture media (Chatot et al 1980, Herken & Hsu 1983), these can prove toxic (Steele 1985 b). The most consistently normal development for both rat and mouse postimplantation embryo culture is obtained using rat serum, prepared by centrifugation immediately after withdrawal from the donor, as the basic culture medium (Steele & New 1974; New et al 1976 a).

Serum prepared in this way (IC rat serum) is not, as far as we are aware, available commercially, so it is necessary for workers to prepare their own. This is in any case desirable, due to the variable quality and high cost of commercial serum. The procedure, briefly, is to anaesthetise the rat with ether, open the abdomen, and to withdraw blood gently (to avoid haemolysis) from the dorsal aorta with a 10 or 20 ml syringe and 0.8 or 1.1 x 40 mm needle. The blood is then placed in a 15 ml centrifuge tube and transferred as rapidly as possible to a bench centrifuge where it is spun at 3000 rpm for at least 5 minutes. This will bring down the blood cells and a fibrin clot will form in the supernatant. The clot is squeezed to remove contained serum, and the tube re-centrifuged, after which the supernatant is decanted, antibiotics added, and the serum stored frozen at -20°C.

Before use the serum is heat-inactivated at 56°C for 30 minutes and whilst it is hot it is advisable to gas it (with whatever mixture will be used for the subsequent culture) to drive off any residual ether.

For the culture of rat embryos pure rat serum may be used or it may be diluted with up to 50% balanced salt solution (Cockroft & Coppola 1977; Tuckett & Morriss-Kay 1985). By contrast, pure rat serum seems to be toxic to eighth-day mouse embryos, which grow better in 50% DMEM, 50% rat serum (Lawson et al 1986). However, older mouse embryos are best cultured in pure rat serum. These media are suitable for many testing purposes, but for more detailed investigative studies, a fully defined medium is highly desirable; unfortunately, however, such a formulation has not yet been developed.

Some success has nevertheless been achieved with partially defined media (Gunberg 1976; Cockroft 1979; Freeman et al 1981), using extensively dialysed rat serum supplemented with vitamins, amino acids and glucose. Further details of the performance of these media will be given in section 3, but because some laboratories have apparently had problems with serum dialysis, further technical details of Cockroft's procedure will be given here.

Visking dialysis tubing (Scientific Instrument Centre Ltd, Eastleigh, Hampshire) has proved consistently reliable. It has a nominal exclusion size of 12-14,000 daltons. All dialysis tubing should be regarded as toxic as supplied, so it is very important to rinse it thoroughly before use. This may most conveniently and effectively be achieved by placing a length of the dialysis tubing, straight, in a measuring cylinder and running tap water down the centre for 24 hours, followed by several, prolonged rinses in distilled water. The serum (IC rat serum) is dialysed in batches of 25-35 ml, and sufficient tubing (at least twice that necessary to contain the original serum volume) should be allowed for the serum to expand during dialysis, as it will do since the recommended balanced salt solution for dialysis (see Cockroft 1979 for formula) has a lower osmolarity than does serum. Naturally, all air should be excluded from the tubing before the final sealing. The serum is dialysed for four days at 4°C against four changes of constantly stirred balanced salt solution, each change being of 500 ml. Because plastic-coated magnetic stirring rods may release toxic substances, it is preferable to use one encased in glass - easily made by sealing a length of iron nail in glass tube. To allow this to rotate freely without interference from the dialysis bag, the latter is supported on a grid made of bent glass rod.

Similar caution about introduction of toxic substances makes it advisable to knot the ends of the dialysis tubing (doubly) rather than use any of the plastic fittings made for this purpose. Although everything else may be sterilized, it is not necessary to sterilize the dialysis tubing, and probably not desirable owing to possible effects of the process on the tubing pore size. Provided that reasonable cleanliness is observed, no problems with infections should be encountered.

To achieve normal embryonic growth, vitamins and amino acids in the formulations for Eagle's Minimal Essential Medium (MEM, Flow Laboratories) and 1.5 mg/ml glucose should be added to the dialysed serum just before use.

Assays

The assays most frequently used in the assessment of postimplantation embryos are growth, usually measured by total protein (Lowry et al, 1951) or by crown-rump length; somite counts; persistence of a heart beat or, more critically, of a blood circulation; and frequency and type of developmental anomalies.

In teratological terms, gross anomalies which *in vivo* would undoubtedly be lethal are of limited interest. Hence morphological analyses which include and categorise more subtle defects such as slight reductions in the size of parts of the brain, or defects of the eyes (Cockroft & New 1978, Cockroft 1984) are to be preferred. In more general terms, a morphological scoring system which takes into account all the most significant developmental parameters of an embryo may be valuable (Brown & Fabro 1981).

EXPERIMENTAL EXAMPLES

Clearly, the possible range of uses and responses of *in vitro* teratological testing is very great, and a variety of protocols and approaches have been discussed by Steele (1985a) and Brown & Fabro (1982). However, this review will concentrate on just three aspects:

(a) the importance of the timing of exposure to a potential teratogen,

(b) the detection of defects not obvious on visual examination, and

(c) embryonic development in partially defined media.

a) Timing of exposure

Prolonged exposure in culture to high levels of D-glucose has previously been shown to cause a high incidence of anomalies in the embryos of both rats (Cockroft & Coppola 1977) and mice (Sadler 1980). The action of this substance on primitive-streak and head-fold stage rat embryos in culture may be used to illustrate the effects of brief exposure to a teratogen at slightly different stages of development (Cockroft 1984).

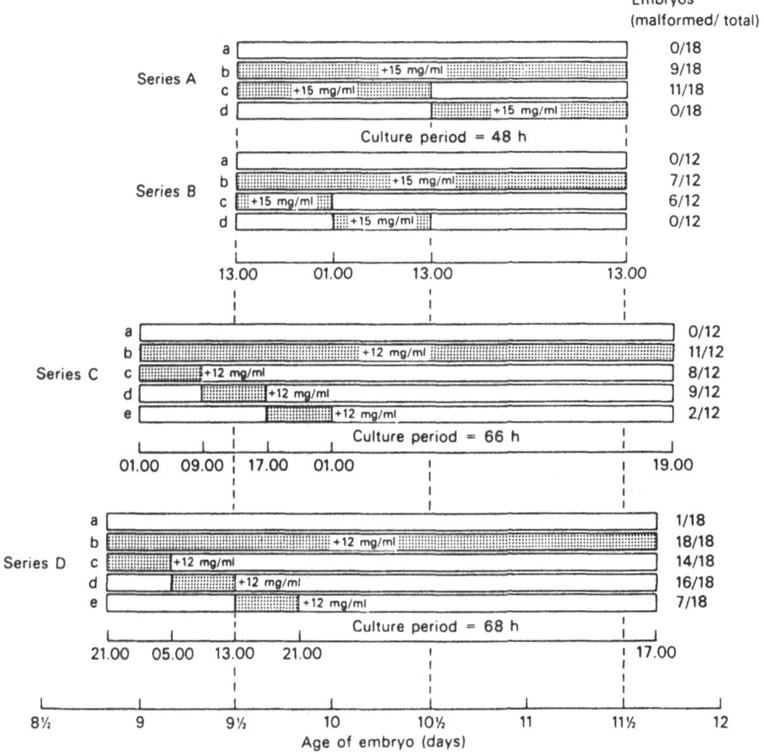

Figure 4. Diagram summarising the results of exposing rat embryos in culture to elevated glucose levels for various periods (hatched in diagram). Periods at normal glucose levels are represented by white bars. (From Cockroft 1984, by permission of the British Journal of Experimental Pathology).

Figure 4 summarises the effect of briefly raising the glucose concentration in the culture medium of rat embryos explanted at precise times between the 9th and 10th day of gestation. In series A, 24h exposure to 15 mg/ml for the first half of a 48h culture had as great a deleterious effect on the embryos as exposure for the entire culture period, whereas elevating the glucose concentration by the same amount during the second half of the culture did not cause malformations.

In series B, it was found that 15 mg/ml glucose for just the first 12h of a 48h culture caused abnormalities in half the embryos, whilst all the embryos thus exposed during the second 12h were normal.

In series C, the embryos were explanted 12h earlier and cultured for 66h, and glucose concentrations were raised by 12 mg/ml for the first, second, or third 8h of culture. Embryos exposed for the first or second 8h periods were mostly malformed, whereas only two of those exposed for the third 8h period were affected. In order to test whether the similar malformation rates in the first and second 8h periods in these cultures reflected a maximum sensitivity of the embryos at the arbitrarily chosen changeover time between these two periods (i.e. 09.00h) or simply a prolonged period of sensitivity, the cultures in series D were started 4h earlier than in series C. The cultures were for a total of 68h, and again exposure to 12 mg/ml exogenous glucose was for the first, second, or third 8h. In this case, the raised glucose levels again had their greatest effect in the first and second 8h periods, with relatively little action in the third 8h period.

In general, therefore, the sensitivity of the embryos to glucose increases with earlier exposure to the teratogen. However, the malformation rate in the second 8h period in both series C and D was slightly higher than in the first 8h, and thus against this trend, suggesting that the latter part of the morning of the tenth day may be, for the rat embryo, a time of particular sensitivity to hyperglycaemia.

Detailed analyses of the anomalies induced in these studies showed that later and more prolonged exposure to high glucose levels (i.e. series A and B) produced very severe malformations in the affected embryos - principally abnormal fusion of the anterior and posterior neural folds to each other, giving the embryo a squirrel-like appearance. It is very unlikely that such embryos would be viable in vivo. However, shorter exposures to lower glucose levels earlier in development (i.e. series C and D) resulted in relatively minor anomalies, principally of the eyes (reduction, malformation or absence) which were affected in two thirds of the embryos exposed to raised glucose levels for the first or second 8h of the cultures in series C and D, but only one sixth of the embryos exposed for the third 8h. The other most common anomaly was microcephaly, which usually manifested itself as reduction of the mid-brain, and this was again most frequently observed in embryos exposed to 12 mg/ml glucose for the first or second 8h of the cultures in series C and D. Similar eye and brain defects could also be induced in embryos cultured over the same 66h period as in series C (i.e. from 01.00h on the tenth day) and exposed to only 6-9 mg/ml exogenous glucose, but throughout the culture period.

These studies thus show that in vitro it is possible to arrange brief and accurately controlled exposure of embryos at known developmental stages to teratogens, and that their response may differ markedly with quite small changes in the conditions of exposure.

b) Detection of Defects

Temporary elevation of deep body temperature resulting from environmental influences or fever occurs in many species, including man. Such hyperthermia may often be harmless, but in the pregnant female it has been implicated as a cause of congenital defects (Edwards & Wanner 1977).

In a study of the effects of hyperthermia on rat embryos in culture (Cockroft & New 1978) it was found that the majority of head-fold embryos cultured for 48h at 40.5 or 41.0°C were grossly abnormal and retarded (Fig. 5). Embryos cultured at 40.0°C, however, were very similar in all respects (i.e. protein content, crown-rump length and somite number) to the controls incubated at 38.0°C and only one out of eighteen was abnormal, with microcephaly. To investigate whether a more widespread effect of culture at 40.0°C could be

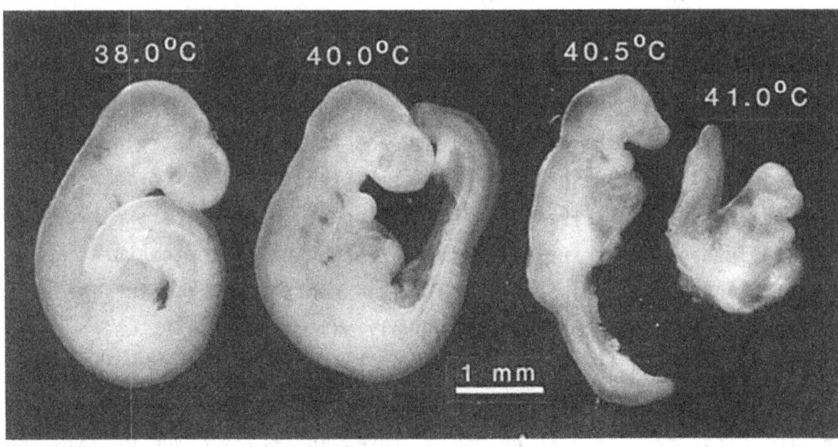

Figure 5. Rat embryos explanted on the tenth day of gestation and cultured for 48h at temperatures of 38-41°C. The general appearance of the embryos cultured at 38 and 40°C is very similar, whilst the embryo cultured at 40.5°C is retarded and abnormal. In the embryo cultured at 41°C, the neural folds of the anterior trunk have partially fused with those of the posterior trunk, and the embryo is also very retarded. (From Cockroft & New 1978).

detected, two further series of experiments were undertaken. In the first, the heads of embryos cultured at 38.0°C and 40.0°C were separated by cutting along a line running just above the auditory vesicle and the mandible (Fig. 6) and the head and body protein contents were determined separately. For each embryo a head/embryo protein ratio was then calculated.

Each embryo cultured at 40.0°C was paired with a control with a similar (within 5 μg) total protein content, and the mean head/embryo protein ratios at the two temperatures were calculated and compared by paired-comparison Student's t-test.

Table 1 - Comparisons of head/embryo protein content ratios of groups of rat embryos matched for total protein content after culture at 38 and 40°C (From Cockroft & New 1978)

Temperature	No. of embryos	Total embryo protein (μg ± SE)	Head/embryo protein ratio (± SE)
38°C	18	167 ± 9	0.295 ± 0.003
40°C	18	167 ± 9	0.278 ± 0.005
			$P < 0.02$

As shown in Table 1, eighteen embryos cultured at each temperature were matched in this way and it can be seen from the standard errors of the means that the head/embryo protein ratio at each temperature was remarkably constant. Moreover, the ratio at 40.0°C was significantly lower than at 38.0°C ($P<0.02$).

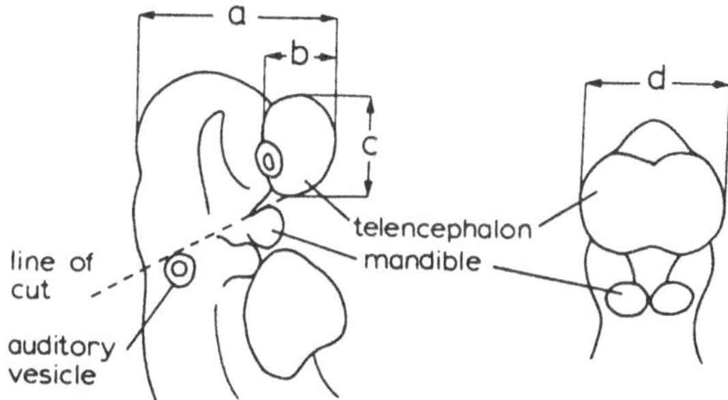

Figure 6. Diagrams showing side view (left) and front view (right) of head region of rat embryo explanted on the tenth day of gestation and grown in culture for 48h. The diagrams show the position of the cut made for separate head and body protein determinations, and the four head dimensions that were measured: a) head length; b) length of telencephalon; c) height of telencephalon; d) width across telencephalon. (From Cockroft & New 1978).

This phenomenon was investigated further by making measurements of various head dimensions, shown in Fig. 6, of embryos cultured at 38.0°C and 40.0°C, and again pairing embryos cultured at the two temperatures, this time on the basis of similar crown rump lengths (within 0.1 mm). The results are shown in Table 2, the length and the height of the telencephalon were found to be significantly less at 40.0°C than at 38.0°C (at $P<0.02$) and so was the length of the head ($P<0.01$). There was no difference, however, in the width of the telencephalon of embryos cultured at the two temperatures.

Thus with suitable analytical techniques it has proved possible to detect statistically defects which could only be suspected in individual embryos.

c) Development in semi-defined media

Table 3 and Figs 7 and 8 show the development of head-fold rat embryos cultured for 48h in whole serum and in extensively dialysed serum containing various combinations of glucose, pyruvate, vitamins, and amino acids.

It can be seen in part A of the table, in which all the dialysed sera were supplemented with vitamins and amino acids, that further supplementation with glucose alone was sufficient to achieve normal growth and differentiation, comparable with that obtained in whole serum. Addition of pyruvate with glucose was detrimental to the embryos, and pyruvate as the sole energy source supported very little development. In part B of the table, all the dialysed sera were supplemented with glucose, and further supplementation with vitamins produced normal growth and differentiation, comparable with development in whole serum. Addition of amino acids with vitamins also gave good development, but amino acids alone supported very little growth.

Further studies were also undertaken in which embryos were cultured in dialysed serum containing glucose and amino acids, but only one vitamin, or in media in which individual vitamins were omitted from otherwise fully-supplemented dialysed serum (Cockroft 1979). These demonstrated that of the eight vitamins present in

Table 2 - Comparison of head dimensions of groups of rat embryos matched for crown-rump length after culture at 38 and 40°C (From Cockroft & New 1978)

Temperature	No. of embryos	Crown-rump (mm ± SE)	(a) length of head (mm ± SE)	(b) length of telencephalon (mm ± SE)	(c) height of telencephalon (mm ± SE)	(d) width of telencephalon (mm ± SE)
38°C	22	3.19 ± 0.04	1.52 ± 0.04	0.63 ± 0.02	0.73 ± 0.02	1.03 ± 0.03
40°C	22	3.19 ± 0.04	1.42 ± 0.02	0.57 ± 0.01	0.66 ± 0.01	1.03 ± 0.02
			$P < 0.01$	$P < 0.02$	$P < 0.02$	

For details of measurements see Figure 6.

Eagle's MEM, only four were necessary for good development. Pantothenic acid had the greatest beneficial effect on growth and differentiation of the embryos, and riboflavin also had a general, though lesser beneficial effect. Inositol did not affect growth, but did prevent failure of closure of the neural tube, whereas the main effect of folic acid was to improve growth.

Thus, although a fully defined medium is not yet attainable, it is possible by dialysis to define and manipulate the micromolecular component of the culture medium for rat embryos.

DISCUSSION

In the preceding sections we have outlined some methods in postimplantation embryo culture and given some examples of their versatility. What remains to be discussed is the extent to which such techniques should supplement or replace more traditional teratological methods. We have already suggested that the greatest contribution that whole embryo culture can make to teratology is likely to be in the detailed investigation of the mechanism of action of substances which have previously been shown to produce malformations *in vivo*. In such studies, the great control afforded by *in vitro* systems outweighs considerations of cost and time, both of which may be greater than for *in vivo* tests.

As discussed in greater detail by Freeman & Steele (1985), embryo culture has few advantages for large scale pre-screening tests (on more than about 5 compounds, say) where cost and time are likely to be the prime considerations. For extensive tests of this type, it is more practicable to use methods such as the micromass cell culture technique described in the chapter by O.P. Flint in this volume. On a smaller scale however, whole embryo culture is being used as a prescreen in teratogenic testing in contract laboratories (Newall et al 1984).

For routine regulatory testing too, embryo culture is not usually considered to be the most suitable approach; it is not clear to what extent *in vitro* tests are predictive of clinical teratogenicity and consequently such techniques do not fall within the

Table 3 - Mean ± s.e.m. protein contents, somite numbers and crown-rump lengths of pre-somite rat embryos cultured for 48h in whole rat serum, or dialysed serum supplemented with various combinations of glucose, pyruvate, vitamins and amino acids (From Cockroft 1979, by permission of the Journal of Reproduction and Fertility)

	No. of embryos	Protein (ug)	No. of somites	Crown-rump length (mm)
(A) Whole serum	12	158 ± 13	26.5 ± 0.3	3.36 ± 0.11
Dialysed serum Δ	12	11 ± 1*	-	0.68 ± 0.03*
Dialysed serum Δ + glucose	12	153 ± 10	26.9 ± 0.3	3.28 ± 0.08
Dialysed serum Δ + glucose + pyruvate	12	108 ± 6*	23.1 ± 0.7*	2.67 ± 0.07*
Dialysed serum Δ + pyruvate	12	28 ± 5*	-	0.62 ± 0.02*
(B) Whole serum	18	177 ± 8	26.4 ± 0.2	3.23 ± 0.07
Dialysed serum ϴ	18	44 ± 6*	-	1.51 ± 0.17*
Dialysed serum ϴ + vitamins	18	172 ± 9	26.1 ± 0.5	3.15 ± 0.08
Dialysed serum ϴ + vitamins + amino acids	18	185 ± 6	27.1 ± 0.2	3.38 ± 0.04
Dialysed serum ϴ + amino acids	18	53 ± 5*	-	1.79 ± 0.15*

* Significantly different from value with whole serum, $P < 0.001$
Δ Including amino acids and vitamins
ϴ Containing 1.5 mg glucose/ml

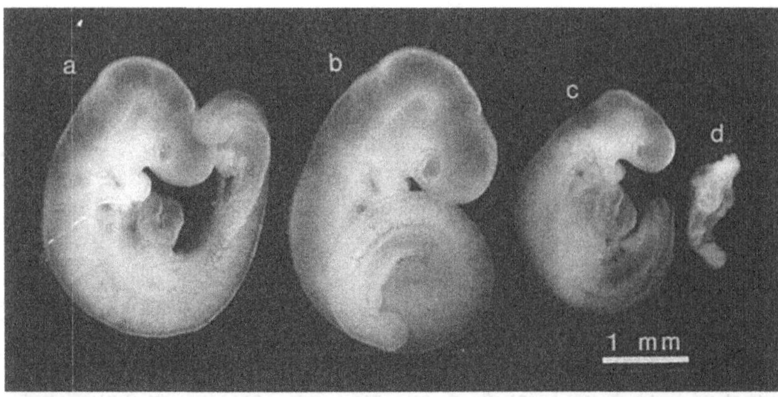

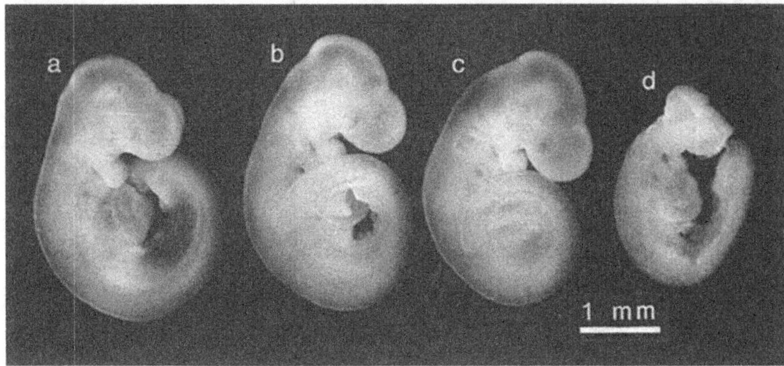

Figure 7. Rat embryos explanted on the tenth day of gestation and cultured for 48h in a) whole rat serum; b) dialysed serum + glucose; c) dialysed serum + glucose + pyruvate; d) dialysed serum + pyruvate. The dialysed sera were also supplemented with vitamins and amino acids. (From Cockroft 1979, by permission of the Journal of Reproduction and Fertility).

Figure 8. Rat embryos explanted on the tenth day of gestation and cultured for 48h in a) whole rat serum; b) dialysed serum + vitamins + amino acids; c) dialysed serum + vitamins; d) dialysed serum + amino acids. The dialysed sera were also supplemented with glucose. (From Cockroft 1979, by permission of the Journal of Reproduction and Fertility).

Government guidelines for teratogenic testing. Nevertheless, from considering the choice of test species, a scientific argument can be made for more extensive use (and regulatory acceptance) of *in vitro* tests. Animals whose physiological and developmental patterns are most similar to man, such as pigs or primates, are extremely expensive, and their use in *in vivo* tests can only be justified in very special cases, such as the testing of substances to which it is known that pregnant women will be exposed - e.g. drugs to relieve morning sickness. In practice therefore, the animals most commonly used for teratogenic testing - rats, mice and rabbits - have come to be chosen mainly from considerations of cost and convenience (i.e. small size, easy breeding, short gestation period, large litters and ease of handling). Postimplantation embryo culture works best with rats and mice, and the use of these species means that, as _in vivo_, large numbers of embryos may be easily and cheaply obtained. _In vitro_, however, there is the additional possibility of adjusting the conditions to more closely resemble the human state, especially if something is known of the metabolism of the test substance.

An idea of what can be achieved physiologically in this respect is provided by the work of Fantel et al (1979) who showed that the activating action of the human liver on cyclophosphamide could be mimicked _in vitro_ by the addition of liver microsomes, NADPH and glucose-6-phosphate to the culture medium of rat embryos. These substances mediated the biotransformation of cyclophosphamide to a teratogenic form, whereas the drug had no effect on embryos cultured in the absence of the activating system. Further studies by Shepard et al (1983) have shown that some substances may be activated _in vitro_, some inactivated and some unaffected. In the particular instance of cyclophosphamide, Klein et al (1980) showed that activation could also be achieved in rats _in vivo_, as serum prepared from animals dosed with the substance was teratogenic, whereas cyclophosphamide added directly _in vitro_ produced no malformations, in agreement with the findings of Fantel et al (1979). The use of embryo culture in combination with an _in vitro_ activation system would be particularly valuable in the testing of substances that might be activated in humans, but not in the commonly used test animals _in vivo_.

Developmentally, the most striking difference between man and the favoured _in vivo_ test species - rats, mice and rabbits - is that the latter all possess an otherwise unique extraembryonic structure, the inverted yolk sac placenta. This provides an alternative and possibly easier route for transmission of drugs to the embryo than via the chorioallantoic placenta, but conversely it may also have a protective function, as it has been shown to sequester certain substances whose transmission to the embryo is thus prevented (Wilson et al 1959; Beck et al 1967). Unfortunately the visceral yolk sac cannot be dispensed with *in vitro* as its placental functions are vital for good development, and it also appears to play an essential role in mediating embryonic nutrition (Freeman et al 1981). However, *in vitro* the great accessibility of the explanted embryos allows precise localisation of the site of administration of a test substance, as has been demonstrated with yolk sac antibody (New & Brent 1972) and phosphoramide mustard (Satish et al 1985), so again there is the possibility of adjusting the *in vitro* rodent condition to mimic that of the human.

Much work still needs to be done to validate whole embryo culture as a routine teratological screening method. However, some *in vitro*/*in vivo* comparisons have produced encouraging results. For example Schmid et al (1983) cultured tenth-day rat embryos for 48h in forty different compounds and compared the results with those obtained for the same compounds *in vivo*. In each system, half the compounds were shown to be teratogenic, and half were not, but only one of the forty compounds gave different results *in vitro* from *in vivo*. However, most of the *in vivo* data were taken from the literature, so this study cannot be considered definitive. A more exhaustive series of validation tests has been proposed (Smith et al 1983), but has yet to be brought to fruition.

A number of studies have combined *in vivo* administration of a teratogen with subsequent explantation and culture of the embryos, thereby ensuring that the drug initially reaches the embryos in the form and by the route that occurs *in vivo*. For example, Steele et al (1983) treated pregnant rats with retinoic acid on the ninth day of gestation and explanted the embryos from one uterine horn of each dosed animal 26h later, whilst the embryos in the contralateral horn were allowed to continue their development *in vivo*. The explanted embryos were cultured for 48h in normal serum and then compared with their littermates *in utero*. It was found that the frequency and types of malformations induced by retinoic acid were very similar for the *in vitro* and *in vivo* groups, suggesting that the fundamental lesion was already present in the relatively undifferentiated embryos at the time of explantation, even though the abnormalities manifested themselves in organ systems which developed during culture.

In a broadly similar study, Beaudoin & Fisher (1981) treated pregnant rats with a range of compounds before explanting the embryos and growing them in culture. These workers found that the correlation between the types of malformations then seen _in vitro_ and those reported previously for the same compounds _in vivo_ was less good than in the study by Steele et al (1983). However, Beaudoin & Fishers' study was less well controlled, because the _in vivo_ data were taken from the literature, rather than from littermates. Other factors that may have influenced the results were that the _in vivo_ treatment of the embryos subsequently grown _in vitro_ was at a later stage, when sensitivity may have been lower, and the culture medium used (fetal calf serum and Waymouth's medium) is inferior to I.C. rat serum. Even so, all the compounds known to be teratogenic _in vivo_ showed some deleterious effect _in vitro_ in this study.

The main disadvantages of whole embryo culture are the limited range of stages to which it is applicable and the maximum culture period of a few days. Fortunately, the stages which grow best encompass the main processes of organogenesis, but the restrictions on culture period mean that effects may only be seen with unphysiological doses of test substances, and care may need to be exercised to detect other than gross malformations. A final point that needs to be made concerns the normality of control cultures: with careful application of the techniques outlined earlier to head-fold rat embryos, a malformed control embryo after 48h in culture should be a rare and remarkable event. If this is not so, something is wrong and cleaning and preparative procedures particularly should be scrupulously examined for the source of the problem.

CONCLUSIONS

In conclusion we hope this review has shown that _in vitro_ teratological testing is a powerful, flexible and sensitive technique, and one whose value is further increased when it is used in conjunction with other established methods and with an understanding of the physiological and biochemical implications of the system.

ACKNOWLEDGEMENTS

Financial support for the experiments described in this chapter was provided by the Medical Research Council (U.K.). We are grateful to Dr. D.A.T. New for his valuable comments on this manuscript.

REFERENCES

Beaudoin, A.R. & Fisher, D.L. (1981). An _in vivo/in vitro_ evaluation of teratogenic action. Teratology, 23, 57-61.

Beck, F., Lloyd, J.B. & Griffiths, A. (1967). A histochemical and biochemical study of some aspects of placental function in the rat, using maternal injections of horseradish peroxidase. J. Anat., 101, 461-478.

Brown, N.A. & Fabro, S. (1981). Quantitation of rat embryonic development _in vitro_: a morphological scoring system. Teratology, 24, 65-78.

Brown, N.A. & Fabro, S.E. (1982). The _in vitro_ approach to teratogenicity testing. In Developmental Toxicology, ed. K. Snell. New York: Praeger Publishers.

Buckley, S.K.L., Steele, C.E. & New, D.A.T. (1978). _In vitro_ development of early postimplantation rat embryos. Devl. Biol., 65, 396-403.

Chatot, C.L., Klein, N.W., Piatek, J. & Pierro, L.J. (1980). Successful culture of rat embryos on human serum: use in the detection of teratogens. Science, 207, 1471-1473.

Cockroft, D.L. (1973). Development in culture of rat foetuses explanted at 12.5 and 13.5 days of gestation. J. Embryol. exp. Morph., 29, 473-483.

Cockroft, D.L. (1977). Postimplantation embryo culture. In Methods in Prenatal Toxicology, Eds. D. Neubert, H.J. Merker & T.E. Kwasigroch pp 231-240. Stuttgart: Georg Thieme.

Cockroft, D.L. & Coppola, P.T. (1977). Teratogenic effects of excess glucose on head-fold rat embryos in culture. Teratology, 16, 141-146.

Cockroft, D.L. & New D.A.T. (1978). Abnormalities induced in cultured rat embryos by hyperthermia. Teratology, 17, 277-284.

Cockroft, D.L. (1979). Nutrient requirements of rat embryos undergoing organogenesis _in vitro_. J. Reprod. Fert., 57, 505-510.

Cockroft, D.L. (1984). Abnormalities induced in cultured rat embryos by hyperglycaemia. Br. J. exp. Path., 65, 625-636.

Copp, A.J., Seller, M.J. & Polani, P.E. (1982). Neural tube development in mutant (curly tail) and normal mouse embryos: the timing of posterior neuropore closure _in vivo_ and _in vitro_. J. Embryol. exp. Morph., 69, 151-167.

Edwards, M.J. & Wanner, R.A. (1977). Extremes of temperature. In Handbook of Teratology, eds. J.G. Wilson & F.C. Fraser. Vol. 1, pp. 421-444. New York: Plenum Press.

Fantel, A.G., Greenaway, J.C., Juchau, M.R. & Shepard, T.H. (1979). Teratogenic bioactivation of cyclophosphamide _in vitro_. Life Sci., 25, 67-72.

Freeman, S.J., Beck, F. & Lloyd, J.B. (1981). The role of the visceral yolk sac in mediating protein utilization by rat embryos cultured _in vitro_. J. Embryol. exp. Morph., 66, 223-234.

Freeman, S.J. & Steele, C.E. (1986). Post implantation whole embryo culture and the study of teratogenesis. Fd. chem. Toxicol., (in press).

Gunberg, D.L. (1976). _In vitro_ development of postimplantation rat embryos cultured on dialysed rat serum. Teratology, 14, 65-70.

Herken, R. & Hsu, Y-C. (1983). Development of mouse embryos grown in human cord serum (HCS) in vitro. Anat. Embryol., 168, 137-150.

Klein, N.W., Vogler, M.A., Chatot, C.L. & Pierro, L.J. (1980). The use of cultured rat embryos to evaluate the teratogenic activity of serum: cadmium and cyclophosphamide. Teratology, 21, 199-208.

Lawson, K.A., Meneses, J.J. & Pedersen, R.A. (1986). Cell fate and cell lineage in the endoderm of the presomite mouse embryo, studied with an intracellular tracer. Devl. Biol. 115, 325-339.

Lowry, O.H., Rosebrough, N.J., Farr, A.L. & Randall, R.J. (1951). Protein measurement with the Folin phenol reagent. J. biol. Chem., 193, 265-275.

New, D.A.T. (1967). Development of explanted rat embryos in circulating medium. J. Embryol. exp. Morph. 17, 513-525.

New, D.A.T. (1971). Methods for the culture of postimplantation embryos of rodents. In Methods in Mammalian Embryology, ed. J.C. Daniel, ch. 22, pp 305-319. San Francisco: Freeman.

New, D.A.T. & Brent, R.L. (1972). Effect of yolk-sac antibody on rat embryos grown in culture. J. Embryol. exp. Morph., 27, 543-553.

New, D.A.T., Coppola, P.T. & Terry, S. (1973). Culture of explanted rat embryos in rotating tubes. J. Reprod. Fert., 35, 135-138.

New, D.A.T., Coppola, P.T. & Cockroft, D.L. (1976a). Improved development of head-fold rat embryos in culture resulting from low oxygen and modifications of the culture serum. J. Reprod. Fert., 48, 219-222.

New, D.A.T., Coppola, P.T. & Cockroft, D.L. (1976b). Comparison of growth in vitro and in vivo of postimplantation rat embryos. J. Embryol. exp. Morph., 36, 133-144.

New, D.A.T. (1978). Whole-embryo culture and the study of mammalian embryos during organogenesis. Biol. Rev., 53, 81-122.

New, D.A.T. & Cockroft, D.L. (1979). A rotating bottle culture method with continuous replacement of the gas phase. Experientia, 35, 138-139.

Newall, D.R., McAnulty, P.A., Tesh, J.M. (1984). Embryo culture as a screen for teratogenic potential. Presentation by Life Science Research, Suffolk, England, at the European Teratology Society Annual Conference, Veldhoven, The Netherlands.

Robkin, M., Shepard, T.H. & Baum, D. (1974). Autonomic drug effects on the heart rate of early rat embryos. Teratology, 9, 35-44.

Sadler, T.W. (1979). Culture of early somite mouse embryos during organogenesis. J. Embryol. exp. Morph., 49, 17-25.

Sadler, T.W. (1980). Effect of maternal diabetes on early embryogenesis: II Hyperglycaemia-induced exencephaly. Teratology 21, 349-356.

Sadler, T.W. & New, D.A.T. (1981). Culture of mouse embryos during neurulation. J. Embryol. exp. Morph., 66, 109-116.

Satish, J., Pratt, B.M. & Sanyal, M.K. (1985). Differential dysmorphogenesis induced by micro-injection of an alkylating agent into rat conceptuses cultured in vitro. Teratology, 31, 61-72.

Schmid, B.P., Trippmacher, A. & Bianchi, A. (1983). Validation of the whole embryo culture method for in vitro teratogenicity testing. Dev. Toxicol. Environ. Sci., 11, 563-566.

Shepard, T.H., Fantel, A.G., Mirkes, P.E. Greenaway, J.C., Faustman-Watts, E., Campbell, M. & Juchau, M.R. (1983).

Teratology testing: I. Development and status of short-term prescreens. II. Biotransformation of teratogens as studied in whole embryo culture. Prog. Clin. Biol. Res., 135, 147-164.

Smith, M.K., Kimmel, G.L., Kochhar, D.M., Shepard, T.H., Spielberg, S.P. & Wilson, J.G. (1983). A selection of candidate compounds for in vitro teratogenesis test validation. Teratogenesis Carcinog. Mutagen., 3, 461-480.

Steele, C.E. & New, D.A.T. (1974). Serum variants causing the formation of double hearts and other abnormalities in explanted rat embryos. J. Embryol. exp. Morph., 31, 709-719.

Steele, C.E., Trasler, D.G. & New, D.A.T. (1983). An in vivo/in vitro evaluation of the teratogenic action of excess vitamin A. Teratology, 28, 209-214.

Steele, C.E. (1985a). The role of postimplantation mammalian embryo culture in the study of teratogenic mechanisms. Prog. Clin. Biol. Res., 163C, 271-276.

Steele, C.E. (1985b). Human serum as a culture medium for rat embryos. Experientia, 41, 1601-1603.

Tam, P.P.L. & Snow, M.H.L. (1980). The in vitro culture of primitive-streak-stage mouse embryos. J. Embryol. exp. Morph., 59, 131-143.

Tarlatzis, B.C., Sanyal, M.K., Biggers, W.J. & Naftolin, F. (1984). Continuous culture of the postimplantation rat conceptus. Biol. Reprod., 31, 415-426.

Tuckett, F. & Morriss-Kay, G.M. (1985). The kinetic behaviour of the cranial neural epithelium during neurulation in the rat. J. Embryol. exp. Morph., 85, 111-119.

Wilson, J.G., Beaudoin, A.R. & Free, H.J. (1959). Studies on the mechanism of teratogenic action of trypan blue. Anat. Rec., 133, 115-128.

SUB-MAMMALIAN AND SUB-VERTEBRATE MODELS IN TERATOGENICITY SCREENING

Stuart J. Freeman, PhD
SK&F Research Ltd., The Frythe, Welwyn, AL6 9AR, England

Nigel A. Brown, PhD
MRC Experimental Embryology & Teratology Unit,
Medical Research Council Laboratories,
Woodmansterne Road, Carshalton, SM5 4EF, England.

INTRODUCTION

The 'multi-tier' approach has been adopted in several areas of toxicity testing, particularly in screening for carcinogens and mutagens. The overall philosophy is to establish a range of test systems of increasing biological complexity, from quick simple pre-screens, such as the Ames test, to highly complex whole mammal tests. An individual test agent is directed through these tests according to test results, likely human exposure and use of the chemical. For example, an environmental pollutant that occurs in very low concentrations and to which human exposure is extremely low and which, by pre-screen, is demonstrably non-toxic, would probably not be referred for further testing. On the other hand, a toxic response elicited in a pre-screen would dictate that further more elaborate test procedures were called for. Similarly, further testing would probably be required of a chemical that, although non-toxic in pre-screen, was relatively abundant in the environment. The major reasons for taking this step-wise approach are that the whole mammal tests routinely used in the past are time-consuming, expensive, require great expertise and are wasteful of all resources, including experimental mammals. The number of untested chemicals far exceeds the capacity to test them by whole-mammal methods. Hence there is a need to reserve these tests for those agents identified by pre-screens as likely to constitute the greatest hazard to man.

The past ten years have seen the development of the multi-tier approach to tackle the problem of teratogenicity testing. Methods have been developed at all levels of complexity from whole pregnant mammal systems to isolated cells (see Brown & Freeman, 1984; Johnson, 1985 for review). In this chapter we consider test methods which have been proposed as first-level screens for teratogens which use sub-mammalian and sub-vertebrate species as the model system. The use of such models in mechanistic teratology studies (see Chapter by Cockcroft and Steele) and in monitoring ecological toxic hazards will not be discussed.

In establishing an *in vitro* screen it is essential to define the aims of the test and to satisfy certain basic design criteria. In teratogenic risk assessment, the three main aims are to provide estimates of the "teratogenic potential", "teratogenic potency" and "teratogenic hazard" of the test agent. These concepts, formulated and discussed in detail by Fabro *et al*. (1982) and Johnson (1981), are defined respectively as follows: Potential - the ability of a test agent, under any circumstances, to induce abnormal development; Potency - the dose or concentration of test agent required to induce abnormalities; Hazard - the ratio of teratogenic dose to general adult or maternally toxic dose.

Estimation of the latter parameter is arguably the most important aim of a pre-screen since it provides an indication of the specificity of the effect of the test agent on the developing organism. Many teratologists agree with 'Karnofsky's Law' that all agents theoretically possess some 'teratogenic potential'. An estimate of 'teratogenic potency' for final risk estimation must be generated from whole animal studies, rather than from *in vitro* tests although data from such tests is useful for comparative purposes.

It is often difficult for screens for teratogenicity that use isolated mammalian embryonic tissues or cells to provide an estimate of teratogenic hazard. In order to do so these tests would require additional data on general (adult) toxicity, and it is unclear which parameter, i.e. LD_{50}, LD_{10}, etc. is most appropriate for hazard estimation and how this data relates to an *in vitro* teratogenic dose. It is in this context that teratogenicity screens using lower animals, non-mammalian vertebrates and particularly invertebrates, may offer advantages, since both adult and embryonic forms can be studied '*in vitro*'.

Other criteria that apply to the use of an *in vitro* screen for teratogens have been described by several authors (Wilson 1978;

Brown & Fabro, 1982; Kimmel et al., 1982; Freeman & Steele, 1986). Essentially, the test must be practicable, that is simple, rapid, reliable and yield interpretable results, and should be well validated with a variety of agents of established teratogenic potential from whole animal studies.

SUB-MAMMALIAN EMBRYO ASSAYS

Chick Embryo Tests

In spite of the published view of the World Health Organization (WHO; 1967) that the chick embryo was unsuitable for the testing of agents for teratogenicity, the chick embryo has continued to be used in studies of experimental teratogenicity. Much of the WHO criticism was directed towards the high non-specific sensitivity of the chick model and hence the large number of false-positive results generated.

Since the WHO report was published, improvements in techniques (see below) and a recognition of the need for toxicological testing of a wider variety of chemicals has led to a greater acceptance of the chick model in teratogenicity screening.

In its most common form, the design of the test follows that outlined by Wilson (1978). Initially, a lethal dose (LD_{100}) of test agent is determined in 30h embryos by injection of several log dilutions of molar solution (group size of 10 eggs) into the sub-germinal yolk. The lowest dose killing all embryos in a group within 3 days is taken as the LD_{100}. Subsequently, fractions of the LD_{100} are administered to groups of sixty 30h fertile eggs, and embryos are assessed on day 10 of incubation. Control eggs are treated with an equal volume of the vehicle. At the dose level of test agent that produces approximately (within 10%) the same number of survivors as the control group, an increase in the percentage of survivors that are malformed indicates a teratogenic effect. When the incidence of malformation at this non-lethal dose is similar to controls, a negative teratogenic effect is scored. In this instance, the experiment is repeated and chicks are allowed to go to hatching. If hatchability, gross-appearance, locomotion and general behaviour in treated chicks does not differ from control, a negative embryotoxic effect is scored.

Inability of the test agent to induce abnormalities at doses equivalent to a reasonable multiple (e.g. 100 times) of levels to which humans are exposed is considered a negative test result. Otherwise, the test is positive, and referral of the test agent to higher levels of testing should be considered.

Using an essentially similar procedure to screen 80 food additives, it has been claimed (Verrett _et al._, 1980) that the chick embryo test is capable of estimating teratogenic potential and does not respond non-specifically to test agents. A refinement of the windowing technique used to expose embryos _in ovo_ (Fisher & Schoenwolf, 1983) has also helped to reduce the induction of non-specific dysmorphogenesis of embryos.

The chick embryo screening test (CHEST) technique developed by Jelinek (1977), quite different in design to the standard tests, also responded to WHO's criticism by using subjects of the same developmental stage (Hamburger-Hamilton Stage 10-11) and administering test agents by intra-amniotic rather than sub-germinal injection. The screen uses the development of the caudal morphogenetic system of the embryo as an index of embryotoxic effects. A small volume (usually 3μl) of test substance solution is injected directly below the caudal region of the embryo through a small window in the egg shell and embryonic development is allowed to continue for a further 24h. At this time, the length of the caudal trunk between the vitelline arteries and the tip of the tail is measured with the use of an eyepiece micrometer in the dissecting microscope to provide a quantitative estimate of embryotoxicity.

The test is relatively easy to perform, has a well-defined endpoint and is economical in terms of bóth time and money. A recent study (Jelinek _et al_; 1985) used a combined CHEST (so-called CHEST I) and standard chick embryo test (so-called CHEST II) to examine the embryotoxic effects of 130 compound. These compounds were biologically and chemically diverse and included industrial and agricultural chemicals (eg. acrylamide, benzidine, nitrovin), as well as pharmaceuticals: analgesics (eg. phenacetin, ibuprofen), antiarrhythmics (eg. cromipranol), antibiotics (eg. tetracycline), antihistaminics, antiparasitics, cytostatics (eg. aminopterin, cyclophosphamide), hormones and vitamins (eg. cortisone, retinoic acid), hypnotics (eg. hexobarbital), and psychotropic drugs (eg. diazepam). For 119 of these, a dose-response relationship was established and discrimination was possible between substances of high and low embryotoxicity, indicating that the test is able to predict teratogenic potency. Although many of these substances have not been studied in mammals, previous smaller scale studies (Jelinek & Rychter, 1979; Vesely et al; 1982) suggest that the screen is reasonably able to rank agents in order of their teratogenic potency in whole mammal systems. Further independent validation is required, however, to substantiate this claim.

Frog Embryo Teratogenesis Assay: Xenopus (FETAX)

The use of this amphibian model for teratogenicity screening has been developed by Dumont and colleagues (Dumont et al; 1982). Although much of its initial use has been concerned with ecotoxicological assessment of industrial wastes, its application has now been extended to include testing of pharmaceuticals and other chemicals.

The test uses blastula-stage embryos which are exposed to test substance for up to four days in static modified amphibian Ringer's (Schultz et al; 1984). At 24h intervals, embryos are examined and dead ones discarded. At the end of the four day test, the motility and pigmentation of tadpoles are scored on a scale from 0 for a lack of either of these parameters to +4, for normal development of these characteristics. In addition, data are collected concerning mortality, incidence, type and severity of malformations, stage of development reached, and embryo length.

Using these data, a quantitative measurement of abnormal development induced by the test agent is provided by the calculation of a teratogenic index, defined as the ratio of the LC_{50} (concentration lethal to 50% of embryos over 4 days) to the EC_{50} (concentration producing a 50% incidence of abnormality). Whilst this is not a true estimate of teratogenic hazard (due to the unknown relationship bewteen embryolethality and adult toxicity), it does provide some indication of the ability of a compound to specifically subvert development without necessarily inducing large scale embryo cell death and hence lethality.

In a preliminary validation of FETAX, reported without data in abstract form (Dumont & Epler, 1984) 34 known mammalian teratogens and 6 compounds thought not to be teratogenic in mammals were tested. A teratogenic index of greater than 1 was considered as positive identification of a teratogen. On this basis, more than 90% of teratogens were correctly identified. However, the yield of false positive results, admittedly based on a sample size of only 6, was greater than 10%.

The further and independent validation required to substantiate the claims of FETAX as an alternative teratogenicity screen is in hand (Courchesne & Bantle, 1985; Sabourin et al., 1985). There can be no doubt that it is an inexpensive and rapid assay, and furthermore, the variety of endpoints, even though some are rather subjective, may increase its ability to detect teratogens.

Other tests that use amphibian subjects have been reported (Birge et al., 1983; Dumpert & Zietz, 1984; Fulton & Chambers, 1985). The application of these tests has so far been confined to ecological toxicity testing, although there is no reason why they could not also be used in estimation of teratogenic risk of drugs and industrial chemicals.

SUB-VERTEBRATE ASSAYS

Drosophila Test

The use of the intact Drosphila embryo as a test subject in teratogenicity screening has been proposed by Schuler and colleagues (1982). In the test, adult wild-type flies are mated under defined conditions of light (12 hour light/dark cycle), temperature (25°C) and humidity (60%). The female flies deposit eggs for up to six days in a nutritive medium comprising fresh instant Drosophila medium, reconstituted in distilled water that also contains test agent, and viable yeast. Within 24h, larvae hatch from the eggs and begin metamorphosis through two further larval stages and a final pupal stage before emerging from the puparium as adult flies. Under experimental conditions, development lasts for 9-10 days. The emerged adult flies are examined, under anaesthesia, daily for 10 days and a thorough assessment of the shape, size and colour of various body parts (head, thorax, wing and abdomen), as observed in several orientations, is made. Additional examination of body part alignment, excess tissue growth and extra or absent body parts makes for a comprehensive analysis of any adverse developmental effects. Although not described by Schuler _et al_, it is assumed that measurement of the size of the flies would provide additional information on the effects on growth of the test agent. Seven compounds, some of unknown teratogenic potential in mammals, were tested with this system and although meaningful validation against mammalian data is not possible, developmental defects were shown to be quite reproducible.

In the original description of the technique, a pre-determined approximate maximum tolerated dose was used to assess effects of a compound on morphogenesis. Adopting such a protocol as standard would be of limited value in predictive teratogenicity tests and the procedure would require modifying to demonstrate dose-response relationship and provide estimates of teratogenic hazard, with a consequent increase in the work involved in the assay. Furthermore, the detailed procedure for morphological assessment of flies would suggest that this is a rather specialist practice, and this may also limit its usefulness.

A similar type of assay, using the cricket _Acheta domesticus_, has proved useful in detecting the teratogenicity of certain impurities in complex mixtures of industrial chemicals (Walton, 1983). Eggs, oviposited in contaminated sand, are allowed to develop for 5 days before being transferred to a petri dish for continued development on moist filter paper. Nymphs begin to emerge on day 12 and embryos exposed to teratogen display a range of abnormalities involving compound eyes, antennae, legs and head. The model appears to be able to distinguish between specific teratogenic effects and general embryotoxic effects, but in its present form does not provide an estimate of teratogenic hazard.

Artemia Tests

The brine shrimp, _Artemia salina_, has been used as the test subject in two independently proposed teratogenicity tests. In the first and simplest of these (Kerster and Schaeffer, 1983), the increase in body length of nauplii (larval form characteristic of crustacea, Figure 1) between 24h and 48h after hatching from cysts is measured and used as an index of teratogenicity. Suitably developed specimens (instar I nauplii) are selected from bulk cultures of cysts,

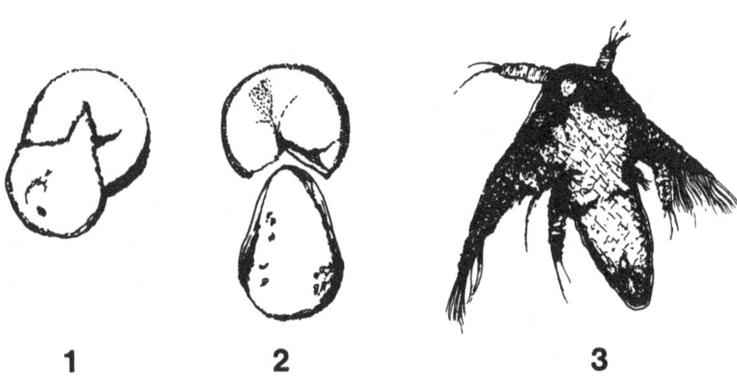

Figure 1. Development of nauplius of Artemia Salina. 1. Emergence of nauplius from cyst following wetting. 2. Completely emerged specimen contained within hatching membrane. 3. Hatched, free-swimming nauplius.

24h after wetting of cysts, and divided into treatment and control groups. Nauplii are cultured in an artificial seawater-based medium containing test agent and their body lengths recorded, to the nearest 30µm with an ocular micrometer, 24h after the start of treatment (48h post-hatching). A statistically significant difference (t=1.96 by Student's t-test analysis) between treated and control groups is considered positive identification of a teratogenic effect. The test has been used with a number of heavy metals (eg. cadmium, mercury, lead, zinc) and organic compounds (eg. bromoform, nitrobenzene, toluene) but no attempt has been made to correlate the effects of these agents on naupliar development with mammalian data.

The second Artemia test (Sleet and Brendel, 1985) also uses instar I nauplii as subjects. The organisms are cultured for 24h, again in an artificial seawater medium, in the presence of test agent. During the 24h culture period, the nauplii develop to the instar IV stage, and this development is reflected in the increase in body length, body water volume and DNA content, and the decrease in protein content. The median concentrations of test agent lethal to 50% (LC_{50}) of nauplii after 6h of culture, and after 24h of culture, are determined. These two time points are chosen as there are considerable differences in naupliar development at these stages. A ratio of the 6h LC_{50} to the 24h LC_{50} yields a number that is claimed to indicate the degree of teratogenic hazard posed by the test agent. If the 6h and 24h LC_{50} values are similar and the ratio approximates to unity, it is considered that the test agent is a general toxicant and does not specificially affect development. On the other hand a large ratio (ie the 6h LC_{50} is much greater than the 24h LC_{50}) apparently indicates a developmental stage-dependent effect of the test agent and therefore a high teratogenic hazard. As discussed below with planaria tests, this is not a true indication of hazard since both parameters measured in providing an index of teratogenicity are derived from differentiating organisms. Only three agents have been tested with this system: cadmium and mercury proving to be hazardous, and sodium azide, which showed no evidence of a specific developmental toxicity.

The scant data available precludes a realistic appraisal of the screen, which must await further extensive validation.

Planaria Tests

In the screen using the planarian *Dugesia dorotocephala*, essentially two tests are employed (Best and Morita, 1982). The first examines the ability of surgical fragments of the flatworm to regenerate into an intact animal in the presence of the test agent and is assumed to model many of the differentiation and development processes that occur in embryogenesis. In this test, decapitated planarians are maintained individually in aerated purified water containing test agent. Normally, regeneration of the head, eyespots and auricles occurs in sequence over a period of 7-14 days. Re-appearance of normal morphology and full pigmentation are indicative of complete regeneration and test agents may act by causing 1) delayed regeneration, 2) a failure of the subject to regenerate all or part of the head process, or 3) regeneration of an abnormal head. Observation of regeneration is a fairly straightforward procedure and the endpoints of the test are well-defined.

The second test takes as its starting material the intact planarian. The morphology of the planarian is maintained by continuous renewal of specialized cell types from differentiating progenitor neoplast cells and thus has certain parallels with regenerative and embryonic development. The experimental protocol for this test is precisely the same as in the surgical frament assay. The endpoint of this test is simply a loss of normal morphology, such as head resorption or development of a serpentine appearance, presumed as a consequence of an action of the test agent on the differentiating neoplast cells. There has been little validation of the planaria tests and although the system identifies deleterious effects on development of well-known mammalian teratogens such as mercury, actinomcycin D, colchicine and ethanol, it is uncertain whether the tests are specifically indicative of developmental toxicity. In a recent study (Sabourin _et al_; 1985), the results from the two planaria tests were combined in an attempt to establish an index of teratogenic hazard of 4 chemicals by calculating the ratio of the LC_{50} (concentration lethal to 50% of subjects) obtained in the intact planaria test to the LC_{50} obtained in the surgical fragment test. However, since the LC_{50} values in the two tests were similar for a given chemical, the teratogenic index approximated in all cases to 1.0. If the target cells in the two assays are, as claimed, the same, _viz_. neoplast cells, then this result is to be expected. However, it does mean that the test is unable to predict teratogenic hazard, and consequently is of restricted value as a screen.

Hydra Assay

Like tha planaria test, the Hydra assay (Johnson _et al_, 1982) is essentially two tests; however, unlike the former the Hydra tests are complementary and are specifically designed to estimate teratogenic hazard.

In the first part of the test, adult polyps of _Hydra attenuata_ are individually maintained in a defined Hydra medium containing test agent to which they are exposed for up to 90h. The toxicological response of the organism follows a characteristic sequence: degeneration and eventual loss of the tentacles followed by a total loss of the normal morphology and the assumption of a rounded shape, the so-called tulip form. Development of a tulip form marks the endpoint of the assay and once this stage is reached normal appearance is almost always irrecoverable. Initially, a dose-ranging experiment is performed at whole-log concentrations of test agent (10^{-3} to 10^{3} mg/l). Once the lowest effective whole-log concentration has been determined a second experiment is performed at concentrations of 0.9 to 0.1 of the lowest effective whole-log concentration. In this way a more exact measure of the lowest effective concentration is determined, and this value is termed "A".

In the second part of the assay, an artificial "embryo" is prepared from adult polyps and its regeneration back into the adult form provides the basis of the assay. The "embryo" is simply a pellet of dissociated adult cells produced by repeated pipetting of polyps. A constant mass of dissociated cells is plated out into the wells of a tissue culture dish in a reaggregation medium that contains test agent. Under control conditions, adult polyps are reformed within 90h. During the course of this period several changes of medium of decreasing osmolarity are necessary to permit reformation of polyps. The toxic endpoint of the test is dissolution of the embryos which can occur at any stage of the developmental sequence. The protocol to establish the minimum concentration of a test agent required to effect dissolution, termed "D", is the same as that used for adult polyps in determining "A". Once the A and D values have been determined for a given test agent, calculation of an A/D ratio provides an index of teratogenic hazard. In general, A/D values that exceed 1.0 are indicative of a specificity of action on the developing organism; the greater the A/D ratio, the greater is the teratogenic hazard.

Independent validation in several centres would seem to be required as preliminary findings (Sabourin _et al_, 1985) suggest that

A/D ratios for a particular chemical can vary widely between laboratories. The assay is simple, inexpensive and rapid to perform and uses subjects available in large numbers. The test is also unique among the systems described herein since it is the only screen that specifically aims to estimate teratogenic hazard.

A slight variation of the Hydra test described above has been introduced by Wilby et al. (1986). In the study of regeneration, rather than use dissociated cells these workers have measured regeneration of the adult polyp from the isolated digestive region of the polyp. Furthermore, a scoring system has been introduced into both parts of the test: toxicity to the adult organism is scored on a scale of 10 (for no effect) to 0 (for complete disintegration of the polyp); toxicity to the regenerating fragment is scored from 0 (for no development) to 10 (for complete regeneration of the adult). The concentration of the test agent in each part of the test at which a mean score of 5 is determined after 72 h incubation is used for the calculation of the teratogenic index. The limited validation data available for this form of the test is unconvincing. While thalidomide, for example, is claimed to demonstrate a high hazard, other teratogens, retinoic acid and methylmercuric chloride, fail to be detected as the hazardous agents they are known to be.

Sea Urchin Test

Embryos of the sea urchin have long been used in studies of developmental biology and this use has now been extended to include test for teratogenicity. A system has recently been described (Hose, 1985) in which the sea urchin embryo is used in a combined embryotoxicity-genotoxicity test. Gametes and embryos are exposed to test agent in sea water maintained at 15°C. Fertilization success is monitored 15 min after combination of sperm and egg by examining the eggs for the presence of a fertilization membrane. Embryos are allowed to develop for a further 48h under test conditions and are then assessed for survival and abnormalities. Normally by this time gastrulation of the embryos is complete. A sample of the embryos is further analysed for mitotic configurations using light microscopy. Mitotic rates of isolated embryonic cells are used as an indicator of general embryonic health. The cells are further analysed for cytologic irregularities such as pycnosis and pleomorphism. This rather detailed examination of the embryos increases the power of the assay to detect embryotoxic effects. However, it does require rather specialist knowledge and technical expertise and therefore may be useful on only a limited scale. Furthermore, the system is yet to be validated. Only a single compound, benzo(α)pyrene, has so far been tested.

Slime Mould Test

In this screen (Durston *et al.*, 1985), the cellular slime mould *Dictyostelium discoideum* is used as the test subject. Although there is little information available, the test appears to be designed to provide an estimate of teratogenic hazard. In the test three values are determined: the lowest concentration of test agent causing an effect on spore yield (A); the lowest concentration causing an effect on morphogenesis (B); the highest concentration at which no cell death is recorded (C). For a given test agent, a value for A or B that is equal to or greater than C indicates a positive result. Using the test, 43 out of 61 tested substances (71%) were correctly identified as 'teratogens' or 'non-teratogens'.

DISCUSSION

It is presently unclear whether embryogenesis and regeneration in sub-mammalian species is a good model for studying the toxicologic response of the mammalian embryo. There are the obvious differences of viviparity and the placental link between mother and fetus in mammals, but it has been argued that some of the basic features of differentiation and morphogenesis are common to phylogenetically diverse species (Best, 1983). Inevitably, no screen, whether it uses invertebrates or cultured cells, is going to detect all agents that are teratoenic in the whole mammal and it is important to stress that the tests described in this chapter are simply pre-screens. By subjecting a test agent to several different pre-screens, the chances of detecting a toxic effect are increasded, whereas using only one or two tests makes it more likely that a teratogen could fail to be detected. Likewise, a test that is based on a whole embryo or regenerating organism contains many more potential targets for a toxin than does a simple cell culture system and may be more likely therefore to detect a toxic effect.

Failure of a test agent to elicit toxicity in a large number of pre-screens might still not preclude it from further testing if human exposure to a substance was likely to be high. Based on this rationale therefore, it is clear that pre-screens are intended to augment standard safety evaluation procedures and not replace them.

A qualitative difference among the pre-screens that have been developed for teratogenicity testing concerns the nature of the endpoints of tests. Some screens, for example the drosophila test, monitor malformation (abnormal morphogenesis) of emerging flies while others, such as the Hydra test, are only able to detect perversion of developmental processes, such as growth and intercellular organisation resulting in the single end-point of disintegration of the organism. The importance of any difference in the two types of endpoints with regard to the prediction of teratogenicity will only become clear when further validation of the tests has been performed.

For all of the tests described in this chapter, considerably more validation is required before they can seriously be considered suitable for widespread use as screens. Precisely what form that validation should take is an important issue. The following points require consideration: 1) <u>Validation must involve comparison of test results with data from standard laboratory animal testing</u>. Since it is to reduce the requirement for the latter form of testing that alternative screens are being developed, it is obvious that these screens must produce data that is generally concordant with the observed teratogenic potency and hazard in whole animal tests. 2) <u>Selection of appropriate chemicals for validation studies is essential</u>. Validation of tests should be performed with a wide range of agents of differing degrees of well-established teratogenic effects in laboratory animals. Progress has been made in this area with the reasoned proposal of about 50 chemicals (Smith <u>et al.</u>, 1983) that would serve this purpose. Validation of different tests with the same test agents would also permit comparisons to be drawn between tests, thus allowing judgement as to the best and most appropriate tests to be used. 3) <u>Validation of tests must be performed in several</u>

independent laboratories. The demonstration of reproducibility of results between laboratories is essential for the establishment of a particular test as routine practice.

On the basis of presently available information, it is uncertain whether any of the non-mammalian screens will gain widespread acceptance. The Hydra test is one of the more popular screens and is now, perhaps prematurely, commercially available. Of the tests described, based on design and validation performed so far, Hydra and possibly FETAX, offer the most promise and might merit inclusion in a battery of screens alongside some of the cell culture tests that have been developed (Brown and Freeman, 1984).

REFERENCES

Best, J.B. (1983). Transphyletic animal similarities and predictive toxicology. In Old and New Questions in Physics, Cosmology, Philosophy and Theoretical Biology, ed. A. Van der Marwe, pp. 549-591. New York: Plenum Press.

Best, J.B. & Morita, M. (1982). Planarians as a model system for invitro teratogenesis studies. Teratogen. Carcinogen. Mutagen. 2, 277-291.

Birge, W.J., Black, J.A., Westerman, A.G. & Ramey, A.B. (1983). Fish and amphibian embryos - a model system for evaluating teratogenicity. Fund. Appl. Toxicol. 3, 237-242.

Brown, N.A. & Fabro, S.E. (1982). The in vitro approach to teratogenicity testing. In Developmental Toxicology, ed. K. Snell, pp. 31-57. London: Croom Helm.

Brown, N.A. & Freeman, S.J. (1984). Alternative tests for teratogenicity. ATLA, 12, 7-23.

Courchesne, C.L. & Bantle, J.A. (1985). Analysis of the activity of DNA, RNA and protein synthesis inhibitors on Xenopus embryo development. Teratogen. Carcinogen. Mutagen. 5, 177-193.

Dumont, J.N. & Epler, R.G. (1984). Validation studies on the FETAX teratogenesis assay (Frog embryos). Teratology 29, 38A.

Dumont, J.N., Schultz, T.W. & Newman, S.M. (1982). A frog embryo teratogenesis assay: Xenopus (FETAX) - a model for teratogen screening. Teratology 25, 37A.

Dumpert, K. & Zietz, E. (1984). Platanna (Xenopus laevis) as a test organism for determining the embryotoxic effects of environmental chemicals. Ecotoxicol. Environ. Safety 8, 55-74.

Durston, A., Van de Wiel, F., Mummery, C. & de Laat, S. (1985). Dictyostelium discoideum as a test system for screening for teratogens. Teratology 32, 21A.

Fabro, S., Shull G. & Brown N.A. (1982). The relative teratogenic index and teratogenic potency: proposed components of developmental toxicity risk assessment. Teratogen. Carcinogen. Mutagen. 2. 61-76.

Fisher, M & Schoenwolf, G.D. (1983). The use of chick embryos in experimental embryology and teratology: Improvements in standard procedures. Teratology 27, 65-72.

Freeman, S.J. & Steele, C.E. (1986). Post-implantation whole embryo culture and the study of teratogenesis. Fd. Chem. Tox. (in press).

Fulton, M.H. & Chambers, J.E. (1985). The toxic and teratogenic effects selected organophosphorus compounds on the embryos of three species of amphibians. Toxicol. Lett. 26, 175-180.

Hose, J.E. (1985). Potential uses of sea urchin embryos for identifying toxic chemicals: Description of Bioassay incorporating cytologic, cytogenetic and embryologic endpoints. J. Appl. Toxicol. 5, 245-253.

Jelinek, R. (1977). The chick embryotoxicity screening test. In Methods in Prenatal Toxicology, Evaluation of Embryotoxic Effects in Experimental Animals, ed. D Neubert, H-J. Merker, T.E. Kwasigroch, R. Kreft & A. Bedfurtig, pp 381-386. Stuttgart: Georg Thieme Publishers.

Jelinek, R., Peterka, M. & Rychter, Z. (1985). One hundred and thirty compounds tested with the chick embryotoxicity screening test (CHEST). Ind. J. Exp. Biol. 23, 588-595.

Jelinek, R. & Rychter, Z. (1982). Morphogenetic systems and the central phenomena of teratology. In Advances in the Study of Birth Defects, Vol 11 Teratological Testing, ed. T.V.M. Persaud, pp 41-67. Baltimore: University Park Press.

Johnson, E.M. (1985). A review of advances in prescreening for teratogenic hazards. Prog. Drug. Res. 29, 121-154.

Johnson, E.M., Gorman, R.M., Gable, B.E.G. & George, M.E. (1982). The Hydra attenuata system for detection of teratogenic hazards. Teratogen. Carcinogen. Mutagen. 2, 263-276.

Kerster, H.W. & Schaeffer, D.J. (1983). Brine Shrimp (Artemia salina) nauplii as a teratogen test system. Ecotoxicol. Environ. Safety 7, 342-349.

Kimmel, G.L., Smith, K., Kochhar, D.M. & Pratt, R.M. (1982). Overview of in vitro teratogenicity testing: aspects of validation and application to screening. Teratogen. Carcinogen. Mutagen. 2, 221-229.

Sabourin, T.D., Faulk, R.T. & Gross, L.B. (1985). The efficacy of three non-mammalian test systems in the identification of chemical teratogens. J. Appl. Toxicol. 4, 227-233.

Schuler, R.L., Hardin, B.D. & Niemeier, R.W. (1982). Drosophila as a tool for the rapid assessment of chemicals for teratogenicity. Teratogen. Carcinogen. Mutagen. 2, 293-301.

Schultz, T.W., Dumont, J.M. & Epler, R.G. (1985). The embryotoxic and osteolathyrogenic effects of semicarbizide. Toxicology 36, 183-198.

Sleet, R.B. & Brendel, K. (1985). Homogeneous populations of Artemia nauplii and their potential use for in vitro testing in developmental toxicology. Teratogen. Carcinogen. Mutagen. 5, 41-54.

Smith, M.K., Kimmel, G.L. Kochhar, D.M., Shepard, T.H., Spielberg, S.P. & Wilson, J.G. (1983). A selection of candidate compounds for in vitro teratogenesis test validation. Teratogen. Carcinogen. Mutagen. 3, 461-480.

Verret, M.J., Scott, W.F., Reynaldo, E.F., Alterman, E.K. & Thomas, C.A. (1980). Toxicity and teratogenicity of food additive chemicals in the developing chicken embryo. Toxicol. Appl. Pharmacol. 56, 265-273.

Vesely, D., Vesela, D. & Jelinek, R. (1982). Nineteen mycotoxins tested on chicken embryos. Toxicol. Lett. 13, 239-245.

Walton, B.T. (1983). Use of the cricket embryo (Acheta domesticus) as an invertebrate teratology model. Fund. Appl. Toxicol. 3, 233-236.

Wilby, O.K., Newall, D.R. & Tesh, J.M. (1986). A Hydra assay as a pre-screen for teratogenic potential. Fd. Chem. Tox. (in press).

Wilson, J.G. (1978). Survey of in vitro systems: their potential use in teratogenicity screening. In Handbook of Teratology, Vol. 4, Research Procedures and Data Analysis, ed. J.G. Wilson & F.C. Fraser, pp 135-154. New York: Plenum Press.

Table 1 Summary of Test Systems

Assay	Approx. number[a] of chemicals studied	Current Use of Assay	Level of skill[b] required	Estimation[c] of hazard	Estimation of potency	Minimum time[d] to test one chemical
Chick Embryo	>100	>10 labs + commercially available	High	Yes	Yes	~2 weeks
CHEST	>100	1 Lab	High	No	Yes	~2 weeks
FETAX	<50	2 Labs	Moderate	Yes	Yes	~1 week
Drosophilia	<10	1 Lab	High	No	Yes	1-2 Weeks
Cricket	<10	1 Lab	Moderate	No	Yes	~2 weeks
Artemia	<10	2 Labs	Moderate	Yes	Yes	<1 week
Planaria	<40	2 labs	Moderate	No	Yes	1-2 weeks
Hydra	<50	3 Labs + commercially available	Low	Yes	Yes	~1 week
Sea Urchin	<10	1 Lab	V. High	No	Yes	>2 weeks
Slime Mould	<50	1 Lab	Moderate	Yes	Yes	~1 week

a Information available in open literature only.
b Includes all phases of test, particularly evaluation of endpoints.
c Those tests that attempt to distinguish between general toxic (embryotoxic) effects and specific developmental effects are for the purpose of this table considered to estimate hazard. This does not necessarily mean that they comply with the strict definition of 'teratogenic hazard' given in the Introduction.
d Includes time taken to produce starting material eg. 30h chick embryo.

Table modified, with permission, from Brown and Freeman (1984).

USE OF IN VITRO TECHNIQUES TO INVESTIGATE THE ACTION OF TESTICULAR TOXICANTS

D.A. Garside,
Smith Kline & French Research Ltd., The Frythe,
Welwyn Garden City, Hertfordshire, AL6 9AR, England.

INTRODUCTION

The testis performs two main functions that are largely complimentary, namely the production of spermatozoa and the production of hormones, principally testosterone. Any perturbations of either of these activities will result in reduced fertility. Generally, damage to testicular function can result from either inhibition of the overall hormonal controlling mechanisms at the hypothalamic - pituitary or testicular level, or by direct action at the testicular cell level. Chemicals and drugs can exert their toxic effects via one or both of these mechanisms.

A number of morphological and functional parameters are employed to assess toxic effects on male reproduction, however the conventional methods used are mainly involved with the overall controlling mechanisms, for example blood hormonal measurements, sperm analysis and fertility profiles. Histopathology and biochemistry provide an insight into events at the testicular level, but there is a need for a further reliable and fast method which will provide more detailed information of events within the testis.

The testes consist of the seminiferous tubules, containing Sertoli cells and germ cells involved in spermatogenesis (which make up over 90% of the testicular mass) and interstitial Leydig cells (Figure 1). The endocrine control of spermatogenesis is very complex (Setchell, 1978; di Zarega and Shervis, 1981) involving hormones from the pituitary (systemic) and intragonadal hormones operating at a local level (paracrine) (Figure 2). The testis is under the influence of the systemic gonadotrophins, follicle stimulating hormone (FSH) and luteinising hormone (LH), both of which bind to specific receptors

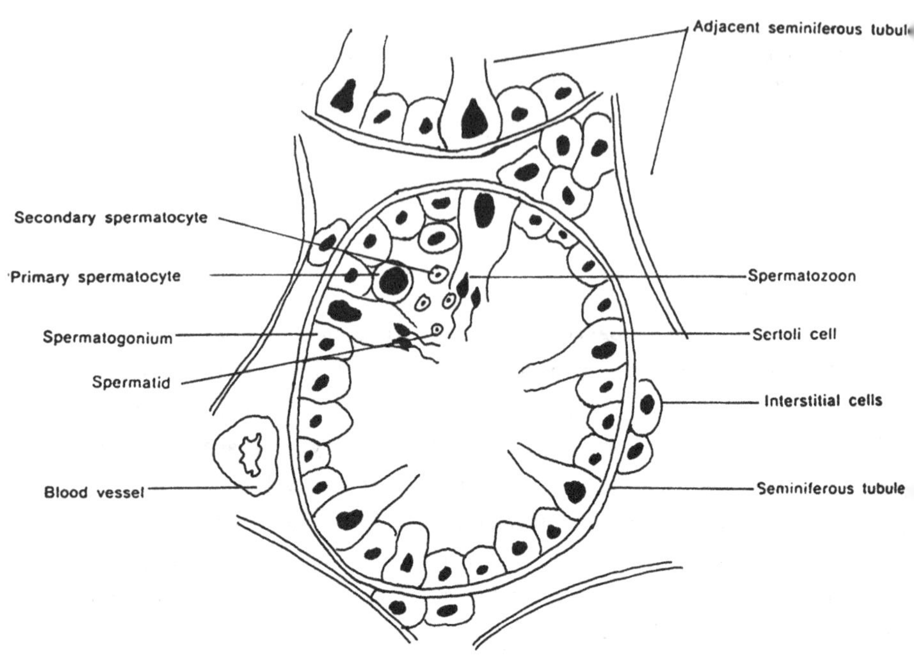

Figure 1. Section through a seminiferous tubule showing the stages of spermatogenesis and the location of sertoli and Leydig cells.

on their target organs, the Sertoli cell (Steinberger et al, 1975) and Leydig cell, respectively (de Kretser et al, 1971).

Luteinising hormone promotes testosterone synthesis from the Leydig cell, which is required for normal spermatogenesis (Steinberger et al, 1973), and to maintain the integrity of male accessory glands (i.e. prostate). Follicle stimulating hormone increases protein synthesis in the Sertoli cell, especially that of androgen binding protein which acts to bind testosterone and facilitate its entry into the seminiferous tubule and inhibin (Le Gac and de Kretser, 1982) which controls follicle stimulating hormone release from the pituitary.

Spermatogenesis starts at puberty with the onset of testis maturation and is maintained almost throughout life. It is a continuous

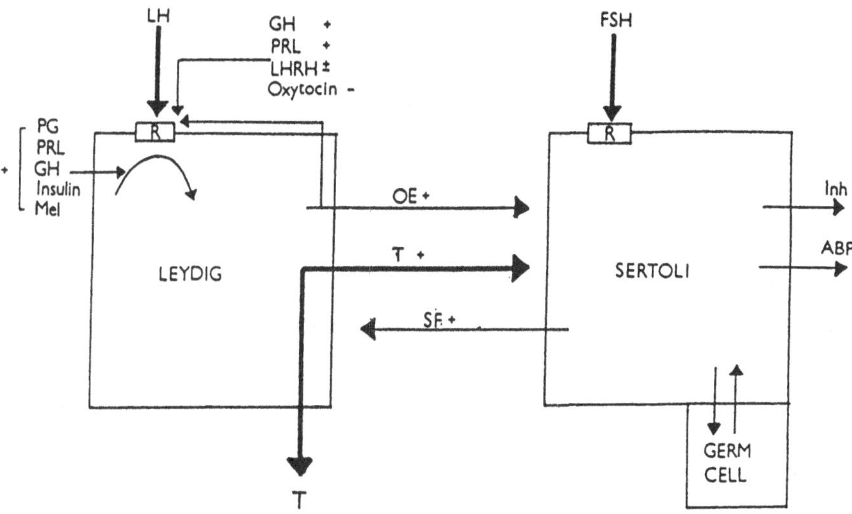

Figure 2. The endocrine control of the testis, the involvement of systemic and intragonadal hormones.

LH - Luteinising hormone
OE - Oestradiol
Inh - Inhibin
FSH - Follicle stimulating hormone
PG - Prostaglandin
Mel - Melatonin
PRL - Prolactin
LHRH - LH releasing hormone
T - Testosterone
SF - Sertoli cell factor
ABP - Androgen binding protein
GH - Growth hormone

rather than a cyclic event, with different stages of spermatogenesis being evident at all times. However, as well as the gonadotrophins, there is recent and convincing evidence that spermatogenesis is also dependent on the local Sertoli-Leydig cell interactions (Rich et al, 1979; de Kretser, 1981; Bergh, 1983). The Sertoli cell produces a factor(s) which controls Leydig cell function _in vitro_ (Verhoeven and Cailleau, 1985; Garside et al, 1985) and damage to seminiferous tubules _in vivo_ results in the loss of this control mechanism leading to the hypertrophy of those Leydig cells adjacent to the damage with a reduction of luteinising hormone receptors (Aoki and Fawcett, 1978; Risbridger et al, 1981). Unilateral disruption of spermatogenesis, for example by heat or cryptorchidism, results in identical Leydig cell changes and reduced testosterone output in the treated testis only (Main and Setchell, 1980; Johnsen et al, 1981).

It is evident, therefore, that the normal function of the mammalian testis is governed by the interaction of intratesticular factors with pituitary hormones; the former modulating the action of the latter on their target organs. Chemicals and drugs that interfere with this interaction will inhibit spermatogenesis.

The recent technique of culturing testicular cell types *in vitro* (Schumacher et al, 1978; Verhoeven et al, 1982) has potential to be an invaluable tool for assessing the mechanisms of testicular toxicity, especially those of intragonadal interactions and spermatogenesis. Moreover, Sertoli/germ cell cultures can provide additional essential information regarding damage to the early stages of spermatogenesis. These tissue culture techniques are the only *in vitro* methods available to assess testicular toxicity and they also fulfil the criteria for a test which is versatile and simple, while able to yield information quickly.

PRACTICAL ASPECTS

The following is intended as a guide to the equipment and methodology necessary for testicular cell culture.

General solutions and equipment

Equipment

- Laminar flow cabinet
- Sterile 1ml pasteur pipettes
- Sterile 10 ml pipettes
- 0.22μ sterile filters
- Sterile culture wells
- Sterile 30 ml Universals
- Haemocytometer
- Eppendorf Multipette
- Eppendorf combitips (sterilised) 5ml
- Sterilised blunt and sharp end scissors
- Sterilised small dissecting scissors
- Sterilised pair fine forceps
- Incubator, carbon dioxide type
- Centrifuge

Solutions — Dissecting media (sterile) 1 litre

Dulbecco's Modified Eagles Medium (DMEM) (x10)	
Bovine serum albumin	0.1%
Kanamycin	0.1 mg/ml
pH 7.4	

Culture media (sterile) 1 litre

DMEM/Hams F12 (1:1 u/v)	
Hepes buffer	10 mM
Bovine Serum Albumin	0.1%
Kanamycin	0.1 mg/ml
$NaHCO_3$	2.4 g/l

(10% Fetal calf serum is included for Sertoli cells only).

Leydig cells

Equipment
- Shaking water bath
- Sterile swinnex 60µm filter
- Sterile 50 ml syringe
- Sterile 50 ml Universal
- Sterile syringe filling tube

Percoll gradients (2)

Earls basic salt solution	2.5 ml
Percoll	21.8 ml
Hepes buffer 1M	0.25 ml
Kanamycin	0.25 ml
Dissection media	25.0 ml
Minipuls 2 pump and tubing (2.90 cc/M)	
Sterile 30 ml Universals (x2)	

Cell dispersal media (sterile)

Trypsin inhibitor	0.1 mg/ml
Collagenase	0.25 mg/ml
Dissection media	7.0 ml

Sertoli cells

Equipment
- Sterile nylon mesh (100 µm and 75 µm)
- Sterile 100 ml beaker (x2)
- Sterile 500 ml stoppered conical flask (x2)
- Sterile petri dishes 50 mm diameter

Cell dispersal media (sterile)

Solution I	Dulbecco's Modified Eagles Medium	- 100 ml
	Trypsin	- 0.25%
	DNAse Type III bovine pancreas	- 10 μg/ml
Solution II	Dulbecco's Modified Eagles Medium	- 100 ml
	Collagenase	- 0.1%

Experimental Procedures

Male rats are sacrificed by Halothane euthanasia and cervical dislocation always at the same time of day, in order to standardise for any possible effects of hormonal diurnal rhythms.

Removal of Testis

The rat is laid on a clean surface on absorbent paper and the scrotum soaked with 70% ethanol. An incision is made with blunt end scissors through the scrotal wall and cremnasteric fascia. A further incision is made through the tunica vaginalis, the testis located and removed using forceps, trimming away as much adherent fat as possible. It is then transferred rapidly to a 30 ml Universal containing dissection medium at room temperature.

Testis dissection

The following procedures are carried out in a laminar flow cabinet, the surfaces of which have been sterilised by swabbing with 70% ethanol. The testis is transferred to a sterile petri dish containing a small amount of dissection media and decapsulated. A small incision is made with sharp dissecting scissors through the tunica vasculosa and albuginea at the appendix of the testis and a longitudinal section made, taking care not to damage the seminiferous tubules. The testicular capsule is teased off gently and discarded.

Leydig cells isolation

Two decapsulated testes (rats 200-300g) are placed in a 30 ml Universal containing 7 ml of Leydig cell dispersal media that has been filtered through a 0.22 μ filter, and incubated longitudinally in a shaking water bath at 37°C until the seminiferous tubules are separated (15-20 mins). 15 ml of dissection media is then added to the tube and inverted slowly 20 times, allowed to settle and the cell suspension decanted off using a sterile 50 ml syringe and filling attachment. The suspension is filtered through a 60 µm filter attached to the syringe and the filtrate centrifuged (100 g) for 5 mins. The supernatant is removed, the cells resuspended and centrifuged as before. After again removing the supernatant, the cells are resuspended in 2 ml of dissection medium and pipetted onto the top of a 0-90% Percoll gradient (Conn et al 1977) (50-60 x 10^6 cells/gradient) and centrifuged (400 g) for 20 mins. The resultant cell bands are isolated using a pasteur pipette and Band III (Leydig cell fraction density 1.070g/ml) collected into a separate 30 ml Universal. The Band III cell suspension is then diluted three times with dissection media and the cells washed to remove all Percoll by centrifuging (100 g) and resuspending three times as previously described. The cells are counted using a haemocytometer and then the cell suspension is drawn up into a 'Combitip' fitted to an Eppendorf Multipette and delivered in 100 µl (50,000 cells) aliquots to each well. The volume of each well is made up to 500 µl with culture medium and the cells incubated at 32°C, in an atmosphere of 10% CO_2, initially for two hours before being used experimentally. At this time, the media is changed and replaced with 500 µl culture medium.

Sertoli/germ cell isolation

Decapsulated testes from 23-30 day old rats are placed in a sterile petri dish, containing dissecting medium at room temperature, in a laminar flow cabinet as before. The seminiferous tubules are minced with small dissecting scissors and incubated at 37°C with cell dispersion media, Solution I (40 testes in 50-100 ml media) for 15 mins, manually shaking once every minute. The cell suspension is then filtered through 100 µm mesh stretched over a beaker and washed through with 50 ml of dissection medium. The filtrate is incubated with cell dispersion medium, Solution II (40 testes in 50-100 ml media) for 8 mins, shaking as before or until small segments of seminiferous tubule can be seen. Wash through a 75 µm mesh with 50 ml dissection media and at this stage, under a light microscope, small cell clumps consisting of Sertoli cells with attached germ cells should be present. In order to count the number of cells, separate the cell clumps in the volume to be counted into single cells by agitating with a pasteur pipette. Using a 10 ml pipette the Sertoli/germ cell clumps are then plated out in a 50 mm petri dish at 15-20 x 10^6 cells in 4 ml culture medium.

Assessment of cell viability

The viability of the cells in culture can be assessed by replacing the media from five wells of cells cultured for 24 hrs each, with 200 µl of phosphate buffered saline containing 1 mg/ml Nitrobluetetrazolium (NBT) and 3 mg/ml NADH. Incubate at 37°C for 30 minutes, after which non-viable cells will have become purple/black in colour. The percentage viability is calculated by counting the number of viable and non-viable cells in several fields of view spanning both diagonals of the well. Control wells (five) do not contain NADH in the saline.

Assessment of steroid producing cells

To determine the number of steroid producing cells in the culture (indication of purity), freeze one drop of cell suspension with one drop of 6% dextran in 0.9% saline. After thawing, allow to dry in air before adding one drop of reaction mix (0.1M Phosphate buffered saline with 2 mg/ml epiandrosterone, 1 mg/ml NBT, 3 mg/ml NAD^+ and 1.6 mg/ml Nicotinamide) and incubate for 30-60 minutes at 37°C. Remove the reaction mix with adsorbent paper and add one drop of dissection media, leave for 2 minutes and remove as before. Fixative (10% formalin) is then added and left for 30 minutes after which the cells are again washed in dissection media (3 minutes). Dry the cells in air and mount in gelatine. Control cells receive the same reaction mix without the epiandrosterone. Steroid producing cells will be blue/purple in colour and the percentage can be calculated as before.

Measurement of testicular cell secretory products

At the end of the incubation period, the medium from individual wells is collected and stored at -20°C until required for assay. Testosterone (Leydig cell) and oestradiol (immature Sertoli cell) concentration in the media is evaluated by radioimmunoassay. Other secretory products of Sertoli cells can also be measured; i.e. androgen binding protein by steady state polyacrylamide-gel electrophoresis (Ritzen et al, 1974) and inhibin by an *in vitro* bioassay system (Scott et al, 1980).

EXPERIMENTAL EXAMPLES

The *in vitro* culture of testicular cell types has so far had limited application to investigative toxicology, however, the Sertoli/germ cell preparation has provoked interest due to the information it can provide as to the toxic effects of chemicals on the early stages of spermatogenesis. The Leydig cell culture system has only recently been used to further the knowledge of the toxic effects of chemicals on testosterone production. For example, it is difficult to assign xenobiotic changes in plasma testosterone levels to the systemic control mechanisms or to a direct effect on the Leydig cells. Laskey et al (1986) have utilised *in vitro* culture of Leydig cells to investigate testosterone biosynthesis in the presence of metal cations. Leydig cells were incubated with various metal ions for 3 hrs in the presence of human chorionic gonadotrophin hCG (to investigate receptor stimulation) and cyclic adenosine monophosphate (cAMP) (for post receptor stimulation of testosterone) after which testosterone output was determined by radioimmunoassay. Several metal cations produced a dose response depression in both hCG and cAMP stimulated testosterone production, indicating that some metal cations alter testosterone biosynthesis by directly exerting an effect on the Leydig cell both at the receptor and post receptor level. Alterations in plasma testosterone levels due to metal cations is therefore partly (at least) due to direct effects.

The Sertoli cell preparation has been increasingly used to investigate the toxic effects of phthalate esters and glycol ethers on spermatogenesis. Glycol ethers are widely used as solvents in industry and are found in inks, dyes and water-based cleaners. They produce, however, varying levels of toxicity due possibly to differences in metabolism or the toxicity of their metabolites and exposure to some (eg. ethylene glycol monoethyl ether (EGE), ethylene glycol monomethyl ether (EGM)) causes testicular damage characterised by the degeneration of primary spermatocytes and spermatids (Foster et al, 1983). The Sertoli cell preparation has been used to facilitate the detection of testicular toxicity and to study the mechanisms of action, as alterations in Sertoli-cell function induced by EGE, EGM or their metabolites could be critical for maintenance of spermatogenesis. Beattie and co-workers (1984) incubated Sertoli cells *in vitro* with EGE or its metabolite methoxyacetic acid (MA) at 0, 3 or 10mM for up to 12 h and showed a significant decrease in Sertoli cell lactate production by MA but not EGE. This would not adversely affect Sertoli cell function but could have detrimental effects on the viability of spermatocytes, which appear to be the primary target of EGE _in vivo_. These data have been substantiated by Gray et al (1985) who also obtained no toxic effects of EGM or EGE at up to 50mM for 72 hours in culture. However, the metabolites MA and ethoxyacetic acid (EA), respectively, caused degeneration of the pachytene and dividing spermatocytes. There was a close correlation between the effects of the glycol ethers and their metabolites _in vivo_ and their toxicity in Sertoli cell cultures, suggesting that the mechanism of action _in vivo_ is similar to that _in vitro_.

The phthalate esters are among the most extensively used industrial chemicals and like the glycol ethers, some of the commonly used (eg. di-(2-ethylhexyl) phthalate, DEHP) produce testicular damage _in vivo_ (see review by Thomas and Thomas, 1984). The effects are again characterised by a loss of the pachytene and dividing spermatocytes and seminiferous tubule atrophy, indicating perhaps a disruption of the interactions between Sertoli and germ cells. Gray and Beamand (1984) have examined the response of Sertoli/germ cell cultures to treatment with phthalate esters. They found that there was an increased rate of germ cell detachment from the Sertoli cells with exposure to monophthalate ester (MEHP) which was concentration dependent, whereas similar concentrations of monophthalates which do not affect the testis _in vivo_, had no effect _in vitro_. DEHP did not produce germ cell detachment _in vitro_. The detachment of germ cells in culture apparently corresponds to the shedding of germ cells into the seminiferous tubule lumen _in vivo_ after dosing with some phthalate esters (Creasy et al, 1983).

The lack of response of Sertoli/germ cell cultures to DEHP seen by Gray and Beamond (1984), may be due to the fact that the toxic effect is again exerted by the metabolite and not the parent compound. Experiments by Sjoberg and co-workers (1986) indicate that only one of the five metabolites of DEHP, mono-(2-ethylhexyl phthalate), produced degenerating spermatocytes and spermatids _in vivo_ and a corresponding germ cell detachment from Sertoli/germ cell cultures. This supports the hypothesis that the toxic effects observed after exposure to many drugs and chemicals are exerted by the relevant metabolites.

Sertoli/germ cell cultures have also been used to investigate the testicular toxicity of 1-,3-Dinitrobenzene (DNB), a chemical intermediate in the synthesis of many organic compounds (Lloyd and Foster, 1985) and cadmium (Clough et al, 1985). DNB produced analogous results *in vitro* to those seen *in vivo*, i.e. Sertoli cell vacuolation and germ cell exfoliation, and cadmium affected the biochemical parameters of Sertoli cell function *in vitro*, which may explain the disruption of spermatogenesis brought about by cadmium *in vivo*.

DISCUSSION AND CONCLUSIONS

Testicular cell cultures are particularly useful in facilitating the understanding of the mechanisms of action involved in testicular toxicity. The Sertoli/germ cell cultures provide a sensitive *in vitro* model for investigating toxic effects on spermatogenesis as shown by the experiments involving phthalate esters and glycol ethers. Testicular toxicity *in vivo* is often characterised by an early detachment of spermatocytes and spermatids, suggesting that there is disruption of the normal interactions between germ cells and Sertoli cells. The cultures of Sertoli/germ cells show a similar shedding of germ cells when treated with known testicular toxicants which correlate well with the *in vivo* studies. There are other similarities between the known effects of testicular toxicants tested *in vitro* and their observed effects *in vivo*. For example, the cultures only exhibited effects with the phthalate esters which caused germ cell detachment *in vivo* and not with those that have not shown testicular toxicity *in vivo*. Also species differences and age dependency of the toxicity of phthalate esters is seen *in vitro*, which is in agreement with that observed *in vivo*. The same was true for the glycol ethers, with the effects in culture appearing to be specific to the same target cell types (pachytene and spermatocyte) as *in vivo*. This close correspondence between the cultures and *in vivo* effects suggests that the toxicants act in a similar mode *in vitro* as *in vivo*. Thus, Sertoli/germ cell cultures can provide a useful means of investigating chemical effects on spermatogenesis.

The Leydig cell cultures are a valuable tool for investigating the action of testicular toxicants on testosterone production and *in vitro* receptor assays could provide a basis for indicating the potential of drugs and chemicals to produce direct hormonal disturbances. Combined with the Sertoli/germ cell cultures, Leydig cells provide comprehensive and detailed information on the action of testicular toxicants at the level of the testis.

However, Sertoli and Leydig cell cultures are limited in their ability to take account of metabolic and pharmacokinetic factors which influence toxicity *in vivo*, such as absorption from the gut and distribution to the testis. Although recently there have been reports of xenobiotic metabolism in Sertoli/germ cell cultures (Lloyd and Foster, 1986). In these experiments it was ascertained that 1-3, Dinitrobenzene was metabolised by the cultures to two more polar metabolites, the production of which was dose and time related. The Sertoli/germ cell cultures have also been invaluable in establishing whether the parent compound or a metabolite is responsible for the toxicity.

In conclusion, testicular cell cultures have an important role to play in assessing the reprotoxic potential of chemicals and drugs, primarily by identifying the site of action and the mechanisms involved. The possible significance of such perturbations to testicular function and the effect in man can then be better evaluated.

REFERENCES

Aoki A and Fawcett D.W. (1978). Is there local feedback to the seminiferous tubule affecting activity of Leydig cells. Biol. Reprod. 19, 144.

Beattie P.J., Welsh M.J. and Brabec M.J. (1984). The effect of 2-methoxyethanol and methoxyacetic acid on Sertoli cell lactate production and protein synthesis in-vitro. Toxicol. and Appl. Pharmacol. 76, 56-61.

Bergh A. (1983). Paracrine regulation of Leydig cells by seminiferous tubules. Int. J. Androl. 6, 57-65.

Clough S.R., Welsh M.J. and Brabec M.J. (1986). Biochemical response of primary rat Sertoli cell cultures to cadmium. The Toxicologist, abstracts of the 25th Anniversary Meeting of the Society of Toxicology Vol.6. Abs. 1160, p289.

Conn P.M., Tsuruhara T., Dufan M., and Catt K.J. (1977). Isolation of highly purified Leydig cells by density gradient centrifugation. Endocrinology 101, 639.

Creasy D.M., Foster J.R. and Foster P.M. (1983). The morphological development of di-n-pentyl phthalate induced testicular atrophy in the rat. J. Path. 139, 309-321.

Foster P.M., Creasy D.M., Foster J.R., Thomas L.V., Cook M.W. and Gangolli S.D. (1983). Testicular toxicity of ethylene glycol monomethyl and monoethyl ethers in the rat. Toxicol. Appl. Pharmacol. 69, 385-399.

Garside D.A., Craig P. and Cooke B.A. (1985). Evidence for the local control of Leydig cell function by Sertoli cells in vitro. J. Endoc. 107, abs 124.

Gray T.J. and Beamond J.A. (1984). Effect of some phthalate esters and other testicular toxins on primary cultures of testicular cells. Fd. Chem. Tox. 22 (2), 123-131.

Gray T.J., Moss E.J., Creasy D.M. and Gangolli S.D. (1985). Studies on the toxicity of some glycol ethers and alkoxyacetic acids in primary testicular cultures. Toxicol. Appl. Pharmacol. 79, 490-501.

Johnsen T., Gordeladze J.O., Haug E. and Hansson V. (1981). Changes in rat testicular adenylate cyclase activity and gonadotrophin binding during experimental cryptorchidism. J. Reprod. Fert. 63, 381-390.

de Kretser D.M. (1982). Sertoli-Leydig cell interactions in the regulation of testicular function. Int. J. Androl. Suppl. 5, 11-17.

de Kretser D.M., Catt K.J., Burger H.G. and Smith G.C. (1969). Radioautograph studies on localisation of I^{125} labelled hLH and GH in immature rats. J. Endoc. 43, 105-111.

Laskey J.W., Phelps P.V. and Laws S.D. (1986). Leydig cell function in-vitro following metal cation treatment. The Toxicologist abstracts of the 25th Anniversary Meeting of the Society of Toxicology, Vol.6, Abs. 344, p86.

Lloyd S.C. and Foster P.M. (1985). 1-3, Dinitrobenzene: toxicity and metabolism in rat testicular cell cultures. Human Toxicology-in press.

Le Gac F. and de Kretser D. (1982). Inhibin production by the Sertoli cell. Mol. Cell. Endoc. 28, 487-498.

Main S.J. and Setchell B (1980). Responsiveness of the pituitary gland to androgens and of the testis to gonadotrophins following damage to spermatogenesis in rats. J. Endoc. 87, 445-454.

Purvis K., Clausen O.P., Brandtzaeg P. and Hansson V. (1978). LH receptors and Leydig cell responsiveness to hCG _in-vitro_. Archs. Androl. _1_, 299-310.

Rich K.A., Kerr J.B. and de Kretser D.M. (1979). Evidence for Leydig cell dysfunction in rats with seminiferous tubule damage. Mol. Cell. Endoc. _13_, 123-135.

Risbridger G.P., Hodgson Y.M. and de Kretser D.M. (1981). Mechanism of action of gonadotrophins on the testis. _The Testis_. Burger, H.G. and de Kretzer, D.M. (Eds), p.195-211. Raven Press, New York.

Ritzen E.M., French F.S., Weddington S.C., Nayfeh S.N. and Hansson V. (1974). Steroid binding in polyacrylamide gels: quantitation at steady state conditions. J. Biol. Chem. _249_, 6597-6604.

Setchell B.P. (1978). _The Mammalian Testis_. New York Cornell University Press.

Schumacher M., Schafer G., Hobtein A.F. and Hilz H. (1978). Rapid isolation of mouse Leydig cells by centrifugation of Percoll density gradients with complete retention of morphological and biochemical integrity. Fed. Europ. Biochem. Soc. Lett. _91_, 333.

Scott R.S., Burger H.G. and Quigg H. (1980). A simple rapid _in-vitro_ bioassay for inhibin. Endoc. _107_, 1536-1542.

Sharpe R.M. (1984). Intratesticular factors controlling testicular function. Biol. Reprod. _30_, 29-49.

Sjoberg P., Bandesson U., Gray T.J. and Ploen L. (1986). Effects of di-(2-ethylhexyl) phthalate and five of its metabolites on rat testis _in-vivo_ and _in-vitro_. Acta. Pharmacol. et Toxicol. _58_, 225-233.

Steinberger E. and Steinberger A. (1974). Hormonal control of testicular function in mammals. Handbook of Physiology. Knobil K. and Sawyer W.H. (Eds.) Vol.4. part 2. pp.325-345. Washington D.C. American Physiology Society.

Steinberger A., Heindel J.J., Lindsey J.N., Elkington J.S., Sanborn B.M. and Steinberger E. (1975). Isolation and culture of FSH responsive Sertoli cells. Endoc. Res. Comm. _2_, 261-272.

Thomas, J.A. and Thomas M.J. (1984). Biological effects of di-(2-ethylhexyl) phthalate and other phthalic acid esters. Crit. Rev. Toxicol. _13_, 283-317.

Verhoeven G. and Cailleau J. (1985). A factor in spent media from Sertoli cell enriched cultures that stimulates steroidogenesis in Leydig cells. Mol. Cell. Endoc. _40_, 57-68.

Verhoeven G., Kaninckx P. and de Moor P. (1982). Androgen and progestogen production in cultured interstitial cells derived from immature rat testis. J. St. Biochem _17_, 319-330.

Vernon R.G., Kopeck B, and Fritz I.B. (1974). Observations on the binding of androgens by the rat testis seminiferous tubules and testis extracts. Mol. Cell. Endoc. _1_, 167-187.

IN VITRO ASSESSMENT OF OVARIAN FUNCTION: A POTENTIAL TOOL FOR INVESTIGATING MECHANISMS OF TOXICITY IN THE OVARY

D.A. Garside
Smith Kline and French Research Ltd, The Frythe,
Welwyn Garden City, Herts, AL6 9AR, United Kingdom.

P.E. McKibbin
Central Toxicology Laboratory, Imperial Chemical
Industries plc, Alderley Park, Macclesfield, Cheshire
SK10 4TJ, United Kingdom.

INTRODUCTION

The survival of a species depends on the integrity of its reproductive system, thus the toxic effects of drugs and environmental chemicals on the human reproductive system is an important health concern. The potential toxicity of such chemicals to the human *in utero*, one of the most vulnerable stages of development, is the focus for most studies in reproductive toxicology and includes assessment of the higher (hypothalamus - pituitary) control of reproductive function, for example blood hormone measurement. However, the incidences of chemically induced germ cell damage and sterility appear to be on the increase, with many chemicals shown to have a direct toxic effect on the female gonads (Harbison and Dixon, 1978).

In female mammals, all germ cells are formed in the ovary before birth. Many of these become atretic so that by puberty only half the initial number of oocytes remain. Therefore, any agent that damages the oocyte will accelerate the depletion of oocyte number, thereby reducing fertility. After birth, the development of all germ cells progresses no further than the primary oocyte stage (diplotene) until just before they ovulate. Thus, in the adult, follicles in various stages of growth can always be found, although only a few achieve maturity and ovulate.

The follicle consists of an inner granulosa cell layer, which extends to surround the oocyte (the cumulus oophorous) and an outer layer, the theca folliculi made up of the theca interna and theca externa (Figure 1). The control of ovarian steroid synthesis and secretion is a complex process involving the interaction of these two follicular compartments as well as a coordinated sequence of actions by the pituitary gonadotrophins, luteinising hormone and follicle stimulating hormone (Erickson, 1983) (Figure 2).

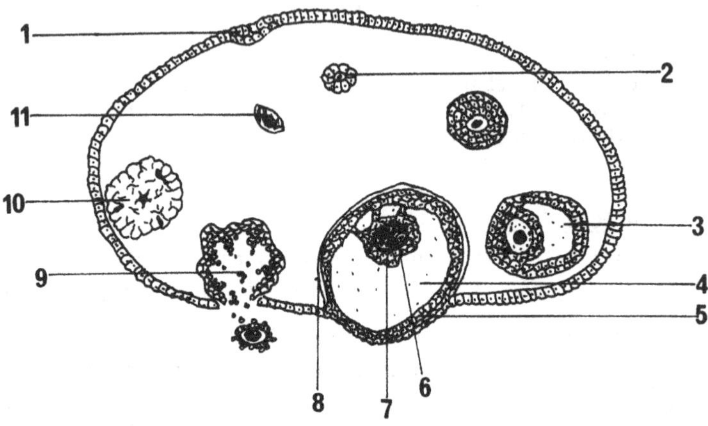

Figure 1. Section through the ovary showing the stages in development of the follicle and corpora lutea formation.

1. Oogonia
2. Primary follicle
3. Preovulatory follicle
4. Graafian follicle (ovulatory)
5. Granulosa cells
6. Oocyte
7. Cumulus oophorous
8. Theca folliculi
9. Developing corpus luteum
10. Corpus luteum
11. Corpora allbicantae (regressing corpus luteum)

Oestrogen and progesterone are produced primarily by the granulosa cell (McNatty, 1981) and there is evidence that these steroids in the follicular fluid act locally to influence cytoplasmic and nuclear maturation of the developing oocyte (Eppig et al, 1983; Osborn and Moor, 1983). Indeed there are indications that human oocytes from follicles containing high follicular fluid levels of oestrogen and progesterone are most likely to undergo fertilisation and normal implantation development _in vitro_ (Carson et al, 1982; Marrs et al, 1983).

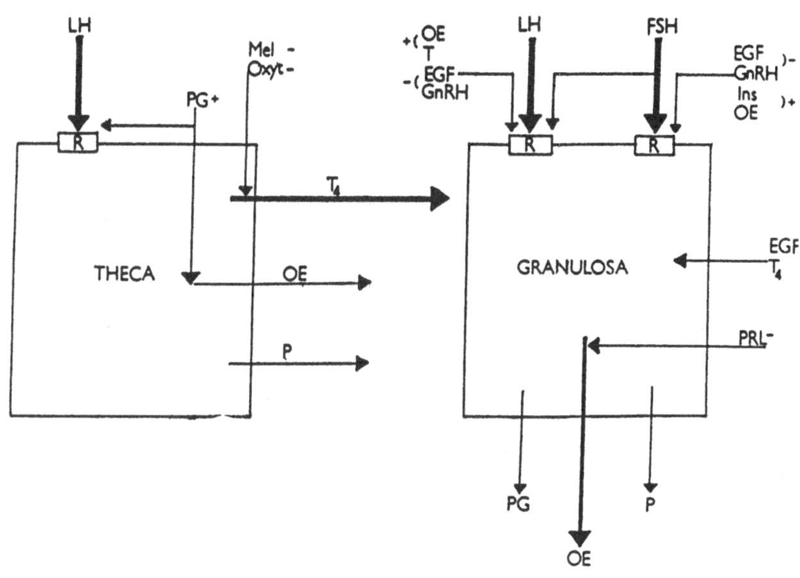

Figure 2. The peripheral and local hormonal interactions between the theca and granulosa cells governing steroid biosynthesis.

LH	- luteinising hormone	Mel	- melatonin
FSH	- follicle stimulating hormone	Oxyt	- oxytocin
OE	- oestradiol	EGF	- epidermal growth factor
P	- progesterone	PG	- prostaglandin
TL	- testosterone	Ins	- insulin
PRL	- prolactin	R	- receptor
GnRH	- gonadotrophin releasing hormone		

In response to luteinising hormone from the pituitary, combined with the facilitatory effect of follicle stimulating hormone and prolactin, ovulation of the mature Graafian follicle is initiated (Schwartz, 1974; Holt et al, 1976; Nalbandov, 1976; Welschen et al, 1980) (Figure 3). The post ovulatory follicular cavity is filled with lymph and blood from ruptured thecal vessels (Nalbandov, 1976) and the gradual hypertrophy and hyperplasia of the granulosa cells results in the eventual obliteration of the follicular cavity and the formation of the corpus luteum (Perry, 1971). Histologically, the corpus luteum is composed mainly of luteinised granulosa cells, but theca cells may also contribute to its formation. The main function of corpora lutea is to secrete progesterone, necessary for the maintenance of pregnancy.

The mammalian corpus luteum is an evanescent structure, regressing at the end of the luteal phase of the oestrous and menstrual cycle or at the termination of pregnancy/pseudopregnancy. The maintenance of the corpus luteum and therefore pregnancy is largely regulated by continuous secretion of a luteotrophic hormone complex, which is either derived only from the pituitary (goat, rabbit, pig) or from the pituitary during the first stages of pregnancy after which a luteotrophic stimulus from the placenta takes over (sheep, rat). Progesterone synthesis in the luteal cell requires the availability of cholesterol, the majority of which is derived from circulating lipoprotein cholesterol (high density lipoprotein) rather than from de novo synthesis (Gwynne and Strauss, 1982), the uptake of which is regulated by prolactin and luteinising hormone (Rajkunar et al, 1985; Murphy et al, 1985).

The functional viability of the theca, granulosa and luteal cells is therefore important for the development of the oocyte and the maintenance of pregnancy and any chemical interfering with their cell metabolism will alter the fertility of the female. The cell metabolism of ovarian cells and their response to hormones can be evaluated by isolating them from the ovary and culturing in-vitro and it has been shown that these cells retain their hormone responsiveness and normal physiological functions in culture (Carr et al, 1981; Erickson, 1983).

At present the culture of ovarian cells in-vitro is little used in reproductive toxicology, however it is already proving to have potential as an in-vitro test for assessing the possible toxicity of chemicals in relation to follicular development, luteal function and fertilisation. With the availability of human ovarian tissue, ovarian cell culture has exciting possibilities as an additional test in reproductive toxicology.

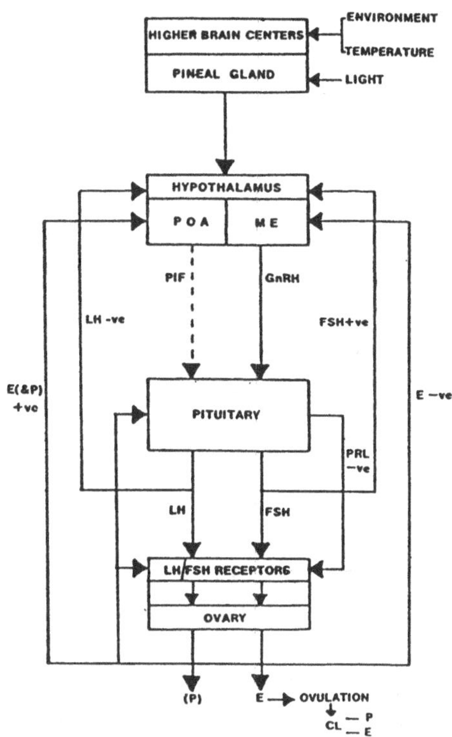

Figure 3 Model for the endocrine control of follicular development and ovulation.
PIF - Prolactin inhibiting factor POA - Preoptic area
E - Oestrogen ME - Median eminence

PRACTICAL ASPECTS

The following is intended as a guide to the equipment and methodology necessary for ovarian cell culture.

General equipment and solutions

Equipment
- Laminar flow cabinet
- Carbon dioxide incubator
- Sterile 1 ml Pasteur pipettes
- Sterile 10 ml pipettes
- Sterile culture wells

Sterile 30 ml Universals
Eppendorf Multipette
Sterile Eppendorf combitips (5 ml)
Haemocytometer
Centrifuge
Sterile petri-dishes. (50 mm diameter)
Light microscope
0.22 µ Millipore filters

<u>Culture Media</u> (1 litre) Dulbecco's Modified Essential Media (DMEM) and Hams F12 (1:1 v/v)

	Bovine serum albumin	- 0.1%
	Kanamycin	- 0.1 mg/ml
	Sodium bicarbonate	- 2.4 g/l.

<u>Theca cells</u>

<u>Equipment</u> Stereomicroscope
Sterile fine forceps
Sterile fine wire loop
Sterile 3 mm knife needle
Sterile sharp dissecting scissors.

<u>Granulosa cells</u>

<u>Equipment</u> Sterile syringes (1 ml and 10 ml)
Sterile needles (1.0 - 1.7 mm dia and 23G)

<u>Solutions</u>	Testosterone	- 10^{-7}M
	Hyaluronidase Type III	- 230 U/ml
	Fetal calf serum	- 10%
	Trypan blue	- 0.5%

<u>Percoll gradients</u> (x2)

Minipuls 2 pump and tubing (2.90 cc/M)
Sterile 30 ml Universals (x2)

DMEM	25 ml

<u>Percoll solution</u>

Earl's Basic Salt Solution	- 2.5 ml
Percoll	21.8 ml
Hepes buffer 1M	0.25 ml
Kanamycin	0.25 ml

Luteal cells

Equipment

Sterile plastic conical flasks
Sterile plastic 12 ml and 30ml centrifuge tubes (tapered)
Sterile plastic LP3/LP4 culture tubes
Siliconised pasteur pipettes
100 μ nylon mesh
Pair fine dissecting scissors
Plastic beakers (25, 50, 100 and 250 ml)
Plastic and glass conical flasks (25, 50 and 100 ml)

Solutions

Culture Media

Eagles Minimum Essential Media (EMEM) (with 0.85 g/l sodium bicarbonate)	- 500 ml
Essential amino acids	- 5 ml
L-glutamine	- 10 ml
Bovine Serum albumin	- 1%
Fetal Calf Serum	- 10%

Collagenase digest solution

EMEM	- 50 ml
Collagenase Type 1	- 125 mg
Bovine Serum albumin	- 1%

All media and solutions should be sterilised before use by passing through a 0.22 μ filter.

EXPERIMENTAL PROCEDURES

Human granulosa cell collection

Preovulatory follicles are aspirated during laparotomy from patients who have given their informed consent. Follicles are aspirated using a hypodermic syringe needle (1.0 - 1.7 mm internal diameter) connected to a 5 ml syringe via a short length of plastic tubing. After the initial aspiration, the follicle is refilled with Ringer's lactate solution and reaspirated. Aspirations for individual follicles are pooled and centrifuged (100 g) for 5 minutes.

Rat granulosa cell collection

Adult female rats (200 - 300 g) are sacrificed by Halothane euthanasia and cervical dislocation in the follicular stage of the oestrous cycle. The animal is laid on a clean surface, covered with absorbant paper and the abdomen swabbed with 70% alcohol. An incision is made with blunt end scissors through the body wall into the peritoneum. The ovaries are then located and removed using sharp scissors and forceps, all adherent fat is removed and they are transferred to a sterile petri dish containing a small amount of culture media at room temperature. In a laminar flow cabinet, the follicles are dissected out using a stereomicroscope and sliced open with a 3 mm knife needle. The expression of granulosa cells is aided by forcing media into the follicle using a sterile 1 ml syringe and needle (23 gauge) and the media from individual rats is pooled and centrifuged (100 g) for 5 minutes.

Granulosa cell isolation and dispersion

All of the following procedures are carried out in a laminar flow cabinet under aseptic conditions. After centrifugation, both human and rat granulosa cells are resuspended in 2 ml media and pipetted onto the top of a 0-90% Percoll gradient (Conn et al, 1977) and centrifuged (400 g) for 20 minutes, in order to purify the cell suspension. The upper of the two bands is isolated (granulosa cells) and placed in a separate 30 ml universal. The lower band containing erythrocytes and damaged cells is discarded (this is sometimes not visible in the rat granulosa cell preparation). To wash the cells of Percoll, dilute the cell suspension with 3 volumes of media and centrifruge (100 g) for 5 minutes, and repeat this step twice. The granulosa cells can be dispersed if necessary by resuspending with hyaluronidase (230 U/ml) and leaving them for 15 minutes at room temperature. The cells are washed twice as described previously, to remove all traces of hyaluronidase and counted using a haemocytometer. The cell suspension is then drawn up into a 5 ml Combitip fitted to the Eppendorf Multipette and delivered in 100 µl aliquots (100,000 cells) to each well and the volume made up to 500 µl/well. Incubate the cells at 37°C, 5% CO_2, initially for 24 hrs with 10% Fetal Calf Serum, after which all traces of the serum should be removed and the cells can be used experimentally. Testosterone is added (10^{-7}M) as an aromatase substrate and the media replaced daily. To assess cell viability and cell purity in-vitro, see the chapter by D.A. Garside in this volume.

Rat thecal cell isolation and dispersion

The thecal shells from the isolated follicles used to collect granulosa cells are gently scraped with a fine wire loop to remove any adhering granulosa cells. Thecae are then washed several times in media and 3 thecal shells incubated per culture well containing 1.0 ml culture media, at 37°C and 5% CO_2.

Luteal cell isolation and dispersion

Female rats at day 16 of pregnancy are sacrificed and the ovaries removed as described previously for granulosa cell collection. In a laminar flow cabinet, the corpora lutea are dissected out into a plastic petri dish using a stereomicroscope. The corpora lutea are cut into quarters with a 3 mm knife needle and washed several times in fresh Hanks Basic Salt Solution, blotted dry, weighed and then minced with sharp fine scissors. The luteal tissue is transferred to a plastic conical flask containing collagenase digest solution (10 ml solution/1g luteal tissue) and the tissue incubated at 37°C for 30 minutes in a shaking water bath. The luteal tissue is dispersed by drawing up and down a siliconised pasteur pipette at 15 minute intervals. A 20 ml aliquot is removed and the number of cells present counted using a haemocytometer. The number of cells required is 0.5 to 1 x 106 cells/ml and if insufficient have been isolated then the collagenase digestion procedure is repeated. When luteal cell dissociation has been completed, the cells are washed thoroughly to remove all collagenase by centrifugation at 100g (5 minutes) and resuspension of the cell pellet in Eagles MEM. This is repeated four times. The cell pellet is finally resuspended in Eagles MEM containing 1% BSA and a substrate for steroidogenesis such as 25-hydroxycholesterol (Toaft et al, 1982), high density lipoproteins or 10% fetal calf serum. The cell suspension can then be sieved through a 100 μ nylon mesh to remove non-cellular debris and a proportion of cells taken in order to determine cell viability (see chapter by D.A. Garside in this volume) which should be 90-100% live cells. The cell suspension is pipetted in 1 ml aliquots (10^6 cells/ml) into LP3 or LP4 plastic culture tubes and preincubated for 30 minutes at 37°C in a shaking water bath in an atmosphere of 95% O_2 and 5% CO_2, after which the cells are centrifuged (100 g for 5 minutes) and the supernatant discarded. This step is incorporated into the procedure as luteal cells secrete excessive amounts of steroids in the first 30 minutes of incubation which are not representative of usual luteal function in-vitro. The cells are then resuspended in Eagles MEM with the steroid substrate and 1% BSA for a period of 2 hours in the conditions previously described, however immediately at the start of this incubation, 10 tubes are centrifuged (100g for 5 minutes) and the pellet and supernatant frozen at -20°C for protein and steroid analysis respectively. These are the zero hour time points. At the end of the 2 hr incubation, the remaining cells are centrifuged (100 g for 5 minutes) and the pellet and supernatant frozen as for the zero hour tubes for subsequent analysis. The amount of steroid production during the incubation period is calculated by subtracting the values for the zero time points from the 2 hour values.

Measurement of ovarian cell steroid biosynthesis

The functional viability of ovarian cell types can be assessed by measuring the steroid output of the cells in culture. Culture the thecal cells with 100 ng/ml luteinising hormone and granulosa cells with 100 ng/ml follicle stimulating hormone (and/or luteinising hormone) for 3 hrs. Controls receive no hormone and at the end of the incubation the medium is collected from individual wells and stored at -20°C until analysis. The oestradiol and progesterone content are measured in the unextracted incubation medium by radioimmunoassay. Luteal cells do not need to be incubated with a stimulatory hormone in order to produce reasonable steroid output, although prolactin and luteinising hormone may be used if necessary, depending on the species and age of corpora lutea.

Experimental Examples

At present there have been no data published using theca or luteal cells for investigating the effects of reprotoxicants on the ovary, although there is increasing interest being shown in their application to toxicology. Granulosa cells however have been used in the study of substituted triazoles and their relationship to delayed ovulation (Wickings et al, 1986; Middleton et al, 1985). It has been demonstrated that a single oral dose of a substituted triazole (1,1-di-(4-fluorophenyl)-2-(1,2,4,-triazol-1-yl)ethanol) can delay ovulation in the rat (Middleton et al, 1984) with a related delay in the preovulatory peaks of plasma progesterone, follicle stimulating hormone and luteinising hormone. Oestradiol levels are depressed and exogenous oestradiol given up to 12 hours after dosing prevented the inhibitory effects of the triazole suggesting an interference with oestrogen feedback perhaps at the level for the hypothalamus/pituitary. The reduction in plasma levels of oestradiol could also be an indication of aromatase inhibition in the ovary especially as the triazole has similar effects to aminoglutethimide, a known inhibitor of aromatase activity. To elucidate further the mechanism of action of the triazole, it has been added to granulosa cells in-vitro in the presence of follicle stimulating hormone (100 mg/ml) and testosterone (10^{-7}M). The triazole produced a dose dependant, specific inhibition of oestradiol production, (94% reduction with 10^{-5}M and 35% with 10^{-7}M) (Middleton et al, 1984), confirming that it inhibits either the induction or activity of granulosa cell aromatase in-vitro, probably in a similar manner to aminoglutethimide i.e. by inhibiting the aromatising enzyme necessary for aromatisation of the steroid ring (Gaunt et al, 1968, Matt and MacDonald, 1984). These observations have been confirmed by Wickings and coworkers (1986, unpublished) who have shown also that the triazole acts as an apparent competitive aromatase inhibitor, as did other structurally related substances (e.g. 4,4-difluorophenyl derivatives).

Granulosa cell cultures have therefore provided evidence that the substituted triazole exerts its effect on the reproductive system primarily at the level of the ovary rather than at the hypothalamus/pituitary, a fact which could not be identified by plasma oestradiol levels alone.

DISCUSSION AND CONCLUSIONS

The *in-vitro* investigation of the hormonal regulation of steroid biosynthesis and the intraovarian mechanisms involved for theca (Silavin & Greenwald 1984), granulosa (see review Hseuh et al, 1983) and luteal cells (see review by Hansel & Dowd 1986) is a recent area of research. The use of the techniques described in this chapter have only recently been applied to the study of reprotoxicants and are in the preliminary stages of assessing their usefulness in reproductive toxicology.

The control of cell metabolism for both theca and granulosa cells is complex. It has been demonstrated that the two exhibit cell-to-cell communication essential for their normal cell function, for example, androgens secreted by the theca cell play an important role in the local (paracrine) control of granulosa cell function (Richards, 1979; Hillier and de Zwart, 1981) and do not only serve as a substrate for granulosa cell aromatase activity (Hillier et al, 1981). For this reason, it is only now with the knowledge of their requirements for cell function that theca and granulosa cells can be cultured satisfactorily and therefore be employed to assess the potential toxicity of chemicals to ovarian cell metabolism and resultant oocyte maturation.

There is recent evidence also that luteal cells can be divided histologically and functionally into two types, namely small luteal cells of thecal origin and large luteal cells mainly of granulosa cell origin (see review by Hansel and Dowd, 1986). The two types of luteal cells both secrete progesterone *in-vitro*, however the small cells are more sensitive to luteinising hormone and it may be that the steroidogenesis of the two types may be controlled by different mechanisms. This is a novel finding and a great deal of research is currently being undertaken to understand these mechanisms and their interrelationships which are important when considering the mechanism of action of toxic compounds on progesterone production and pregnancy maintenance.

In practice, the culture of ovarian cell types could be used as an *in-vitro* screen in reproductive toxicity, especially when there is an indication that the chemical may interfere with fertility. The test can be carried out by one person within one week, including repeat tests and assaying the incubated medium for steroids. As previously mentioned, the availability of human ovarian cell tissue enhances the attractiveness of this technique in reproductive toxicity investigations. The _in-vitro_ assessment of ovarian function will provide a valuable test as an indication to the mechanism of action of toxic chemicals on infertility and pregnancy maintenance although it has as yet to be correlated with _in-vivo_ studies.

References

Cann P.M., Tsuruhara T, Dufau M. and Catt, K.J. (1977). Isolation of highly purified Leydig cells by density gradient centrifugation. Endocrinology 101, 639.

Carr B.R., Sadler R.K., Rochelle D.B., Stalmach M, MacDonald P.C. and Simpson E.R. (1981). Plasma lipoprotein regulation of progesterone biosynthesis by human corpus luteum tissue in organ culture. J. Clin. Endocrinol. Metab. 52, 875-881.

Carson R.S., Trounson A.O. and Findley J.K. (1982). Successful fertilisation of human oocytes in-vitro; concentration of oestradiol 17ß, progesterone and androstenedione in antral fluid donor follicles. J. Clin. Endoc. Metab. 55, 798-800.

Eppig F.F., Freter R.R., Ward-Bailey P.F. and Schultz R.M. (1983). Inhibition of oocyte moturation in the mouse; participation of cAMP, steroid hormones and a putative maturational inhibiting factor. Dev. Biol. 100, 34-49.

Erickson G.F. (1983). Primary cultures of ovarian cells in serum free medium as models of hormone dependant differentiation. Molec. Cell. Endoc. 29, 21-49.

Gaunt R., Steinetz B.G. and Chart J.J. (1968). Pharmacologic alteration of steroid hormone functions. Clin. Pharmacol. Ther. 9, 657-681.

Gwynne J.T. and Strauss J.F. (1982). The role of lipoproteins in steroidogenesis and cholesterol metabolism in steroidogenic glands. Endoc. Rev 3, 399-329.

Hansel W. and Dowd J.P. (1986). New concepts of the control of corpus luteum function. J. Reprod. Fert. 78, 766-768.

Harbison R.D. and Dixon R.L. (1978). Proceedings of symposia on target organ toxicity. Gonads-reproductive and genetic toxicity. Environ. Health Perspect. 24, 1-128.

Hillier S.G. and de Zwart F.A. (1981). Evidence that granulosa cell aromatase induction/activation by FSH is an androgen receptor-regulated process in-vitro. Endoc. 109, 1303-1305.

Hillier S.G., Reichert L.E. and Van Hall E.V. (1981). Control of preovulatory follicular oestrogen biosynthesis in the human ovary. J. Clin. Endoc. Metab. 52, 847-856.

Hseuh A.J., Jones P.B., Adashi E.Y., Wang C., Zhuang L-Z and Welsh T.H. (1983). Intraovarian mechanisms in the hormonal control of granulosa cell differentiation in rats. J. Reprod. Fert. 69, 352-342.

Mars R.P., Vargyes J.M. and Lobo R. (1983). Comparison of the intrafollicular hormonal mileau with fertilisation of human oocytes in-vitro. Proceedings of 65th Annual Meeting of Endocrine Society. June 8-10. San Antonio T.X. Abst 847.

Matt D.W. and MacDonald G.J. (1984). In vitro progesterone and testosterone production by the rat placenta during pregnancy. Endocrinol. 115, 741-747.

McNatty K.P. (1981). Hormonal correlates of follicular development in the human ovary. Aust. J. Biol. Sci. 34, 249-268.

Middleton M.C., Watson S.C., Milne C.M., Wickings E.J. and Hillier S.G. (1984). Inhibition of ovarian aromatase and its relationship to a delay in ovulation in the rat. Biol. Reprod. 30(1), Abst. 84.

Middleton M.C., Watson S.C., Hasmall R.L. and Milne C.M. (1985). Inhibition of ovarian oestradiol production by a substituted triazole and its relationship to delayed ovulation in the rat. Toxicologist 5, 186.

Milne C.M., Hasmall R.L. and Middleton M.C. (1985). Studies with an inhibitor of ovulation in the rat. Toxicologist 5, 119.

Murphy B.D., Rajumer K., McKibbin P.E., MacDonald G.J., Buhr M.M. and Grinwich D.L. (1985). The effects of hypophesectomy and administration of pituitary hormone on luteal function and the uptake of high density lipoproteins by luteinised ovaries and adrenal in the rat. Endoc. 116, 1587-1597.

Nalbandov (1986). 'The mechanism of ovulation'. In Reproductive Physiology of Animals and Birds. 3rd Edition. Freeman & Co., San Fransisco. p. 169.

Osborn J.C. and Moor R.M. (1983). Role of steroid signals in the maturation of mammalian oocytes. J. Steroid Biochem. 19, 133-137.

Perry J.S. (1971). The structure and function of the female reproductive system in The Ovarian cycle of Mammals. Eds Oliver and Boyd. Edinburgh Press.

Rejkumar K., Couture R.L. and Murphy B.D. (1985). Binding of high density lipoproteins to luteal membranes: the role of prolactin luteinising hormone and circulating lipoproteins. Biol Reprod. 32, 546-555.

Richards J.S. (1979). Hormonal control of ovarian follicular development; a 1978 perspective. Rec. Prog Horm. Res. 35, 343-373.

Silavin S.L. and Greenwald G.S. (1984). Steroid production by isolated theca and granulosa cells after initiation of atresia in the hamster. J. Reprod. Fert. 71, 387 - 392.

Short R.V. (1964). Steroids in the follicular fluid and corpora lutea of the mare - a two-cell type theory of ovarian steroid synthesis J. Endoc. 24, 59.

Toaff M.E. Schleyer M. and Strauss J.F. (1982). Metabolisms of 25-hydroxycholesterol by rat luteal mitochondria and dispersed cells Endoc. 111, 785-1790.

Wickings E.J., Hillier S.G. and Middleton M.C. (1986). Non-steroidal inhibition of granulosa cell aromatase activity in-vitro - unpublished data.

Conclusion

CONCLUSION

C.K. Atterwill and C.E. Steele
SK&F Research Ltd., Welwyn, AL6 9AR England

In this book a wide variety of techniques has been described by experts in the various fields and we would now like to outline how they now or in the future might fit into the process of compound development. In general, *in vitro* models such as these are employed for several reasons. Firstly, to perform mechanistic work of an applied nature in parallel with, and subsequent to, routine *in vivo* toxicity studies. Secondly, in the commercial environment they are increasingly being used for pre-development screening of potential development compounds. Finally, they have been, and will be, used empirically for obtaining new and fundamental background knowledge on biochemical/cellular toxicology phenomena. This will undoubtedly encompass many of the biotechnological and molecular biology advances and will continue to provide new information and techniques for the practitioners of applied *in vitro* toxicology.

We have chosen some of the more familiar systems currently used in *in vitro* toxicology and have taken a different approach from earlier works in that we have concentrated exclusively on viable cell/tissue/organ preparations which maintain functional capacity *in vitro*. By reference to the topics discussed at recent symposia and in the scientific literature it is evident that there are still other systems to be considered such as gut, bone, smooth muscle etc. Inevitably this list will expand as technology advances and we look forward to updating and expanding the current volume for later editions.

With reference to the chapters in this book it is difficult to classify each model into distinct 'use categories' since all could be adopted for a variety of uses. It is evident, however, that various techniques are at different stages of validation and thus certain uses would have to be precluded. For example, techniques such as the micromass technique (O. Flint) and the thyrocyte cultures (C. Brown) have clearly been well validated and can be employed as pre-screens. Others such as the isolated rat heart (A. Cockburn) and whole embryo culture (D.L. Cockroft and C.E. Steele) do not lend themselves to large-scale screening procedures but are clearly useful for empirical, mechanistic studies. Many of the models (e.g. cultures of the brain, ear, kidney and lung) will be used more widely in the future as validation ensues. It must be remembered, as clearly pointed out in the Introduction by G.B. Leslie and P. Johnson, that as far as regulatory submissions for specific development compounds are concerned _in vitro_ data cannot stand alone and must be considered in the context of _in vivo_ data - a good example of this would be the mutagenicity tests used to predict genotoxic potential in man.

The role of _in vitro_ techniques in association with tests performed _in vivo_ can be well illustrated by our own experiences of drug design and development candidate selection (i.e. pre-screen) in the pharmaceutical industry. This complex process is summarised in Fig.1.

FIGURE 1

ROLE OF IN VITRO & IN VIVO INVESTIGATIVE TOXICOLOGY IN COMPOUND DESIGN & CANDIDATE SELECTION.

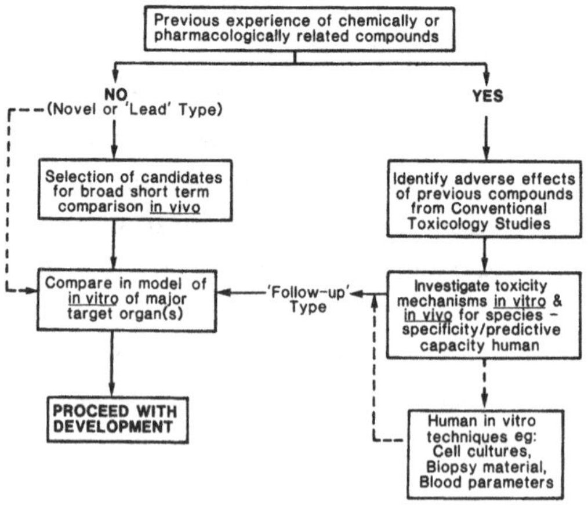

Previous experience of chemically or pharmacologically related compounds

NO (Novel or 'Lead' Type)

YES

Selection of candidates for broad short term comparison _in vivo_

Identify adverse effects of previous compounds from Conventional Toxicology Studies

Compare in model of _in vitro_ of major target organ(s)

'Follow-up' Type

Investigate toxicity mechanisms _in vitro_ & _in vivo_ for species - specificity/predictive capacity human

PROCEED WITH DEVELOPMENT

Human in vitro techniques eg: Cell cultures, Biopsy material, Blood parameters

It is, however, not a unique route of candidate selection and can be modified according to the nature and number of the compounds and potential target organs. For example, if no background information ofa class of compounds was available an alternative to preliminary in vivo testing would be simply to establish relative cytotoxicity (enzyme leakage, cell death) before proceeding to more sophisticated parameters and specific endpoints with more relevance to the specific target organ (ion translocation, receptor function etc). Well validated tests (in terms of in vivo comparability of response) are usually necessary unless for example the in vitro test is used as a mechanistic adjunct to a much larger series of in vivo tests. In both instances validation of the measured endpoints is necessary. If regulatory authorities are to accept in vitro techniques then not only well-validated but also appropriate and well understood endpoints should be selected.

The advantages and disadvantages of each technique have been considered by each author and are also frequently discussed in the literature and at specialised in vitro toxicology meetings. However, for those who are relatively new to this field of research we feel this book would be incomplete without a final restatement of this aspect of in vitro toxicology. In brief, the advantages and disadvantages which are summarised in Table 1, include one or more of the following categories: 1. Quality of information.
2. Cost/Time benefits.
3. Ethical considerations.

Table 1

MAJOR ADVANTAGES (+) AND DISADVANTAGES (-) OF IN VITRO STUDIES

. Direct manipulation of drug concentration and duration of exposure (+).
. Conservation of resources (animals, time, compound) (+).
. Study specific cell population in isolation from others (+).
. Complements in vivo studies and ethically more acceptable (+).
. Elimination of effects of absorption, distribution, metabolism and excretion (+/-).
. Limited duration of viability and functional activity (-).
. Inability to detect delayed/chronic toxicity (-).
. Absence of organ interactions (+/-).

Finally, we believe that continual interaction between academic toxicology and biotechnology departments and the private sector is desirable for the development and improvement of *in vitro* toxicology techniques and that this process will ensure the rapid and ethical development, and not the suppression (by either the company or regulatory agencies), of safe compounds of benefit to mankind.

INDEX